UPDATED TOPICS IN MINIMALLY INVASIVE ABDOMINAL SURGERY

Edited by **Ahmed AbdelRaouf ElGeidie**

Updated Topics in Minimally Invasive Abdominal Surgery
Edited by Ahmed AbdelRaouf ElGeidie

Published by InTech

Janeza Trdine 9, 51000 Rijeka, Croatia

Publishing Process Manager Martina Blecic

Technical Editor Teodora Smiljanic

Cover Designer InTech Design Team

Additional hard copies can be obtained from orders@intechopen.com

Updated Topics in Minimally Invasive Abdominal Surgery,
Edited by Ahmed AbdelRaouf ElGeidie
p. cm.
978-953-307-773-4

For EU product safety concerns:
IN TECH d.o.o., Prolaz Marije Krucifikse Kozulić 3, 51000 Rijeka, Croatia,
info@intechopen.com or visit our website at intechopen.com.

Meet the editor

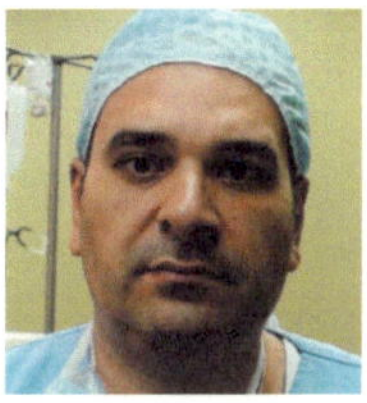

Dr. Ahmed AbdelRaouf ElGeidie is an Assistant Professor of Surgery, Gastroenterology Surgical Center, Mansoura University, Egypt. He is a well recognized expert in advanced laparoscopic surgery in Egypt. He is the author of more than 50 professional publications. He is a member of many local and international society of laparoscopic surgery. He received the MD degree from Mansoura University, Egypt. He is a reviewer of many surgical journals. He supervised many MD and master thesis. He shared in over 20 international conferences as a speaker, and also in many local conferences and meetings. He holds many prizes for his work.

Contents

Preface

It goes without saying that the introduction of laparoscopy, with its well-known advantages, changed the face of surgery. Big surgeons make big incision is now proved to be incorrect dictum. Now surgeons can work via key holes to reach areas considered to be very difficult to reach in open surgery. No more ugly big wounds, no more adhesions, less pain, rapid recovery .... and many more. For all these benefits, patients ask their surgeons for laparoscopy. However, laparoscopy is not that easy. It requires new skills and talents that differ from those required in open surgery. It is more difficult and needs more experience and training.

We tried in this book to present evidence-based up-to-date information in laparoscopic surgery. This book does not cover all minimally invasive abdominal surgery; only included selected topics covering a variety of medical conditions. Each chapter is written by an expert in laparoscopy. The book is geared not only toward surgical residents in-training, but also to expert surgeons who seek for a recent solution of some controversies.

I would like to dedicate this book to my wife Reham, my daughter Salma and my son Omar. Undertaking this book steals time from family, and I very much appreciate their support.

I believe you will find this book up-to-date and a useful read that could help you in growing your surgical knowledge about laparoscopy for the sake of your patients.

Ahmed AbdelRaouf ElGeidie
Gastroenterology Surgical Center, Mansoura University,
Egypt

Part 1

Laparoscopic Biliary-Pancreatic Surgery

1

Transcylindrical Cholecystectomy for the Treatment of Cholelithiasis and Its Complications: Cholecystectomy Under Local Anesthesia

E. Javier Grau Talens, Julio Horacio Cattáneo,
Rafael Giraldo Rubio and Pablo Gustavo Mangione Castro
Siberia-Serena Hospital, Talarrubias (Badajoz)
Extremadura University
Spain

1. Introduction

Cholecystectomy is the primary treatment of cholelithiasis. But the prevention of the formation and the dissolution of the stones were popular in the 80's . The clinical use of the chenodeoxycholic and after the ursodeoxycholic acid emerged in the 70's, when proved that this acids reduced biliary cholesterol saturation in bile. Important aspects were significant but reversible hepatotoxicity in 3%, diarrhea in 8%, abandonment of treatment in 15% and a similar proportion of abdominal pain. Probably, more important was the increase in total serum cholesterol and low density lipoprotein during treatment with chenodesoxycholic acid. In general, ursodeoxycholic acid appears to have fewer side effects, works faster and causes less liver damage. In patients with small cholesterol stones and floating radiolucent treated with ursodeoxycholic acid, for 6-12 months, partial or complete dissolution can be expected in 40-55% of cases.

The direct dissolution of cholesterol gallstones using methyl tert-butyl ether (MBTE) requires the insertion of a percutaneous transhepatic catheter in the gallbladder. The MBTE (5-10 mL) should be infused in a manner that involves the calculi but does not flow into the common bile duct and duodenum. In 4-16 hours the stones are dissolved. The patient should stay overnight in the hospital. Side effects include pain and nausea; haemolysis and duodenitis are serious consequences of the spilling of the solvent into the duodenum . Transabdominal mechanical lithotripsy is another treatment modality, which leads to fragmentation of the stones in selected cases in almost 100% of patients.

All of these treatments have in common the recurrence of stones (from 45% to 70% at 5 or 7 years of follow-up), due to persistence of a place for the precipitation of cholesterol crystals (gallbladder) and bile prone to precipitate (lithogenic bile). A report by Gilliland and Traverso in 1990 settled any doubts about the alternatives in the treatment of cholelithiasis (Gilliland & Traverso, 1990) These authors reviewed outcomes of 671 cholecystectomy patients during the years 1982-1987 and found no mortality and 2.2% of complications. They conclude that open cholecystectomy is a definitive treatment for symptomatic cholelithiasis with minimal risk to the patient and a high degree of cure of the symptoms.

The first truly major surgery on the biliary tract was performed in 1867 in Indiana (USA). John S. Bobbs, professor of surgery at the Medical College of Indiana, operates a tumor in the right upper quadrant in a 30 year old woman, at home and under general anesthesia, resulting in the diagnosis of gallbladder hydrops which was evacuated and drained. It was the first cholecystostomy performed in the history.

Fifteen years later, in 1882, Carl J. Langenbush of Berlin performed the first cholecystectomy by lithiasis, after exercising cholecystectomy in cadavers for several years. However, as more than a century later would happen with the laparoscopy and in the same Germany, Langenbush's communication in the German Congress of Surgery of three cases of cholecystectomy that evolved successfully, was received with apathy and without due consideration that the time reserved.

1.2 Development of mini-lap (small-incision) cholecystectomy

Minilaparotomy was used for several decades for the diagnosis of obstructive jaundice. Through a small incision is valued, in addition to the aetiology, the operability by palpation of the gallbladder and hilum liver and usually the diagnosis included a cholecistocholangiography.

In 1982 F. Dubois and B. Berthelot (Dubois & Berthelot, 1982) published the first paper on the minilaparotomy for operations on the bile duct, performing the procedure in 1500 patients, including alongside cholecystectomy, some cases of choledochotomy, sphincterotomy and choledochoduodenostomy. All these interventions were carried out with a transverse or oblique skin incision 3 to 6 cm in length, but the duration of surgery, the authors say, was "twice that of a normal operation". Intervention was carried out with the help of an autostatic (if no more than one assistant was available), a vaginal valve for retraction of the liver, a malleable valve for retraction of the hepatic flexure of the colon and the positioning of two packs for the separation of the colon and stomach, referenced with a tape.

The description of the intervention with this procedure and its duration arise a suspicion of some difficulty with exposure of the structures and the easement of the procedure. However, the authors describe: a minimization of cosmetic damage, solidness of the wall closure an a reduction of pain and postoperative ileus.

Moss, in 1983, published the first cases of cholecystectomy with stay less than 24 hours, and in 1986, 100 cases. Later, he operates 160 patients by midline laparotomy, with an incision that "barely allows the surgeon's hand", which were discharged the day after surgery without receiving narcotics, tolerating food intake between 8 and 18 hours and only 3 readmissions. The author concluded in 1996 that the benefits of laparoscopy may be more related to the enthusiasm and expectations for the new technology that in the technique by itself (Moss, 1996).

In 1985, Morton (Morton, 1985) performs a cost containment study of cholecystectomy with intraoperative cholangiography in 96 patients through an incision of 4 to 5 cm with a mean operating time of 45 minutes. The average stay was 2.5 days and analgesic requirements were lower than in the classical subcostal incision. The period of sick leave decreased significantly.

Goco and Chambers in 1988 (Goco & Chambers, 1988) studied the impact of mini-cholecystectomy in the management of health expenditure, considering the reduction of hospital costs compared to traditional cholecystectomy. The authors conclude, by analyzing 450 interventions, that a 4-cm incision produces an average stay of 1.22 days and that the savings stay was 4.78 days per case. Rating the daily cost at $ 200 USA in 1988, it is easy to see the savings produced by minilaparotomy, especially if applied to the 600,000 cholecystectomies performed annually in the United States.

Despite these and further studies, minilaparotomy was never popular. For example, out of seven standard textbooks: Norton al al., (Harris, 2008). Sabiston (Arendt & Pitt, 2004), Schwartz (Schwatz 1989), Doherty (Doherty, 2010), Maingot (Karam & Roslyn, 1997), Marlow & Sherlock (Dawnson, 1985). Morris & Malt (Britton & Bickerstaff, 1994), only the latter describes the technique of cholecystectomy by minilaparotomy.

1.3 Laparoscopic cholecystectomy - Eric Mühe

Laparoscopy has not only caused a revolution in the treatment of cholelithiasis, but that has changed an old surgical proverb: "a large incision, a great surgeon." It seems reasonable to assert that "a smaller incision, less abdominal wall trauma and better aesthetic results." The era of minimally invasive surgery began and laparoscopy has been extended to almost all abdominal surgical operation and almost any procedure has been performed by laparoscopic approach, including resections and all types of gastrointestinal suture.

Interestingly, laparoscopic cholecystectomy was not well received by the German Surgical Society when E. Mühe reported the first operation in 1986. On September 12, 1985, Mühe selected with great care the first patient to perform the first laparoscopic cholecystectomy, almost five years after the first laparoscopic appendectomy by Semm. Like him, Mühe performed the pneumoperitoneum with the Veress needle, inserted the trocar and introduced his own "galloscope" through the umbilicus. Two hours later he concluded successfully the first laparoscopic cholecystectomy (Litynski, 1996). His presentation at the congress was not published and only a summary appeared in Langenbecks Archiv für Chirurgie 1986 (Mühe, 1986). However, with subsequent amendments Mühe concluded that inserting the laparoscope (galloscope) as close as possible to the gallbladder the "cumbersome" pneumoperitoneum could be avoided. After several cholecystectomies without gas, trying to simplify and adapt the technique to be used by most surgeons, he realized that the optical instrument was not necessary, "with or without galloscope, the magic surgical approach could be the same". Soon operated through sheath of the galloscope without the optical instrument with the advantages of minimal incision:

- The abdominal musclulature is not cut
- Little postoperative pain that disappears in two or three days
- short Immobilization(even elderly patients need to be in bed only the day of operation)
- Short hospital stay (4-5 days)
- Quick return to work (50-75% earlier than with traditional surgery)

This outlined the bases of minimally invasive surgery. Sadly, Mühe didn´t publish the evolution of his technique for cholecystectomy in any international journal and we haven´t hat notice of it until 1996 with the Litynski´s. book.

Many reasons can be considered to explain the success of laparoscopic cholecystectomy:

1. It is obvious that the ports, about 1 cm, scattered in the upper abdomen and a umbilical opening for the introduction of optic, produce a minimal aesthetic disorder.
2. The trauma to the abdominal wall caused by an incision about 15 cm is large and has a well-known impact on the respiratory physiology, a greater possibility of formation of adhesions, hernias and, above all, pain.
3. The acceptance by the patient has been quick, because it was publicized with all of the above advantages. The charisma of laparoscopic technology is undeniable, its elegance, too.

4. The commercial pressure has been relentless. Technological research has been overturned in the design and implementation of increasingly sophisticated and safer instruments. Sponsoring of the learning of the technique to the interested surgeons was a strategic objective.
5. Finally, the health financier had an opportunity to reduce hospital stays.

Given all the above mentioned facts it is obvious that the introduction of the technique is an undeniable fact and that, at present, nobody doubt that laparoscopy is the technique of choice for cholecystectomy. However, the advantages of laparoscopic cholecystectomy have been put in evidence, deliberately, with the open cholecystectomy with a generous wound of about 15 cm. But what if the comparison is made against a technique that uses an incision of 5 cm or smaller? It is possible that the above mentioned advantages were less obvious and that the assessment had to be made over other aspects than aesthetics, postoperative pain, parietal trauma, hospital stay, re-employment, etc., entering the field of cost, security and benefits to the patient.

2. Laparoscopic vs. small-incision cholecystectomy

A review in 1993 (Olsen, 1993) concluded that there are no good studies comparing conventional cholecystectomy by minilaparotomy or by laparoscopy. However, it was apparent that the small incision was better than the big one and that the length of the incision appears to be associated with hospital stay and return to the workplace. The ultimate goal is to achieve a safe surgery with the maximum benefit for the patient, and the keys are: knowledge of anatomy, good surgical view and a proper exposure. This last key to safety, exposure, is a limiting factor for minilaparotomy, which leads the question of how small an incision can still provide a exposure to perform the cholecystectomy safely. For Olsen, the answer is the laparoscopy, which allows for smaller incision, but it is noteworthy that the sum of the incisones made for the insertion of four trocars is about 4 cm and two-dimensional view. An incision of this size can provide adequate exposure for cholecystectomy under direct three-dimensional vision.

An overview of the Cochrane Hepato-Biliary Group reviews in January 2010 (Keus et al., 2010) revealed the evidence to date of the revisions that assess the effect of differents techniques of cholecystectomy: open, small-incision, or laparoscopic. A total of 5246 patients in 56 randomized trials are included. Total complications of laparoscopic cholecystectomy and small-incision were similar (17%), hospital stay and convalescence were not significantly different, small-incision cholecystectomy operative time was shortest (16.4 minutes) and is less costly. In our study of 1998 (Grau-Talens et al., 1998) small-incision cholecystectomy was $ 1003 U.S less costly than laparoscopic. The effects of anesthesia and surgery on lung function have been well studied (Lindell & Hendenstierna 1976). There is a reduction in FVC (Forced Vital Capacity) and FEV1 (Forced Expiratory Volume in one second) to 75% of baseline for a separate incision without cutting the muscles, while reducing down to 40-55% in the subcostal incisions and midline laparotomy. An incision that spares the muscular section can prevent postoperative pulmonary complications. The restrictive pattern of lung dysfunction in postoperative abdominal surgery is influenced by several factors and is not well understood. The size, location and direction of the incision are responsible for the alteration of mechanical ventilation, by themselves and the pain. Kind of anesthetic agent and diaphragmatic dysfunction are also involved (Craig 1981).

In some studies, laparoscopic cholecystectomy has shown lower spirometric reductions when compared to open cholecystectomy (Frazee et al., 1991) and to mini-lap (McMahon et al., 1994) although the latter with incisions between 5 and 10 cm. Presumably, a reduction in the length of the incision could be rewarded by a smaller reduction in the impairment of lung physiology, ie, an incision of 4.5 cm, uniform to all layers of the abdominal wall could improve postoperative spirometric results as happened in our study (Grau-Talens et al.,1998) wich shows that the reduction of spirometrics values were similar in laparoscopic and small-incision cholecystectomy, ie over 20% of preoperative value for FVC and 25% for FEV1. The results obtained by keus et al. are similar to ours (Keus et al 2008).

3. Treatment options in biliary lithiasis complications

3.1 Acute cholecystitis

Early cholecystectomy is the best treatement for acute cholecystitis. Laparoscopic cholecystectomy was a relative contraindication in acute cholecystitis, but now is the preferred aproach for most patients. The first articles appear in the early 90´s (Cooperman, 1990) (Yamashita et al., 2007). However, in our experience, cholecystectomy in this way was not easy: the difficulties are related to the inflammatory process, with greater difficulty for dissection and recognition of structures, the possibility of further contamination of the cavity (not the surgical wound), the need for instruments to 10 mm in diameter, greater difficulty in haemostasis and, of course, a greater proportion of conversions (35%) and duration of the intervention.
With these preliminary considerations we began to operate the acute cholecystitis by early transcylindrical cholecystectomy (within 72 hours or more of admission), thinking that the abdominal wall injury should not be higher than laparoscopy, even using the cylinder of 5 cm in diameter, that manipulation of the gallbladder (gripping, aspiration, recovery of stones etc.) could be done in a simpler way than by laparoscopy, and that contamination of the surgical wound could be avoided by the protective and insulating effect of the cylinder. We have only found an article of acute cholecystitis treated by minilaparotomy in the context of a randomized study comparing minilaparotomy with conventional laparotomy (Assalia et al., 1997). The authors show figures contrasting results in a very favourable way, not only with traditional laparotomy, but with the laparoscopic approach. In this article the average time (+ /-SD) of the intervention was 69.1 (+ / - 17.0) minutes and mean hospital stay was 3.1 days.

3.2 Choledocholithiasis

The choledochotomy was first performed in 1884 by Kummel and in 1889 by Thornton and Abbe, who made the first ideal suture of the choledochotomy. In the late nineteenth and early twentieth century the common bile duct exploration was guided by the subjective clinical impression of the surgeon, until the introduction of intraoperative cholangiography by Mirizzi in 1937. In the Massachusetts General Hospital (Bartlett & Waddell, 1958) were reviewed 1000 choledochotomy for suspected choledocholithiasis with a mortality of 1.8% (three times higher than simple cholecystectomy) and 16% global choledocholithiasis. In the presence of previous pancreatitis, stones were found at choledochotomy in 12% of the patients; in the presence of jaundice or a reliable history of jaundice, 35%; in the previous situation more palpable stone in 99%; with bile duct larger than 1 cm diameter, 58%;

jaundice and only cystic dilated (greater than 4 mm), 50%; when occurred only jaundice and small stones (<0.5 cm) in 34%. In patients without jaundice, the presence of stones in the choledochotomy was as follows: If calculation palpable, 89%; if dilated common bile duct, 53%; if the cystic duct dilated, 29%; and in the presence of small stones, 16%.

With the arrival of cholangiography the negative common bile duct exploration decreased from 50% to 6%, the incidence of retained stones also fell from 25% to 11%. Moreover, although it was not popular until the 70, the introduction of rigid choledochoscope in 1941 by McIver reduced the incidence of retained stones. A big progress in the treatment of retained stones was the introduction of endoscopic sphincterotomy in 1974 by german and japanese authors (Classen &Demling, 1974) with a success rate of 95%, 15% morbidity and mortality from 0.2 to 1.5% (Escorrou et al., 1984), relativized the problem of retained stones and its treatment and compared favourably with surgical sphincterotomy, whose mortality was 2.9 to 4.4%.

With the introduction of laparoscopic cholecystectomy, surgery for gallstones changed and preoperative endoscopic retrograde cholangiography became the rule in the care of patients suspected of gallstones in the bile duct to avoid open choledochotomy. In experienced centres, the success rate of ERCP in the extraction of common duct stones is 90% but 1% overall mortality and complication rate of 6% to 10% (Fink, 1993). The risk of mortality and morbidity should be added to the subsequent laparoscopic cholecystectomy. If we accept a risk of death of 0.3% and 5% complication rate for laparoscopic cholecystectomy, the overall mortality of the sum of the two procedures can be 1.3% and morbidity of 11 to 15% (Tomkin, 1997).

Other notable aspects of this sequence of treatments (first ERCP and posterior cholecystectomy) are: the cost and the negative ERCP, ie, discriminating which patients have choledocholithiasis preoperatively. A study by Koo and Traverso (Koo &Traverso, 1996) revealed that the history is the best predictor of choledocholithiasis, but was only able to predict 45% of cases, surpassing the biochemistry of liver function and ultrasound. For this reason, preoperative ERCP is rewarded with the discovery of choledocholithiasis in no more than 50% of cases, which are obviously exposed to morbidity and mortality, and raise the cost of surgical practice. In another recent study, ERCP was performed only if the patient had any of the following criteria: dilatation of the bile duct by ultrasound, gallstone pancreatitis or abnormalities of liver function tests (Katz et al., 2004). ERCP was performed in 41 patients and stones were found in 22 (53.7%). The authors conclude that dilatation of the bile duct along with liver function abnormalities are the most useful, with a yield of 82% correct in detecting choledocholithiasis.

In the last decade has improved radiological assessment of patients with suspected common bile duct stones. Transabdominal ultrasounds are not very sensitive in detecting common bile duct stones, but if ultrasounds are negative and liver function is normal, the chances of choledocholithiasis are minimal. Magnetic resonance cholangiopancreatograpy and endoscopic ultrasonography have high sensitivity and specificity (grater than 90%) and are the best options as preoperative assessment (Werbesey & Birkett 2008). There are different diagnostic and therapeutic options to address the common bile duct, but not an algorithm that can be considered the standard criterion. The management of this disease depends on the experience and the possibilities of available technology of each working group. The therapeutic approaches are:

- Preoperative ERCP and later laparoscopic cholecystectomy
- Laparoscopic surgery and rendezvous

- Laparoscopic cholecystectomy and, if necessary, laparoscopic common bile duct exploration
- Transcylindrical cholecystectomy and, if necessary, transcylindrical common bile duct exploration
- Conventional open surgery
- Laparoscopic cholecystectomy more postoperative ERCP

The first option does not seem reasonable for the reasons already discussed, the last remains reserved for the failures of laparoscopic choledochotomy and retained stones. Conventional open surgery may remain as an option, but at the much higher wall trauma, the greater number of stays, the worse aesthetic outcome and greater disability after surgery. A randomized study demonstrated a greater benefit for the treatment of choledocholithiasis with laparoscopic common bile duct exploration than with postoperative ERCP (Rhodes et al., 1998).

Laparoscopic exploration of common bile duct has been developed in the 90's, almost simultaneously with laparoscopic cholecystectomy, and is performed through the cystic duct or choledochotomy. Laparoscopic choledochotomy is technically demanding, is a difficult procedure that requires a great deal of laparoscopic skill (Kroh & Chand, 2008). In this sense, a simple technique, as is the transcylindrical approach, can have a place in the common bile duct exploration.

In our Hospital this is the algorithm for suspected choledocholithiasis:

Patient with:
Acute pancreatitis, or abnormal liver fuction tests, or jaundice

↓

Transabdominal ultrasound:
Cholelithiasis. Dilated or not bile duct

↓

Operating room for transcylindrical cholecystectomy and intraoperative cholangiography:
If choledocholithiasis

↓

Transcylindrical choledochotomy

4. Transcylindrical cholecystectomy

In 1992, we started laparoscopic cholecystectomy in the Hospital Verge del Toro (Mahon, Menorca, Spain) after a training period at another hospital. The technique quickly settled in the hospital, in a time of full discussion of the validity of this approach and the need for prior training. We conducted a series of 11 laparoscopic cholecystectomy, until the absence of capnography and other circumstances prevented continuation of the procedure The laparoscopic view of Calot's triangle, with the camera close enough to the structures, as it's set to perform the dissection, does not focus more than a few square centimetres area, which is where the dissections and sections between clips of the cystic duct and cystic artery are performed. It crossed our minds that this limited field, but sufficient for the laparoscopic dissection, could be constructed in a straightforward manner, without camera, with a cylindrical or tubular separator that prevented the interposition of intraperitoneal mobile structures between the surgeon's eyes and structures hepatocystic triangle. Of course, the dissection should be performed through the cylinder with material that could be used in laparoscopic or open surgery. With these premises we entrust the construction of the first steel cylinder, 5 cm in diameter and 10 in length, with a polypropylene plunger, like a piston, which protruded from the distal end, with the purpose of helping to introduce and reject the intraperitoneal mobile structures, which could interpose and hinder the hepatocystic triangle. The first time we use it (August 1993) we were rewarded with the success of an intervention without mishap. With the cylinder of 5 cm in diameter were obtained an incision 6-7 cm in length, which could be reduced by a smaller diameter cylinder, therefore, we inquired the construction of another cylinder, 3.8 cm in diameter and with the same length. The choice of length is based on measurements made in emergency surgery, from skin to the triangle hepatocystic. Cholecystectomy with the new cylinder was still easy, but with an incision 4.5 cm length uniform in all the layers of the abdominal wall, aesthetics and a smooth postoperative period where they drew more attention to nausea and vomits than pain. Hepatocystic triangle dissection and recognition of the structures left us less uncertainty than in the laparoscopic approach, we could ensure the identity of the structures and fingertip exploration of the consistency of the organs. We considered it a safe, as it allowed the steps of the classical open cholecystectomy. We decided to call the technique *transcylindrical cholecystectomy*. The first communication in a conference dates back to 1994 when we presented a video communication with the first 20 cases in "The X Surgical Day of District Hospitals" (Tarragona, May 6, 1994). That same year it was admitted to the "XX National Congress of Surgery of the Surgical Spanish Association" Madrid, November, 1994 (Grau-Talens et al., 1994).

The review of the literature on minilaparotomy cholecystectomy and the method used by the authors showed no results of a technique similar to ours, although other types of separators or optical instruments have been developed (O´Dwyer et al.,1990), (O´Kelly et al., 1991) (Rozsos et al.,2003) (Russell & Shankar, 1987) (Shumacher & Kohaus 1994). Rozsos et al., 1997 distinguish between: microlaparotomy, where the incision is less than 4 cm in length, modern minilaparotomy, where it comes to 4-6 cm incision and classical minilaparotomy, with 6-8 cm.

The first operation of transcylindrical cholecystectomy under local anesthesia and sedation dates to 1996, in a patient with low body mass index and followed by other cases performed sporadically. The experience accumulated over 15 years and 387 interventions (Grau-Talens & Giner, 2010) showed us the safety and applicability of transcylindrical cholecystectomy and was applied to realization of the technique in outpatient surgery in the Hospital Siberia-Serena (Talarrubias, Badajoz, Spain), where we offer the transcylindrical cholecystectomy under local anesthesia and sedation to all patients with almost no exceptions (Grau-Talens et al., 2010). Patients greatly appreciate the possibility of not being entirely deprived of consciousness and not to be connected to a respirator during cholecystectomy perhaps resulting in a reduction of preoperative anxiety and stress.

4.1 Selection of patients for transcyndrical cholecystectomy in hospitalization and day-case surgery under local anesthesia plus sedation

Between 1993 and 2008 the patients with symptomatic cholelithiasis, recovering from mild/moderate acute biliary pancreatitis or acute cholecystitis were treated by transcylindrical cholecystectomy. Since 1996 we treat choledocholithiasis in this way.

Informed consent was requested for each patient explaining both the novelty of the transcylindrical cholecystectomy and its rationality, like a minilaparotomy, for aesthetic and functional benefits of a small incision, in order to prevent biliary colic and complications of lithiasis (acute cholecystitis, pancreatitis or recurrent pancreatitis and gallbladder cancer), with emphasis on uncertainty about other symptoms such as headache, dyspepsia, bitter taste, abdominal pain not related to gallstones and food intolerance. All possible and reasonable complications are listed in the informed consent of the Asociación Española de Cirujanos (Spanish Association of Surgeons), the patient read and sign before being included in the surgical waiting list.

With the exception of a randomized study period for comparison with laparoscopic cholecystectomy this series of cases should be considered consecutive. In this way, 387 patients have been included in the study.

Although the 3.8 cm cylinder has been used in most cases, the 5 cm cylinder was used, primarily, in the following situations: diagnosis of acute cholecystitis, strong suspicion of choledocholithiasis (medical history jaundice, common bile duct dilatation greater than 12 mm) and when doubt exists in the identification of structures of the hepatocystic triangle with the cylinder of 3.8 cm. This was used in light of the diagnosis of biliary colic, regardless of the ultrasound findings (normal gallbladder or sclerotic) and in patients recovering from acute pancreatitis. Intraoperative cholangiography was performed selectively.

From 2008 to the present day we exercise our practice in the Hospital Siberia-Serena (Badajoz, Spain), a public community hospital with short-stay and ambulatory surgical facilities. All of our patients are referred to us for elective surgery. The surgical emergencies are translated to de District General Hospital in the area, nevertheless, we accept hospitalized patients with complications of biliary lithiasis and are operated as a as soon as possible. Include patients with cholelithiasis, acute cholecystitis, acute pancreatitis before discharge and choledocholithiasis. We have 4 beds for patients who require hospitalization for short stay surgery.

Patients scheduled for day-case surgery must meet the general criteria of suitable personal and familiar environment and distance from the centre of not more than 45 minutes, together with the ASA I-III.

The selection of patients who would undergo transcylindrical cholecystectomy under local anesthesia plus sedation was done under the following assumptions:

1. Acceptance by the patient to undergo the procedure under local anaesthesia, and the possibility that it will be converted to general anaesthesia if necessary
2. Assessment by the surgeon that the patient meets the general requirements to be involved in ambulatory surgery
3. The assessment by the anaesthesiologist in charge of the case, the degree of patient anxiety, which might conspire with the necessary cooperation of the latter in the case of sedation and local anaesthesia, in addition to the usual pre-anaesthetic evaluation.

4.2 The cylinders

Initially we have designed and constructed a stainless steel cylinder with a polypropylene perforated plunger, like a piston, which protrudes from one end. It is 10 cm long and 3.8 cm

in diameter providing a surgical field area of 11.33 cm2, and another which is 10 cm long but 5 cm in diameter providing to surgical field area of 19.62 cm2 . These sizes have been based on the distance between the wall and the hepatocystic triangle, measured in open surgery, and the minimally area necessary for the identification and dissection of its structures.
We currently use a transparent methacrylate plunger that there exercises an effect of magnifying glass and once introduced into the abdomen allows visualization of the surgical field before unplugging (figure 1).

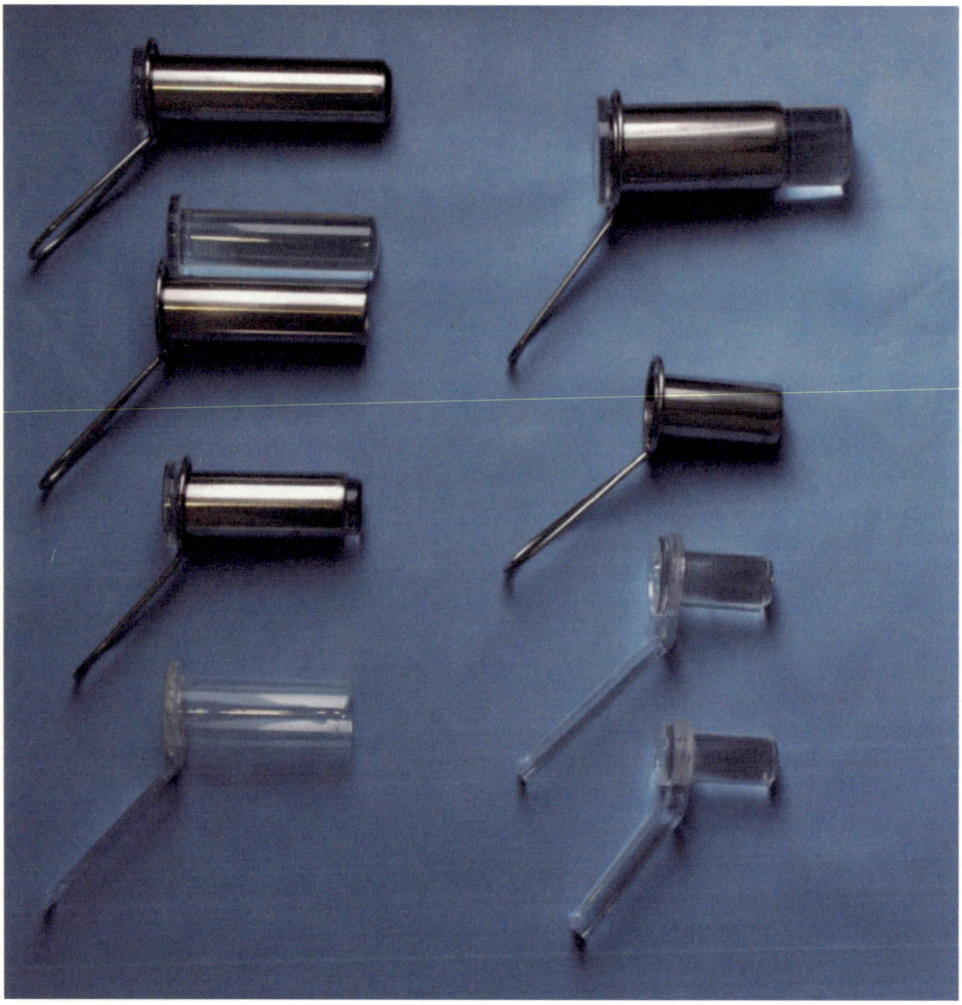

Fig. 1. Cylinders used in Transcylindrical cholecystectomy

The cylinder commonly used is made of stainless steel, though we occasionally use a cylinder totally made in methacrylate to facilitate intraoperative cholangiography. The size of cylinders is always 10.0 cm long and either 3.8 or 5 cm in diameter. But we have cylinders 12 and 14 cm in length, rarely needed in the bigest patients or abnormal liver depth under the ribs in the subdiaphragmatic space. In young people, the use of a cylinder of 2.8 cm in diameter produces an almost imperceptible scar (Figure 2, 3).

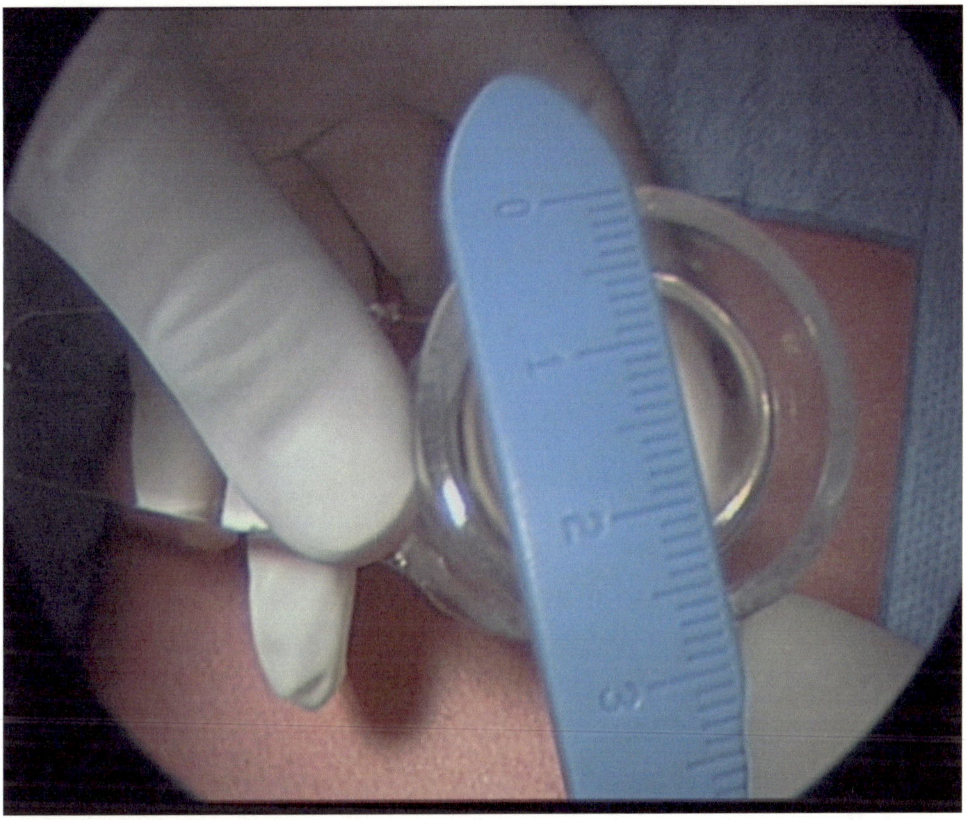

Fig. 2. Methacrylate cylinder, 2,8 cm in diameter

4.3 Technique and equipment

To introduce the 3.8-cm cylinder one makes a right transversal-epigastric incision of 4.5 cm two fingerbreath lateral to the midline, approximately at the seventh or eighth costochondral cartilages level. One then proceeds with a longitudinal incision of the rectus sheath, splitting the muscle and cutting the posterior leaf and peritoneum. This is an uniform 4.5 cm section of all the abdominal wall layers. A suture of polypropylene (No. 1) is then passed through the whole thickness of the wall (not including the skin) on both side of the incision, which helps to guide the introduction of the cylinder. We make sure that there is nothing adhering and check the normality of neighbouring organs by two finger exploration.

Once it is past the surface of the skin it is softly slided and enters without difficulty to its full extent towards the hepatocystic triangle. While we are inserting the cylinder we are seeing the intraperitoneal structures through the transparent plunger, especially the white appearance of the anteromedial aspect of the gallbladder and Hartmann's pouch and we can see, with a little pressure , the cystic duct and common bile duct (Figures 4, 5). Any gallbladder adherence to the hepatic flexure of the colon or omentum can be freed.

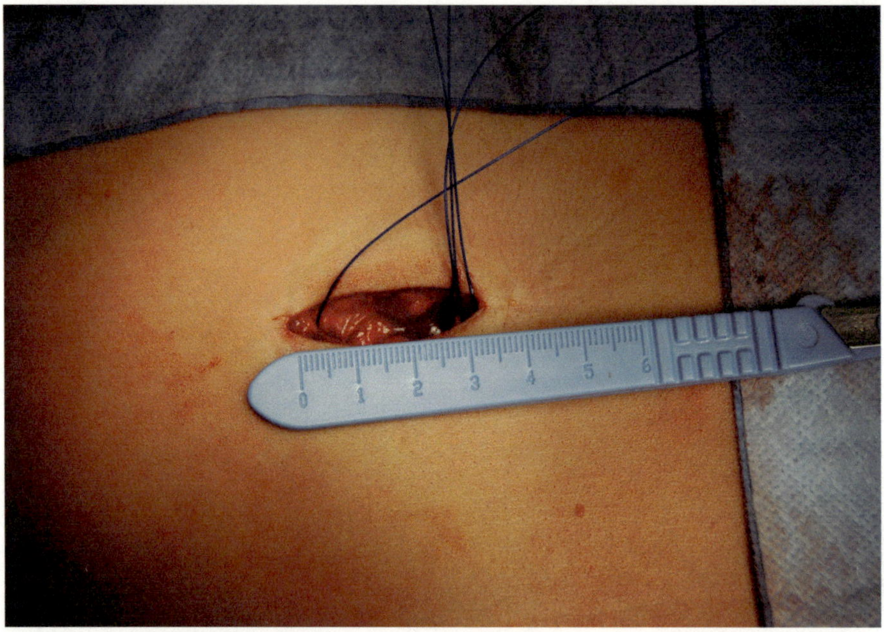

Fig. 3. Incision of 3,5 cm in length

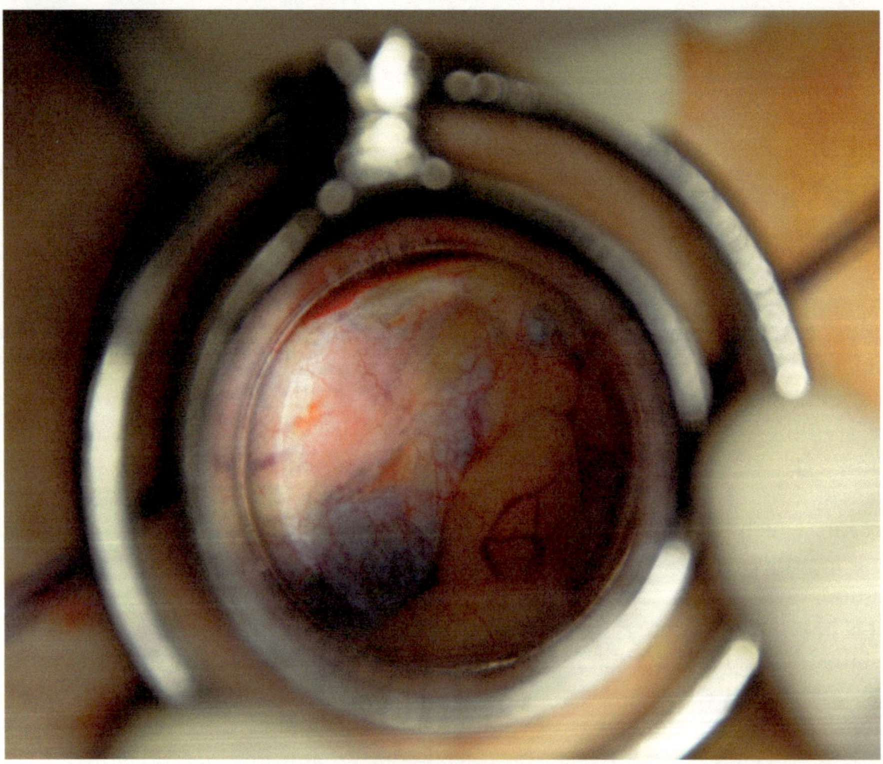

Fig. 4. Cylinder bottom through the methacrylate plug

Before reaching a working position of the cylinder, this is gently moved inside of the abdomen. The blunt shape of the plunger end, slightly protruding from the intra-abdominal side of the cylinder, facilitates this movement. The plunger can be withdrawn and reintroduced as many times as necessary to identify anatomical structures. Lamp lights usually suffice to illuminate the operative field, but a cold light may be of help occasionally.

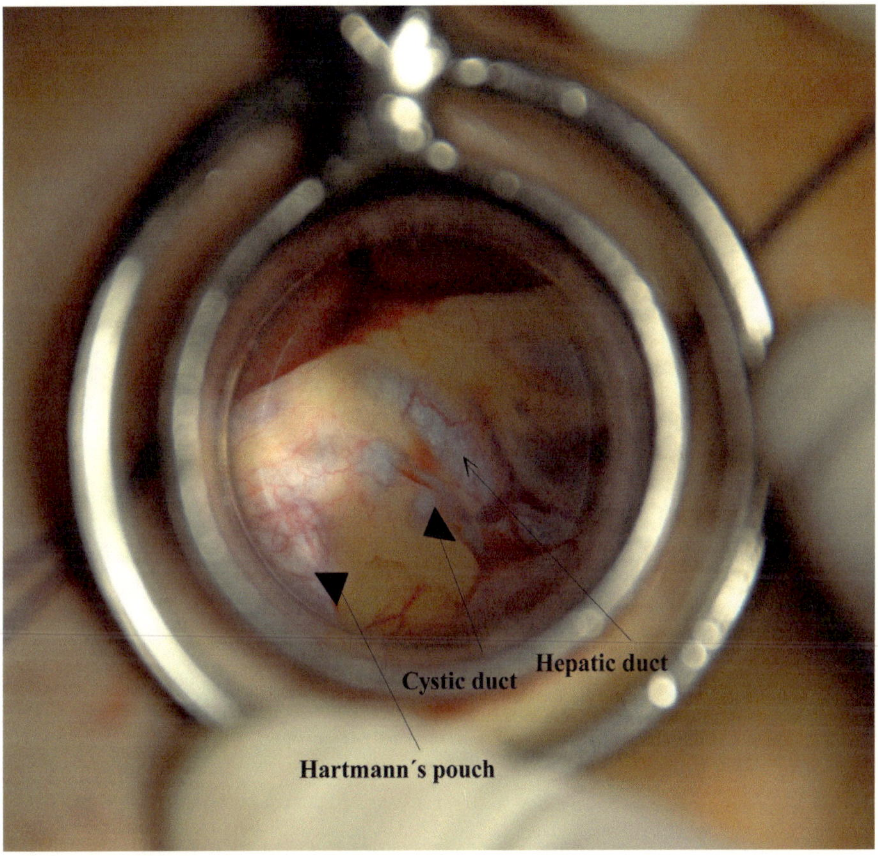

Fig. 5. View of the hepatocystic triangle through the plug

Part of the gallbladder with its infundubulum is visible at the bottom of the cylinder, as well as the omentum, duodenal bulb or colon. The infundibulum or Hartmann Pouch is grasped with tissue Foerster forceps and is drawn anterior and laterally and a medium swab inside the cylinder is used to displace the organs that impede the sight of the angle between the gallbladder and the hepatoduodenal ligament. Afterwards the hepatocystic triangle is dissected using conventional material (Figure 6).

The peritoneum is incised on the hepatocystic triangle, close to the gallbladder neck, and the fat is carefully dissected away on the free edge of the angle between the infundibulum and the hepatoduodenal ligament using gauze pledget held in an other Foerster forceps, until the cystic duct (Figure 7) and common bile duct are clearly defined (no always this later). Afterwards, we check that the cystic duct follows clearly from the gallbladder neck. If the cystic duct lymph node and cystic artery are not yet visible, the dissection is done gently upwards to discover the cystic artery, which will be followed up to its entrance into the gallbladder (a right angle dissector is required). The cystic artery can be sectioned between two distal clips and a proximal one.

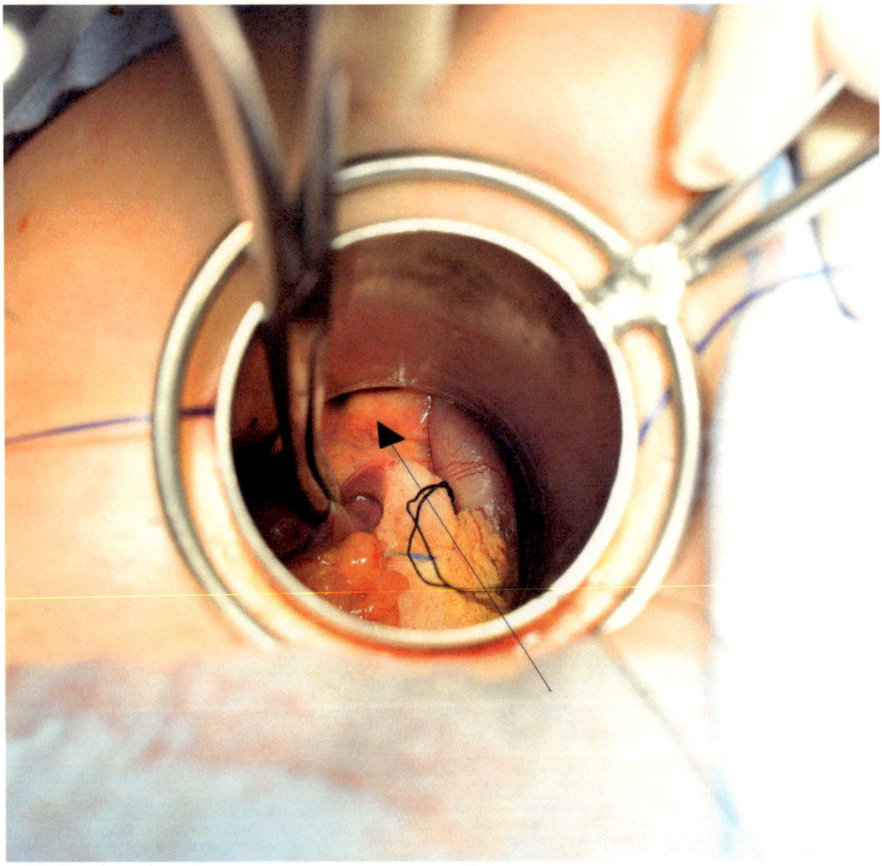

Fig. 6. Calot's triangle (as shown by the arrow) after extracting the plug

At this time, surgeon and assistant must agree on the identity of the visible anatomic structures and make sure that there are no more tubular structures above the cystic duct, other than the cystic artery. Accessory extrahepatic ducts and ductus subvesicularis have to be taken into account, as well as the double cystic artery or any abnormal situation or origin. Once the cystic duct has been identified, a silk ligature is passed around it and prepared for cholangiography (performed selectively) and sectioned with two distal clips. To finish the dissection of the hepatocystic triangle we retract the infundibulum or corpus with the help of a pledget gauze, as much as we can, from its bed in the liver, keeping the dissection close to the gallbladder wall (to avoid structures of the hilum). Separation of the gallbladder from the hepatic bed follows in a retrograde fashion using electrocautery. Perhaps, this is de more laborious part of the procedure because we needs to change the point of traction to free the corpus and fundus that are attached to the liver in a somewhat posterior position. The puncture and emptying of the gallbladder helps freeing it and, finally, we extract it from the interior of the cylinder.

We check out the hepatocystic zone and the gallbladder bed by means of the reintroduction of the cylinder and check for oozing and bile spill from the gallbladder bed. Bleeding can be restrained by gentle pressure of a moist gauze pad through the cylinder or electrocautery. The subhepatic space is irrigated with saline solution through the cylinder and after closing the posterior wall (polydioxanone sulphate) the wound is irrigated again.

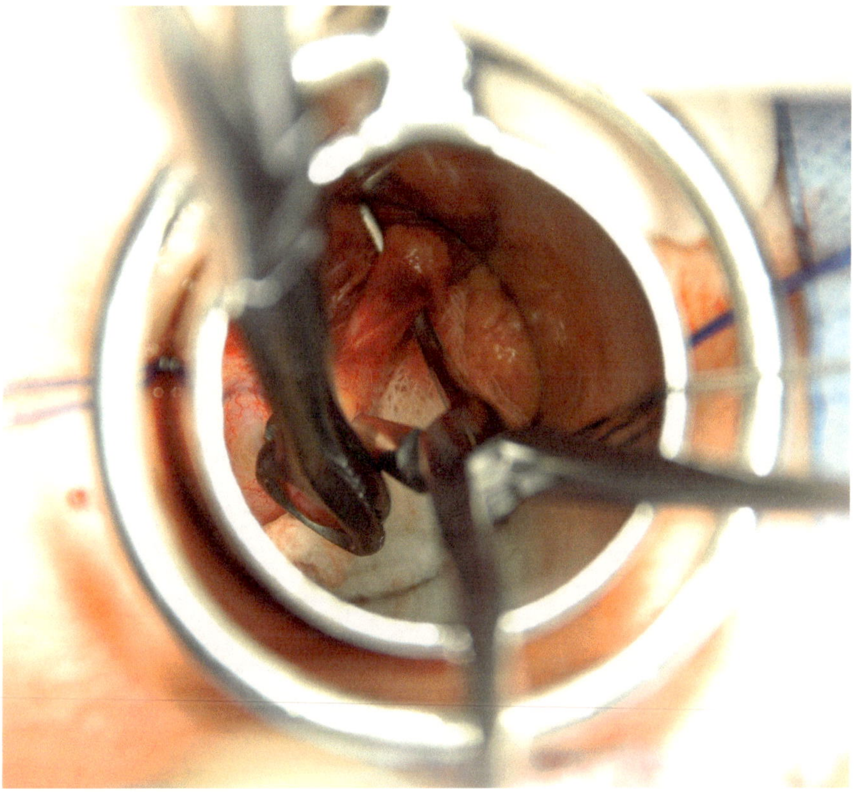

Fig. 7. Cystic duct with right angle dissector

4.4 Transcylindrical cholecystectomy under local anaesthesia plus sedation

All patients were fitted to the following protocol:

1. In the preparation area an intravenous cannula was placed, vital signs were monitored, and was given 50 mg ranitidine and metoclopramide 10 mg intravenously.
2. Once in the operating room after the patient monitor ECG, pulse oxymetry (SpO2), BIS (bispectral index) and noninvasive blood pressure we proceeded to the supply of oxygen with nasal cannula with the end tidal CO2 (ETCO2), Midazolam 0.05 mg/kg/ev and initiation of infusion of remifentanil in doses of 0.05 mcg/kg/min to 0.1 mcg/kg/min.

The objective was to obtain a sedation 2-3 on the Ramsay scale and/or a BIS value of 70 to 85 before the application of local anesthesia. For anesthesia of the abdominal wall surgical area was used 300-500 mg of mepivacaine 1% was used. The infiltration began in the line previously marked for incision, which is located in the epigastrium about 4 cm to the right of the midline and 3 cm from the costal margin. Follows the infiltration of the muscular plane and transverse oblique, lateral to the incision site with the intention of blocking the intercostal nerves VII-IX in the lateral costal margin. Finally we infiltrate the rectus muscle of abdomen in the epigastric region right under the incision line (Figure 8). Once the cylinder has been introduced the triangle of Calot is infiltrate with 2-4 cc of 2% mepivacaine (Figure 9). At the end of surgery and subcutaneous muscle planes were infiltrated with 10-20 ml of bupivacaine 0.25%.

Before leaving the operating room the patients receives: paracetamol 1g/ev, dexamethasone 8mg/ev, ondansetron 4mg/ev and ketorolac 1mg/kg, although the latter was avoided in patients 70 years or older.

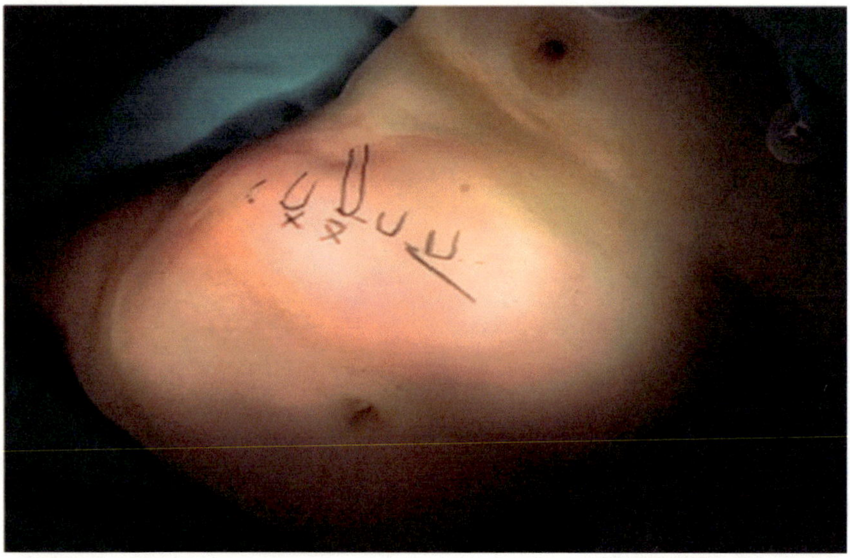

Fig. 8. Local anesthesia on intercostals nerves IX-VII and incision planes

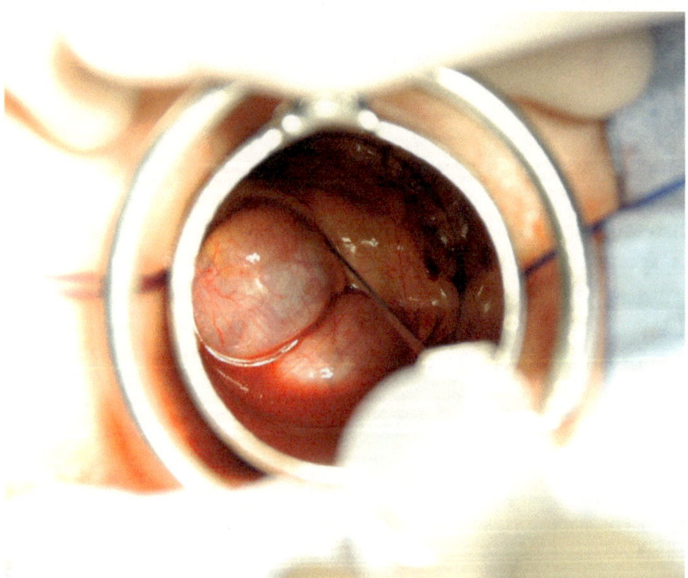

Fig. 9. Infiltration with mepivacaine 2% of the hepatocystic triangle

All patients were assessed for pain after the procedure and were discharged when they met the criteria (pain control, oral tolerance, no bleeding, nausea or vomiting, etc.), and follow analgesia regime alternating paracetamol 1g/6 h and metamizole 1g/6h orally at home.
At 24 hours, through a telephone call, we assessed the pain at rest and with movement (scale of Andersen). In the fifth day, in outpatient visit, we check for the general status, the sate of the wound and the pain is assessed with a visual analog scale (VAS).

4.5 Surgical technique in acute cholecystitis and choledocholithiasis

In acute cholecystitis we always use the 5 cm cylinder, the gallbladder is emptied with the help of an aspirator and a bile sample is send for culture. The dissection of the Calot triangle is done with a swab and if there are difficulties in closing the cystic duct is we use a ligature or stitch of poliglycolic acid. The cystic artery is treated in the same manner as above. The haemostasis of the liver may require more time. A Jackson-Pratt drain by counterincision is the norm in acute cholecystitis and common bile duct exploration.
If the intraoperative cholangiogram shows the presence of stones and a dilated bile duct (Figure 10), we prepare the field for a transcylindrical choledochotomy if the stone could not be pushed through the papilla with a Fogarty catheter. After the cholecystectomy and haemostasis of the liver, we proceed to vary the angle of the cylinder to direct medially, to put it in the hepatoduodenal ligament, taking as reference the cystic duct stump. Once in the position, the bile duct is seen on the lateral border of the ligament once the fat is cleared away with blunt dissection.

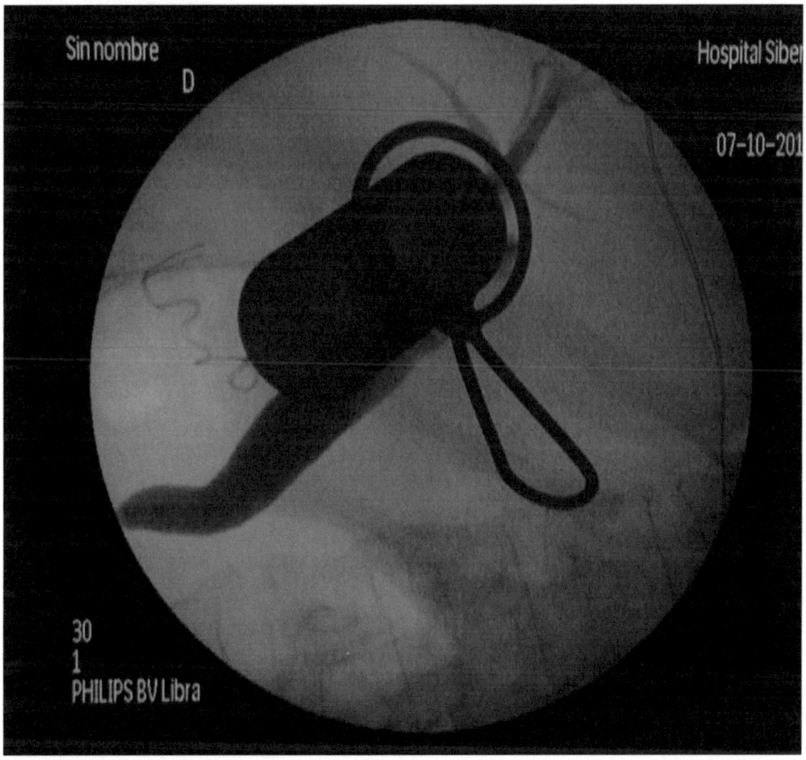

Fig. 10. Cholangiography with cylinder in place

We must ensure that we are below the confluence of the cystic duct (the duodenum can be see in the field), which will expose the common bile duct (keep in mind that the confluence may be low). Two stay sutures using polyglactin 3-0 are located on both sides of the midline of the common bile duct to pull at the time of a vertical choledochotomy as short as possible (2-3 cm), but enough for the manoeuvres of stone removal (Figure 11).

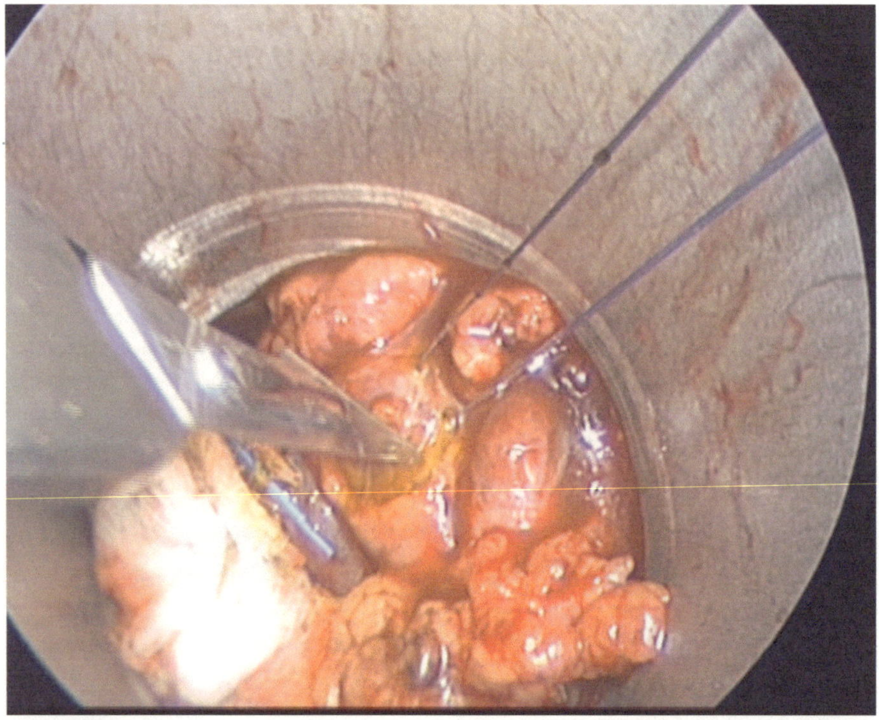

Fig. 11. Coledocotomy about to be performed. Two stay sutures pull the common bile duct.

Randall stone forceps can not be used, but the Fogarty catheter, catheter irrigation and flexible choledochoscope are used. Before performing any manoeuvre, we introduce a gauze ball referenced with a thread at the proximal end of the choledochotomy, to prevent the displacement of the stone proximal to the hepatic duct when dragging with the Fogarty catheter rather than externalized through the incision of choledochotomy. Finally, we introduce the flexible choledochoscope and confirm the absence of calculations. The closure of the choledochotomy we do it with polyglactin 3/0 on a Kehr T tube.

Between the fifth and seventh postoperative day a control cholangiogram is performed, and the patient discharged. The T tube is left in place for 14 days.

4.6 Results

We have to distinguish between two clearly defined periods in the evolution of the implementation of transcylindrical cholecystectomy. A first period, from 1993 to 2008, of the beginning of the technique and treatment of patient in hospitalization and a second period since 2008 until today as outpatient surgery and short stay, mainly under local anesthesia plus sedation. in total we performed 633 operations: 387 belonging to the first stage and 247 to the second.

The results of surgery of the first stage have already been published. In summary:

Total no. of patients	387
Completed transcylindrical	364
Ampliation to open cholecystectomy, no. (%)	23 (5.9)
Duration of simple cholecystectomy, mean (SD)	43,5 (13.3)
Length postoperative hospital stay mean (range), days	2.0 (1-6)
Postoperative complications	
Bile leakage, no. (%)	2 (0.5)
Reoperation for bleeding, no. (%)	2 (0.5)
Bile Duct injury, no. (%)	0
Death, no. (%)	1[1] (0.3)

[1]Death from multiple organ dysfunction syndrome due biliary peritonitis

Table 1. Overall results of cholecystectomy between 1993-2008

The 3.8 cm cylinder was used in 261 cases and the 5 cm in 103 as first choice or an alternatively because of difficulties in recognition of the structures. The main cause of enlargement to open surgery was the fibrotic alteration triangle hepatocystic. The number of conversion is not negligible, but our philosophy has been not to subject the patient to the risk of intervention with uncertainty in identifying the structures of the hepatocystic triangle in order to prevent complications. For that we have not hesitated to convert to a classic laparotomy when facing at a reasonable difficulty.
A survey of satisfaction with the aesthetics of the procedure yielded a 90% satisfied or very satisfied.

4.6.1 Transcylindrical cholecystectomy under local anesthesia plus sedation in day-case surgery

Today we are performing the majority of our cholecystectomies as day-case surgery. Local anesthesia and sedation is the anesthetic technique that we offer at all our patients and that we use unless the patient's preference for general anesthesia. A pilot study of 60 cases was published in Endoscopy (Grau Talens et al., 2010), but now we have performed the procedure in 222 patients, highlight a patient with choledocholithiasis too operated under local anesthesia and sedation, excellently tolerated; while that in 25 other general anesthesia was used for suspected acute cholecystitis (8 patients), suspected choledocholithiasis (3 patients) and specifically stated preference for the patient in the other cases (14 patients).
Local anesthesia was initiated in 222 patients with demographic and anthropometric characteristics in Table 2.

Patients, no.	222
Men/woman	55/167
Age, mean (range) years	55.2 (17-90)
BMI[1], mean (range) kg/m^2	29.9 (19-46)
Height, mean (range) cm	160.5 (140-185)
Eight, mean (range) kg	77.0 (43-122)
Acute pancreatitis, no.	21
Acute cholecystitis previous[2]	34

[1]Body mass index
[2]Acute cholecystitis with a Hospital General admission

Table 2. Demographic and clinical characteristics of patients operated under local anesthesia plus sedation

As it can be seen our patients are obese in almost half the cases and 35 patients had a BMI equal to or greater than 35 (15.8%). Previous acute cholecystitis was detected in 18 of 55 men (33%), but only in16 of 167 women (9%).
Convalescent patients of acute pancreatitis were operated on before hospital discharge and an intraoperative cholangiography was performed.The results of surgery can be read in Table 3.

No. Patients in day-case program	197
Postoperative hospitalization. No. (%)	15 (7.6)
Converted to general anaesthesia. No. (%)	69 (31)
Converted to open surgery. No. (%)**	7 (3.1)
Duration. Mean (SD)	49.4 (22.4)
Intraoperative cholangiography. No. (%)	17 (7.6)
Common bile duct exploration. No.	2*
Wound infection. No. (%)	5 (2.2)
Subhepatic collection. No. (%)	1 (0.4)
Visual Analog scale. Mean (range)	2.0 (0-8)

* a surgery completed under local anesthesia and sedation
** An open surgery for carcinoma of the gallbladder

Table 3. Results of 222 patients scheduled for transcylindrical cholecystectomy under local anaesthesia plus sedation

Nausea and vomiting have virtually disappeared. Pain at rest on the fifth postoperative day is almost nonexistent, while the pain with the movements of sitting or standing is mild and all the patients are able to self care.

Only 6 patients have expressed some discomfort during the operation, but the procedure was well tolerated and there was satisfaction in all cases, even where they were converted to general anesthesia.
The 5 cm cylinder was used in 2 cases of suspected choledocholithiasis and thirteen cases of postinflammatory anatomical distortion that hinders the recognition with the 3.8 cm cylinder
The vast majority of cases that required intubation (Table 4) was due to poor anatomical conditions related to persistent inflammation or scarring, but it is also true that a patient with a bulky or potent abdominal muscles (even with normal BMI) is a factor in consideration, since the absence of relaxation of the abdominal wall increases distance from the skin to the hepatocystic triangle and the cylinder of 10 cm length can be short.

Scarring or inflammatory anatomy	46
Big or muscular patient	16
Poor tolerance	6
Respiratory depression	1

Table 4. Causes of conversion to general anesthesia

In some cases we have changed the cylinder of 10 to 12 cm with satisfactory results. As previously mentioned, in 34 cases, of our patients had suffered a hospital admission for an attack of acute cholecystitis with ultrasound which showed a thickened gallbladder wall. Despite having passed more than 8 weeks after hospital discharge and be asymptomatic, we have found during the intervention that the process is not cured and present frank acute cholecystitis in 7 cases (20%). Of the 69 patients converted to general anesthesia, 29 were men in a series with 55 men. Obviously, the male sex is a definite risk factor for conversion to general anesthesia, as gallstone disease seems more severe in men while the abdominal muscles are larger. In our series both the height and weight is significantly higher in males, but not BMI which is slightly below the average (28.9 kg/m2).
In cases of conversion to a classical laparotomy incision the bad anatomy can also blame as responsible, in fact, five of seven cases converted belong to patients with acute cholecystitis previous and three of the 7 are male. In one case cystic clips were dislodged while reviewing the operative area.
However it is, starting the procedure under local anesthesia and sedation does not produce a significant delay in time, only a few minutes, since the decision to intubate the patient is taken quickly and everything is ready for this eventuality, but it is likely that in the future the general anesthesia be used from the begin in the men who have had an admisssion for acute cholecystitis.

4.6.2 Transcylindrical cholecystectomy in the treatment of acute cholecystitis and choledocholithiasis

In total 99 patients were operated for acute cholecystitis: 45 suspected prior to the intervention and operated in emergency basis or in the first 72 hours after admission (but not from the onset of symptoms, because in our experience, half of the patients came in a mean of 36 hours after the pain). The operation for acute cholecystitis is more laborious, with and greater needs of conversions to classic laparotomy, which in our series occurred in 13 cases. In all cases except one that ended with a cholecystostomy, the gallbladder has been removed. The duration of the intervention is significantly higher than cholecystectomy for

uncomplicated lithiasis is related to the need for more time for dissection and hemostasis. Two superficial wound infections, 2 postoperative subhepatic collections and a third at 9 months after surgery treated by percutaneous puncture and a biliary leak through drainage for 15 days with spontaneous closure are noteworthy complications. At least 3 days of hospitalization and antibiotic treatment follow the surgery.
In our experience, common bile duct exploration presents no special difficulties except juxtapapillary interlocking stone, making it difficult to remove. The location of the bile duct, dissection, and preparation is as simple as in open laparotomy. In 30 cases we performed transcylindrical choledochotomy with an average of 119 minutes, with a range between 70 and 182 minutes of the proceedings. A stone inpacted in a dilated common bile duct required a choledochoduodenostomy. One patient experienced postoperative bleeding requiring intervention without finding the bleeding point.

5. Conclusion

Despite technological advances and the practice of surgery becoming more expensive, we developed a technique for the treatment of gallstones and its complications achievable with natural view of the structures and conventional reusable material. The technique has proven to be fast simple and safe, applicable to all patients. Local anesthesia and sedation provides a quick recovery and many patients lose the fear of the intervention. Both in acute cholecystitis in choledocholithiasis we have obtained good results. The patients suspected of choledocholithiasis are operated and an intraoperative cholangiography is made. The transcylindrical exploration of the common bile duct is performed whenever introperative cholangiography demonstrated stones.

6. References

Arendt, SA. & Pitt, HA. (2004) Biliary Tract. In: *Sabiston Textbook of Surgery: The Biological Basis of Modern Surgical Practice.* Townsend, CM., Beauchamp, RD., Evers, BM., & Mattox, KL., editors, pp. 1597-1641. 17th edition. Elsevier Saunders, ISBN 0-8089-2295-5, Philadelphia.

Assalia, A., Kopelman, D., Hashmonai, M. (1997). Emergency minilaparotomy cholecystectomy for acute cholecystitis: prospective randomized trial--implications for the laparoscopic era. *World J Surg* 1997, Vol. 21, No. 5, pp. 534-9. ISSN 0364-2313.

Bartlett, MK., & Waddell, WR. (1958). Indications for common duct exploration. Evaluation in 1000 cases. *New Eng J Surg* 1958, Jan 23, Vol. 258, no. 4, pp. 164-7, ISSN:0028-4793.

Britton, J., & Bickerstaff, KI (1994). Benign Diseases of the Biliary Tract. In: *Oxford Textbook of Surgery* Morris, PJ., & Malt, RA., editors. Oxford University Press, pp. 1209-1241. ISBN 0192626035, New York.

Classen, M., & Demling, L. (1974). Endoscopic sphincterotomy of the papilla of vater and extraction of stones from the choledochal duct. *Deutsch Med Wochenschr* 1974, Mar 15, Vol. 99, N0.11, pp. 496-7, ISSN 0012-0472.

Cooperman, AM. (1990). Laparoscopic cholecystectomy for severe acute, embedded, and gangrenous cholecystitis. *J Laparoendosc Surg* 1990, Vol. 1, No. 1, pp. 37-40. ISSN 1052-3901.

Craig, DB. (1981). Postoperative recovery of pulmonary function. *Anesth Analg*, Jan 1981, vol 60, No. 1, pp. 46-52, ISSN 0003-2999.

Dawnson, JL. (1985). Colecistectomía. En: *Cirugía de la vesicular y vías biliares,* Marlow, S., & Sherlock, S., editores, pp. 319-335, Salvat Editores S.A., ISBN 84-345-2263-21985, Barcelona

Doherty, GM. (2010). *Current diagnosis and treatment surgery.* 13th edition, Lange Medical Books/McGraw-Hill, ISBN 978-0-07-16389-4, New York.

Dubois, F. & Berthelot, B. (1982) Cholécystectomie par mini-laparotomie. *Nouv presse Med,* April 1982 3;Vol.11, No. 15, pp.1139-41, ISSN 0301-1518, OCLC 9262901.

Escorrou, J., Cordova, JA., Lazortes, F., Frexinos, J., & Ribet A (1984). Early and Late complications after endoscopic sphincterotomy for biliary lithiasis with and without the gallbladder "in situ" . *Gut,* Jun 1984, Vol. 25, No. 6, pp. 598-602, ISSN 0017-5749.

Fink, AS. (1993). To ERCP o not to ERCP: that is the question. *Surg Endosc* 1993, Vol. 56, pp. 375-376, ISSN:0930-2794.

Frazee, RC., Roberts, JW., Okeson, GC., Symmonds, RE., Snyder, SK., Hendricks, JC., & Smith, RW. (1991). Open versus laparoscopic cholecystectomy. A comparison of pulmonary function. *Ann Surg,* Jun 1991, Vol. 213, No. 6, pp. 651-3, ISSN 0003-4932.

Gilliland, TM., & Traverso, LW. (1990). Modern standards for comparison of cholecystectomy with alternative treatments for symptomatic cholelithiasis with emphasis on long term relief of symptoms. *Surg Gynecol Obstet,* Jan 1990, Vol.170, No 1, pp. 39-44. ISSN 0039-6087.

Goco, IR. & Chambers, LG. (1988). Dollars and cents: minicholecystectomy and early discharge. *South Med J,* Feb 1988, vol. 81, No. 2, pp. 161-3. ISSN 0038-4348.

Grau-Talens, EJ., & Giner, M. (2010) Transcylindrical gas-free cholecystectomy for the treatment of cholelithiasis, cholecystitis, and choledocholithiasis. *Surg Endosc,* Sep 2010, Vol. 24, No. 9, pp. 2099-104, ISSN 0930-2794.

Grau-Talens, EJ., Cattáneo, JH., Giraldo, R., Mangione-Castro, PG. & Giner, M. (2010) Transcylindrical cholecystectomy under local anestesia plus sedation. A pilot study. *Endoscopy,* May 2010; Vol. 42, No. 5, pp. 395-9, ISSN 0013-726X.

Grau-Talens, EJ., García-Olives, F., & Rupérez-Arribas, MP. (1998). Transcylindrical cholecystectomy: new technique for minimally invasive cholecystectomy. *World J Surg,* May 1998; 22, No. 5 pp.153-8, ISSN 0364-2313.

Grau-Talens, EJ., Pérez-García, G., & Rupérez-Arribas, MP. (1994). Colecistectomía transcilíndrica. *Cirugía Española,* Noviembre 1994, vol. 56, Suplemento 1, p.297, ISSN 00-9739-X.

Harris, H W. (2008). Biliary system, In: *Surgery. Basic science and clinical evidence,* Norton, JA., Barie, PS., Randal Bollinger, R., Chang, AE., Lowry, SF., Mulvihill, SJ., Pass, HI., & Thompson, RW., Editors, pp. 911-942, Second Edition, Springer Scoience+Business Media,LLC, ISBN 978-0-387-30800-5, New York.

Karam, J. & Roslyn, JL. (1997). Colelithiasis and Cholecystectomy. In: *Maingot´s Abdominal Operations,* Zinner, MJ., Schwartz, SI., & Ellis, H, editors.. Tenth edition. McGraw-Hill, pp.1717-1738. ISBN 0-8385-6106-3, New York.

Katz, D., Nikfarjam, M., Sfakiotaki, A., & Christophi, C. (2004). Selective endoscopic cholangiography for the detection of common bile duct stones in patients with cholelithiasis. *Endoscopy,* Dec 2004,Vol. 36, No. 12, pp. 1045-9. ISSN 0013-726X.

Koo, KP., & Traverso, LW. (1996). Do preoperative indicators predict the presence of common bile duct during laparoscopic cholecystectomy? Am J Surg, May 1996, vol 171, No. 5, pp.495-9. ISSN 0002-9610.

Kroh, M., Chand, B. (2008). Choledocholithiasis, endoscopic retrograde cholangiopancretography, and laparoscopic common bile duct exploration. Sur Clin N Am, Dec 2008, Vol. 88, No. 6, pp. 1019-1031. ISSN0039-6109.

Lindell, P., & Hendenstierna, G. (1976). Ventilation efficiency after different incisión for cholecystectomy. *Acta Chir Scand* 1976, Vol.142, No. 8,pp. 561-5, ISSN 0301-1860

Litynski, G. (1996). *Highlights in the history of laparoscopy. The development of laparoscopic techniques. A cumulative effort of internists, gynecologist and surgeons.* Barbara Bernert Verlag, ISBN 3-9804740-6-2, Frankfurt/Main.

McMahon AJ, Russell IT, Ramsay G, Sunderland G, Baxter JN, Anderson JR, et al (1994). Laparoscopic and minilaparotomy cholecystectomy: a randomized trial comparing postoperative pain and pulmonary function. *Surgery,* May 1994, Vol.115, No. 5 pp. 533-9, ISSN 0039-6060.

Morton, CE. (1985). Cost containment with the use of "mini-cholecystectomy" and intraoperative cholangiography. *Am Surg,* Mar 1985, Vol 51, No. 3, pp. 168-9. ISSN 0003-1348.

Moss, G. (1996). Raising the outcome standards for conventional open cholecystectomy. *Am J Surg,* Oct 1996, Vol. 172, No. 4, pp. 383-5. ISSN 0002-9610.

Mühe, E. (1986). Die erste cholecystektomie durch das laparoskop. *Langenbecks Arch Chir* 1986; Vol. 369, No.1, p.804. ISSN 1435-2443

O'Kelly, TJ., Barr, H., Malley, WR., & Kettlewell, M. (1991). Cholecystectomy through a 5 cm subcostal incision. *Br J Surg;* Jun, Vol. 78,N0. 6, p. 762, ISSN:0007-1323.

O'Dwyer, PJ., Murphy, JJ.,& O'Higgins, NJ (1990). Cholecystectomy through a 5 cm subcostal incision. *British J Surg,* Oct 1990, Vol. 77, No. 10, pp. 1189-9, ISSN 0007-1323.

Olsen DO (1993). Mini-Lap cholecystectomy. *Am J Surg,* Apr 1993, Vol. 165, No. 4, pp 440-3, ISSN 0002-9610.

Rhodes, M., Sussman, L., Cohen, L., & Lewis, MP. (1998). Randomised trial of laparoscopic exploration of common bile duct versus postoperative endoscopic retrograde cholangiography for common bile duct stones. *Lancet,* Jan 17, 1998,Vol. 351(9097), pp.159-61, ISSN 0140-6736.

Rozsos, I., Ferenczy, I., & Rozsos, T. (1997). The surgical technique of microlaparotomy cholecystectomy. *Acta Chir Hung* 1997, Vol. 36, (1-4), pp 294-296, ISSN:0231-4614.

Rozsos, I., Ferenczy, J., & Schmitz, R. (2003). Micro and mini-cholecystectomies in the 21st century *Orv Hetil* 2003, Vol. 144, pp. 1291-1297, ISSN 0030-6002.

Russell, RCG., & Shankar, S. (1987). The stabilized ring retractor. A technique for cholecystectomy. *Br J Surg,* Sep 1987, Vol. 74, No. 8, pp. 826, ISSN:0007-1323.

Schumacher, FJ., & Kohaus, HM. (1994). Cholecystectomy via a surgical tube in 800 patients. *Chirurg,* Apr 1994, Vol 65, No. 4, pp. 373-6, ISSN 0009-4722.

Schwarts, SI. (1989). Gallbladder and Extrahepatic Biliary System. In: *Principles of Surgery* Schwarts, SI. Shires, GT. Spencer, FC. & Husser, WC, editors. pp. 1381-1412, Fith edition, McGraw-Hill Book Company, ISBN 0-07-055822-1, New York.

Werbesey, JE., Kirkett DH. (2008). Common bile duct exploration for choledocholithiasis. *Surg Clin N Am* 2008, Dec, Vol. 88, No. 6, pp.1315-28. ISSN 0039-6109.

Yamashita, Y., Takada, T., Kararada, Y et al (2007). Surgical treatment of patients with acute cholecystitis: Tokyo guidelines. *J Hepatobiliary Pancreat Surg* 2007; Vol. 14, No. 1, pp. 91-7, ISSN 0944-1166.

Zeus, F., Gooszen, HG., & Van Laarhoven, CJ. (2010). Open, small-incision or laparoscopic cholecystectomy for patients with symtomatic cholecystolithiasis. An overview of Cochrane Hepato-Biliary Group reviews. *Cochrane Database Syst Rev* 2010,Jan 20; Issue 1, CD008318, ISSN 1469-493x, 1361-6137.

2

Laparoscopic Cholecystectomy in High Risk Patients

Abdulrahman Saleh Al-Mulhim
King Faisal University
Saudi Arabia

1. Introduction

High risk patients who are candidates for laparoscopic cholecystectomy differ from the patients who have no existing risks and comorbidities in terms of the methods to be used as well as the expected outcomes. In order to recognize the safety of laparoscopic cholecystectomy, different cases of high risk patients undergoing laparoscopic cholecystectomy were gathered which demonstrate their conditions during laparoscopic cholecystectomy. These articles focused on patients with cardiopulmonary diseases, diabetes mellitus, sickle cell diseases, renal diseases, liver cirrhosis, during pregnancy and in the elderly. The results of the different cases showed that laparoscopic cholecystectomy is a safe procedure to be utilized and it is therefore recommended as the treatment of choice, as long as it is done cautiously and skillfully in all the high risk groups. The consequences of this technique including the bile duct injury, influence of pneumoperitoneum on cardiorespiratory system and other complications are outweighed by the benefits that the patients acquire after the surgery.

Patients who are high risk and undergo traditional cholecystectomy carries high morbidity and mortality as compared to laparoscopic cholecystectomy. The introduction of laparoscopic cholecystectomy has decreased the number of contraindications in the past recent years and in which more studies are focused on the constant modifications in terms of the assessed risks as well as the indications for the procedure.[1]

Patients who have past or recent medical conditions who are at risk of presenting perioperative complications and those who cannot survive an operation are the ones classified as high risks patients.[2] The issue that is always brought up for patients with such conditions is whether the benefits of laparoscopic cholecystectomy offset the risks involved especially with the new methods used in the procedure such as CO_2 insufflation and pneumoperitoneum.[3]

There are collated cases which demonstrate the conditions of the high risks patients during laparoscopic cholecystectomy. These articles focused on patients with cardiopulmonary diseases, diabetes mellitus, sickle cell diseases, renal diseases, liver cirrhosis, during pregnancy and in the elderly.

2. Patients with cardiopulmonary diseases

Hemodynamic and respiratory effects of the pneumoperitoneum are the most common hazards of surgical intervention in cardiac and pulmonary disease patients. Popken[1] stated that the advantages of laparoscopic cholecystectomy are more rapid recovery of lung function and a shorter stay in hospital. Catani [4] declared that changes in cardiovascular function due to the insufflation are characterized by an immediate decrease in cardiac index and an increase in mean arterial blood pressure and systemic vascular resistance.

2.1 Cases

Popken et al [1] published a study regarding patients with cardiopulmonary impairment where they used laparoscopic cholecystectomy in 19 high-risk patients (ASA IV) and 465 patients with a lower operative risk (ASA I-III). The authors state that out of 484 patients, there were 5 percent who suffered intraoperative cardiopulmonary complications. There were three who belonged to the high-risk group (15.8%) and 21 to the lower risk groups (4.5%). There were general postoperative complications that occurred in 14 cases (2.9%). The authors noted that the number of days spent in hospital was 4.96 to 7.6 in average days in the high-risk group versus 2.23 to 4.8 days in groups ASA I-III. They concluded that high-risk patients shows a raise perioperative rate of complications in laparoscopic cholecystectomy but they also stated that it is not basically a contraindication for this operative method.

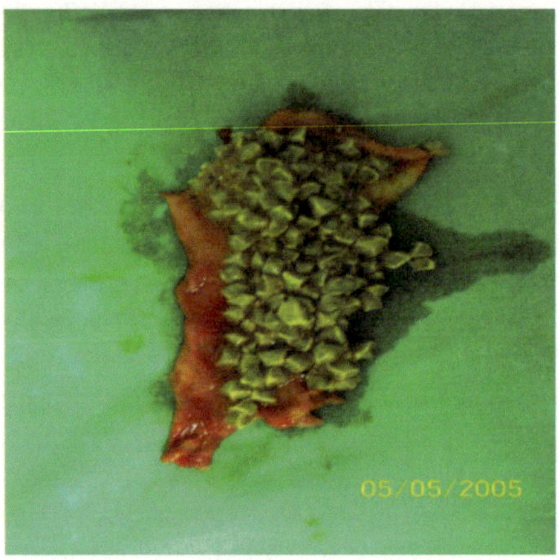

Tillman et al. [2] also investigated their laparoscopic cholecystectomy cases in 17 patients with severe cardiac dysfunction. They reported that there were three of the 17 patients who required administration of nitroglycerin to maintain the MAP and SVR within the accepted limits while one also required administration of dobutamine to maintain CI. There was no myocardial morbidity or mortality in the perioperative period according to their report. They concluded that laparoscopic cholecystectomy in patients with severe cardiac dysfunction results in significant hemodynamic changes.

3. Patients with diabetes mellitus

It has been believed that patients with diabetes mellitus is considered before as a risk factor in patients who undergo laparoscopic cholecystectomy commonly because of symptomatic gallbladder stones.[5] This is due to reports (Chang,M.D)[6] that a high plasma glucose level is associated with a poor neurologic recovery score in patients after cardiopulmonary

resuscitation. Researchers said that even if consciousness is restored, neurologic deficit may remain in hyperglycemic patients. [5] Therefore it is important to maintain an adequate plasma glucose level (120-180 mg/dl) during anesthesia as well as in the pre-operative period.
Specialists agree that in order to achieve strict plasma glucose control, the plasma glucose level is checked and controlled with hypoglycemic agent such as insulin regularly and frequently which helps prevent acute and chronic complications of DM. They said that stress caused by surgery and anesthesia induces hyperglycemia causing higher blood glucose levels in DM patients who underwent surgery than in patients who did not have surgery. [5]

3.1 Cases

Bedirli et al. [8] gathered the data for their laparoscopic cholecystectomy cases where there are eight hundred sixty-two patients with symptomatic gallbladder stones who underwent laparoscopic cholecystectomy. They took into consideration the age, sex, risk classification of the American Society of Anesthesiologists (ASA), laboratory tests, operative records, morbidity and length of hospital stay for each patient. They noted that almost half of their cholecystectomies which comprised 111 patients were performed as acute surgery due to cholecystitis. There were conversions to open surgery which were required in 16% of the diabetic patients undergoing LC. They concluded that when feasible, LC was a safe procedure in diabetes.

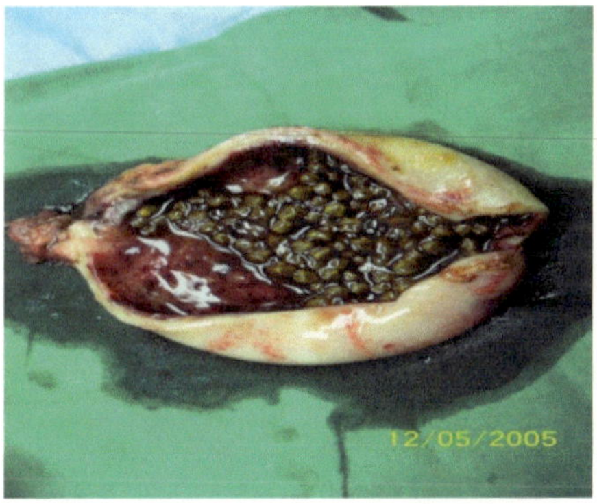

Paajanen et al [9] studied 2,548 consecutive patients (1,581 LC, 967 OC) with symptomatic gallstones who underwent cholecystectomy. They summed up that from 1995 and 2008, they operated 227 patients with diabetes 45 of these patients had type 1 diabetes. They made a comparison with the preoperative data and the operative outcome of the diabetic patients who underwent laparoscopic cholecystectomy and open cholecystectomy. They had observed that more complications occur in the open cholecystectomy group than in the laparoscopic cholecystectomy group. Upon their analysis they stated that comorbidities of diabetes were associated with an elevated risk for complications but obesity or acute surgery was not independently associated with postoperative complications. The authors concluded that laparoscopic cholecystectomy is a safe procedure in diabetic patient as compared to open cholecystectomy where there is a significant reduction in operative risks and complications.

4. Patients with sickle cell diseases

Among the genetic disorders, sickle cell disease is the most common around the world. People who are affected are at an increased risk of developing pigmented gallstones [10] and it is said that this risk increases with age. Perioperative and postoperative complications which are mainly vaso-occlusive crises (VOC) may occur as a result of surgeries for symptomatic stones. Minimal risks have been associated with the introduction laparoscopic cholecystectomy because of its advantages over the traditional open surgeries.

4.1 Cases

It is believed that minimally invasive therapy can reduce morbidity and mortality in sickle cell disease patients. The safety of laparoscopic cholecystectomy in such patients has already been recognized. Rachid et al [10] reported the results of their experience on laparoscopic cholecystectomy in sickle cell disease patients in Niger, which is included in the sickle cell belt. Their study covered 45 months and included 47 patients operated by the same surgeon. The average age was 22.4 years (range: 11 to 46 years) and eleven (23.4%) of them were aged less than 15 years. The types of sickle cell disease found were 37 SS, 2 SC, 1 S beta-thalassemia and 7 AS. The indications for their surgeries were biliary colic in 29 cases (61.7%) and acute cholecystitis in 18 cases (38.3%). Their mean operative time was 64 minutes. Reports from the authors states that there were conversions to open cholecystectomy in 2 cases (4.2 %) for non recognition of Calot's triangle structures. They reported four cases of postoperative complications of vaso-occlusive crisis and one case of acute chest syndrome. Their mean postoperative hospital stay was 3.5days (range: 1 to 9 days). There was no mortality encountered. The authors concluded that laparoscopic cholecystectomy is a safe procedure in sickle cell patients and that it should be a multidisciplinary approach and involve the haematologist, anaesthesiologist and a surgeon.

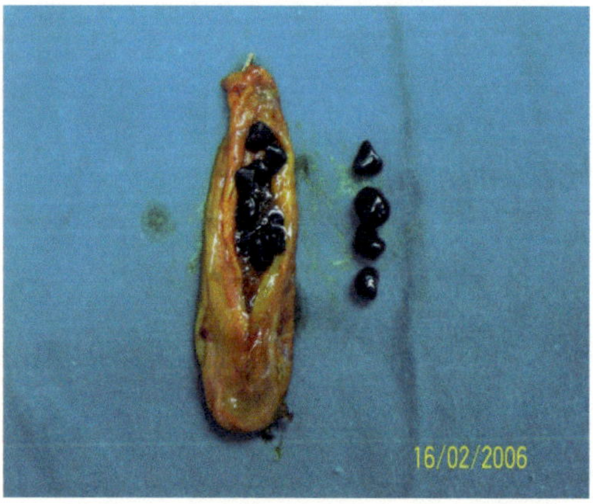

Haberkem et al [12] studied a group of 364 patients who underwent cholecystectomy. There were ninety-eight percent of their patients who had symptomatic cholelithiasis. Their total perioperative morbidity was 39% and they reported that while total morbidity is not affected by preoperative transfusion, the incidence of specific sickle cell events is higher in those patients who were not transfused preoperatively than in those who were. Laparoscopic cholecystectomy was accompanied by shorter hospitalization time (6.4 days)

than the open cholecystectomy (9.8 days) and noted that perioperative outcomes were the same with both techniques. The authors concluded that conservative preoperative transfusion and use of the laparoscopic technique are necessary for patients with sickle cell disease who will be undergoing cholecystectomy to prevent further complications.

5. Patients with renal diseases

Management of gallstones in renal transplant patients was always questioned because of the related complications. It has been found out that patients with renal disease have a higher incidence of coronary artery disease (CAD) and peripheral vascular disease (PVD) compared to the general population because they have the traditional risk factors for CAD such as advanced age, diabetes, hypertension and lipid disorders as well as a high prevalence of such as hyperhomocysteinemia, abnormal calcium phosphate metabolism, anemia, increased oxidative stress and uremic toxins.[27]

5.1 Cases

Ekici et al [25] conducted a study where they assessed laparoscopic cholecystectomy (LC) in patients with end-stage renal disease treated with continuous ambulatory peritoneal dialysis. There were eleven patients receiving peritoneal dialysis treatment and 33 patients without end-stage renal disease who had undergone an elective LC were compared. They reviewed all their medical records and the laboratory values as well as the outcomes and results. Their peritoneal dialysis group showed a higher frequency of associated disease and previous abdominal surgery, a lower hemoglobin and platelet count and elevated alkaline phosphatase, blood urea nitrogen and creatinine values. There was one procedure in each group that was converted to an open cholecystectomy. There were no other catheter-related complications that occurred. The authors concluded that laparoscopic cholecystectomy may be performed with low complication rates in patients undergoing continuous ambulatory peritoneal dialysis with an experienced team.

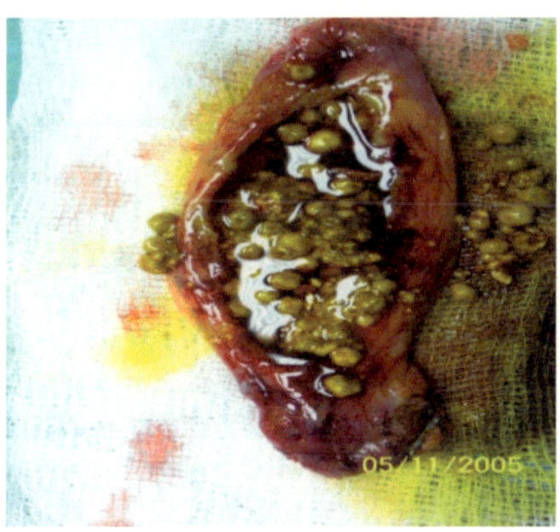

Banli et al [26] evaluated the outcomes of laparoscopic cholecystectomy in renal transplant patients with symptomatic gallstone disease. They reviewed the records of 155 kidney transplant patients, including 16 patients who underwent laparoscopic cholecystectomy. They found out that the shortest interval time between transplantation and cholecystectomy was 2 years. Surgical morbidity were seen in two of the patients with no mortality and no graft loss. They concluded that laparoscopic cholecystectomy can be performed safely with low morbidity in renal transplant patients who have symptomatic gallstone disease.

6. Patients with cirrhotic diseases

Liver diseases are always considered risk factors in operations due to increase risks of complications and sometimes can even be the cause of death. Liver decompensation is also one reason why clinicians are hesitant to recommend surgeries due to the possible occurrence of abnormal clearance of proteins, abnormal excretion, ascites and portal hypertension. [11]

There are also factors being considered such as the patients Child-Pugh score, the length and extent of the surgery as well as postoperative complications.[23] The Child-Pugh score is used to evaluate and assess the condition of a patient with liver disease as well as predict mortality during surgery. Nowadays it is also used to establish the prognosis and the required treatment for the disease. [23]

Another recent assessment tool is the Model for End-Stage Liver Disease, or MELD, a scoring system for assessing the severity of chronic liver disease. This system uses the patient's values for serum bilirubin, serum creatinine, and the international normalized ratio for prothrombin time (INR) to predict the patient's survival after surgery. [11]

6.1 Cases

Cucinotta et al [7] accumulated the records of 22 laparoscopic cholecystectomies which they performed in patients with cirrhosis Child-Pugh A and B. These data were gathered from January 1995 to July 2001. There was no death reported and the average duration of the surgeries were 115 minutes and were noted that they were shorter than the usual open cholecystectomy. They also stated that blood transfusion was not required in all the surgeries and that the intraoperative complications that occurred were liver bed bleeding. They also noted some postoperative morbidities such as hemorrhage, wound complications, cardiopulmonary complications and intraabdominal collections in 36% of the patients but reported that they were all controlled. They observed the length of hospital stay in patients with an average of 4 days. The authors concluded that with laparoscopic cholecystectomy having lower morbidity, shorter operative time and with reduced hospital stay, it can be safely done in patients with cirrhosis Child-Pugh A and B who are carefully selected and screened as to their need for surgery.

Another study was also done by Delis et al [15] from January 1995 to July 2008 where they performed 220 laparoscopic cholecystectomies in patients Child-Pugh class A and B patients with MELD scores ranging from 8 to 27. Their indications for the said operations were symptomatic gallbladder disease and cholecystitis. They reported that no deaths occurred and observed that there were postoperative morbidities that occurred such as hemorrhage, wound complications and intra-abdominal collections but they were controlled. They stated that intraoperative difficulties due to liver bed bleeding were experienced in 19 patients. There was a necessity to convert 12 of their cases to open cholecystectomy. Their median operative time was 95 minutes while their median hospital stay was 4 days. They reported that patients with preoperative MELD scores above 13 showed a tendency for higher complication rates postoperatively. The authors concluded that laparoscopic cholecystectomy can be performed safely in selected patients with cirrhosis Child-Pugh A and B and symptomatic cholelithiasis with acceptable morbidity.

Leone et al [16] presented their cases between January 1994 and December 2000 where there were 1,100 laparoscopic cholecystectomies for symptomatic gallbladder diseases. They reported that there were 24 cirrhotic patients who had well-compensated cirrhosis (Child's class A or B). The authors reported that there were no operative mortality and the postoperative complication rates were 20.8%. They estimated that the intraoperative blood loss was 37.08 ml in average. Their average hospital stay 3.61 days. The authors concluded that laparoscopic cholecystectomy in patients with compensated cirrhosis is safe and should be the treatment of choice for these patients. They further stated that laparotomy should be applied only if the surgeon considers the operation inadequate to be continued laparoscopically.

7. Patients who are pregnant

Diseases in the abdomen requiring surgical intervention during pregnancy present unique challenges to their diagnosis and management [17]. These are said to be due to the changes in physiology and abdominal anatomy characteristic of pregnancy. These changes make laparoscopic surgery technically more difficult, the obstetrician must determine the status of pregnancy such as gestational age, viability and inform the patient about the risks related to pregnancy and surgery itself [18].

There are several mechanisms that have been proposed by specialists for increased fetal morbidity and mortality associated with laparoscopic surgery during pregnancy including direct uterine trauma, fetal trauma, intraamniotic CO_2 insufflation, trauma to maternal abdominal organs and vessels, decreased uterine blood flow and oxygen delivery, teratogenic effects of anesthetic drugs, fetal acidosis due to CO_2 pneumoperitoneum, adverse effects of anesthesia on maternal hemodynamic and acid-base balance, increased risk of thromboembolic disease, the effect of underlying abdominal pathology, manipulation during surgery and effects of postoperative medications [18,20] Therefore laparoscopic cholecystectomy has been used cautiously in pregnant women. This is due to the possible mechanical problems related to the pregnant uterus and the other is fear of fetal injury resulting from instrumentation or the pneumoperitoneum.

7.1 Cases

To assess the effects of laparoscopic cholecystectomy on both the mother and the unborn fetus, Abuabara et al [19] reviewed their surgical experience over a 5-year period where 22 patients ranging from 17 to 31 years underwent laparoscopic cholecystectomy during pregnancy. They noted that the gestational ages ranged from 5 to 31 weeks where there are two patients who are in their first trimester, 16 in the second and four in the third. Their indications for surgery were persistent nausea, vomiting, pain, and inability to eat in 17 patients, acute cholecystitis in three and choledocholithiasis in two. The surgeons established pneumoperitoneum in all patients and their results were all 22 patients survived the surgical procedure without complications and there were no fetal deaths or premature births related to the procedure. The authors concluded that laparoscopic cholecystectomy during pregnancy is safe for both the mother and the unborn fetus and if at all possible, when laparoscopic cholecystectomy is indicated, it should be performed either in the second trimester or early in the third.

Wishner et al [21], members of the Norfolk Surgical Group, gathered their data for the laparoscopic cholecystectomy cases from May 1991 to June 1994 where they performed the operations on 1,300 patients. There were six of these patients who were operated on during pregnancy. They were able to successfully perform the operation on all the six patients and observed that the overall course of the operation is the same with non-pregnant patients. They reported that there were no significant complications to either the patient or the fetus. It was reported later that all the six patients delivered healthy babies and noted no signs of complications. The authors concluded that laparoscopic cholecystectomy can be performed safely in pregnant patients and that it should be considered in any patient who presents with symptomatic cholelithiasis during pregnancy.

8. Elderly patients

Age is one of the critical factors affecting the mortality and morbidity rates after open cholecystectomy for both acute and chronic cholecystitis [2, 3]. Several series of open cholecystectomy [4, 5] report death as a complication occurring almost exclusively in patients over 60 years of age [6]. Smith and Max [7] found that the morbidity-mortality rate after open cholecystectomy was 25% for patients aged 60-69 as opposed to 50% for patients over 70.
Ageing patients with symptomatic cholelithiasis frequently have associated medical disorders. They may be at higher risk of postoperative complications. Evaluation of the results of the laparoscopic approach in the aged would allow patients and surgeons to make decisions on the most appropriate treatment for symptomatic cholelithiasis.

8.1 Case

Brunt et al[22] gathered their laparoscopic data for 421 patients from 1989 to 1999 which were extremely elderly or older than 80 years to determine whether extremely elderly patients, age 80 years or older, were at higher risk for adverse outcomes from laparoscopic cholecystectomy than patients younger than 80 years. The patients were divided into two groups: group 1 (age 65-79 years; n = 351) and group 2 (age, 80-95 years; n = 70). The authors noted that the advanced age (group 2) was associated with a higher mean American Society of Anesthesiology (ASA) class and a greater incidence of common bile duct stones, as compared with those of younger age (group 1). Mean operative times in group 2 were 45-106 minutes as compared with 38 to 96 minutes in group 1, a difference that is not significant. The authors noted that the extremely elderly group had a four times higher rate of conversion to open cholecystectomy and a longer mean postoperative hospital stay of 1.4 to 2.1 days. They also stated that Grades 1 and 2 complications were more common in group 2. They reported that one patient in group 1 had a myocardial infarction 13 days postoperatively, and two deaths occurred in the extremely elderly group within 30 days postoperatively. The authors concluded that laparoscopic cholecystectomy in the extremely elderly is associated with more complications and a higher rate of conversion to open cholecystectomy than in elderly individuals younger than 80 years. The greater chance of encountering a severely inflamed or scarred gallbladder and common bile duct stones as well as increasing comorbidities likely account for these differences in outcome.
Mayol et al[24] gathered the outcome of all their laparoscopic cholecystectomy patients between 60 and 70 years of age and patients over 70 who underwent laparoscopic cholecystectomy for symptomatic non-malignant gallbladder disease. They found out that the operative time and conversion rates were similar with both groups. They noted that the overall morbidity rate was 14.5% and there was no perioperative mortality that occurred. There was a recurrent biliary surgery done in two patients from the above 70 group. There were also postoperative endoscopic retrograde cholangiography and sphincterotomy that

was done in four patients from the below 70 group. They also found out that the mean postoperative stay was longer for older patients above 70 years of age. The authors concluded that simple laparoscopic cholecystectomy is safe in the aged even for patients over 70. They stated that this procedure is associated with a short hospital stay and low rates of re-admission and recurrent biliary surgery.

9. Conclusion

With the success of laparoscopic cholecystectomy on different high risk patients, it is therefore recommended as the treatment of choice. The consequences of this technique including the bile duct injury, influence of pneumoperitoneum on cardiorespiratory system and other complications are outweighed by the benefits that the patients acquire after the surgery and these consequences can be prevented by performing the operation cautiously and skillfully in all the high risk patient groups.

10. References

[1] Popken F, Küchle R, Heintz A, Junginger T. [Laparoscopic cholecystectomy in high risk patients]. Chirurg. 1997 Aug;68(8):801-5. German. http://www.ncbi.nlm.nih.gov/pubmed/9522071

[2] H.A.Tillmann Hein, MD, Girish P. Joshi, MB BS, MD, FFARCSI, Michael A.E. Ramsay, MD, L.George Fox, MD, Bradley J. Gawey, MDab§, Christopher L. Hellman, MD, John C. Arnold, MDa

[3] Wahba RW, Béïque F, Kleiman SJ. Cardiopulmonary func- tion and laparoscopic cholecystectomy. Can J Anaesth. 1995 Jan;42(1):51-63. Review. PubMed PMID: 7889585.

[4] Catani M, Guerricchio R, De Milito R, Capitano S, Chiaretti M, Guerricchio A, Manili G, Simi M. ["Low-pressure" laparoscopic cholecystectomy in high risk patients (ASA III and IV): our experience]. Chir Ital. 2004 Jan-Feb;56(1):71-80. Italian.

[5] Hawthorne GC, Ashworth L, Alberti KG. The effect of laparoscopic cholecystectomy on insulin sensitivity. Horm Metab Res. 1994 Oct;26(10):474-7.

[6] Chul Ho Chang, M.D., Yon Hee Shim, M.D., Youn-Woo Lee, M.D., Yong Beom Kim, M.D., and Yong-Taek Nam, M.D. , Pain Medicine, Yonsei University College of Medicine, 134, Sinchon- dong, Seodaemun-gu, Seoul 120-752, Korea.

[7] Cucinotta E, Lazzara S, Melita G. Laparoscopic cholecystect omy in cirrhotic patients. Surg Endosc. 2003 Dec;17(12):1958-60. Epub 2003 Oct 28. Review.

[8] Bedirli A, Sözüer EM, Yüksel O, Yilmaz Z. Laparoscopic cholecystectomy for symptomatic gallstones in diabetic patients. J Laparoendosc Adv Surg Tech A. 2001 Oct;11(5):281-4. PubMed PMID: 11642663.

[9] Paajanen H, Suuronen S, Nordstrom P, Miettinen P, Niskanen L. Laparoscopic versus open cholecystectomy in diabetic patients and postoperative outcome. Surg Endosc. 2010 Jul 27. [Epub ahead of print] PubMed PMID: 20661751.

[10] Sani Rachid, Lassey James Didier, Mallam Abdou Badé, Chaibou Maman Sani, Abarchi Habibou. Laparoscopic cholecystectomy in sickle cell patients in Niger. The Pan African Medical Journal. 2009;3:19

[11] Kamath PS, Wiesner RH, Malinchoc M, Kremers W, Ther neau TM, Kosberg CL, D'Amico G, Dickson ER, Kim WR (2001). "A model to predict survival in patients with end-stage liver disease". Hepatology 33 (2): 464–70.

[12] Friedman LS. The risk of surgery in patients with liver dis ease. Hepatology 1999; 29:1617-23.
[14] Charles M. Haberkern, Lynne D. Neumayr, Eugene P. Orringer,Ann N. Earles, Shanda M. Robertson, Dennis Black, Miguel R. Abboud, Mabel Koshy, Olajire Idowu, Elliott P. Vichinsky, and the Preoperative Transfusion in Sickle Cell Disease Study Group. Blood, Vol. 89 No. 5 (March 1), 1997: pp. 1533-1542
[15] Delis S, Bakoyiannis A, Madariaga J, Bramis J, Tassopoulos N, Dervenis C. Laparoscopic cholecystectomy in cirrhotic patients: the value of MELD score and Child-Pugh classification in predicting outcome. Surg Endosc. 2010 Feb;24(2):407-12. Epub 2009 Jun 24. PubMed PMID: 19551433.
[16] Leone N, Garino M, De Paolis P, Pellicano R, Fronda GR, Rizzetto M. Laparoscopic cholecystectomy in cirrhotic patients. Dig Surg. 2001;18(6):449-52. PubMed PMID: 11799294.
[17] Modrzejewski A, Lewandowski K, Pawlik A, Czerny B, Kurzawski M, Juzyszyn Z. [Gall bladder stones during pregnancy in the age of laparoscopic cholecystectomy]. Ginekol Pol. 2008 Nov;79(11):768-74. Review. Polish. Machado NO, Machado LS. Laparoscopic cholecystectomy in the third trimester of pregnancy: report of 3 cases. Surg Laparosc Endosc Percutan Tech. 2009
[18] Comitalo JB, Lynch D. Laparoscopic cholecystectomy in the pregnant patient. Surg Laparosc Endosc. 1994 Aug;4(4):268-71.
[19] Abuabara SF, Gross GW, Sirinek KR. Laparoscopic cholecystectomy during pregnancy is safe for both mother and fetus. J Gastrointest Surg. 1999 Jan-Feb;1(1):48-52; discussion 52.
[20] Reyes-Tineo R. Laparoscopic cholecystectomy in pregnancy. Bol Asoc Med P R. 1997 Jan-Mar;89(1-3):9-11. Review.
[21] Wishner JD, Zolfaghari D, Wohlgemuth SD, Baker JW Jr, Hoffman GC, Hubbard GW, Gould RJ, Ruffin WK. Laparoscopic cholecystectomy in pregnancy. A report of 6 cases and review of the literature. Surg Endosc. 1996 Mar;10(3):314-8. Review.
[22] Brunt LM, Quasebarth MA, Dunnegan DL, Soper NJ. Outcomes analysis of laparoscopic cholecystectomy in the extremely elderly. Surg Endosc. 2001 Jul;15(7):700-5. Epub 2001 May 2. PubMed PMID: 11591971
[23] Pugh RN, Murray-Lyon IM, Dawson JL, Pietroni MC, Williams R (1973). "Transection of the oesophagus for bleeding oesophageal varices". The British journal of surgery 60 (8): 646–9.doi:10.1002/bjs.1800600817
[24] Julio Mayol, Javier Martinez Sarmiento, Francisco J. Tamayo, Jesus Alvarez Fernandez Represa. Age Ageing (1997) 26 (2): 77-81.doi: 10.1093/ageing/26.2.77
[25] Ekici Y, Karakayali F, Yagmurdur MC, Moray G, Karakayal H, Haberal M. Laparoscopic cholecystectomy in patients undergoing continuous ambulatory peritoneal dialysis: a case-control study. Surg Laparosc Endosc Percutan Tech. 009 Apr;19(2):101-5. PubMed PMID: 1939027
[26] O. Banli, N. Guvence, H. Altun Transplantation Proceedings.June 2005 (Vol. 37, Issue 5, Pages 2127-2128)
[27] Yeh CN, Chen MF, Jan YY. Laparoscopic cholecystectomy for 58 end stage renal disease patients. Surg Endosc. 2005 Jul;19(7):915-8. Epub 2005 May 3. PubMed PMID: 15868265.

3

Gallbladder Surgery, Choice of Technique: An Overview

E. Nilsson, M. Öman, M.M. Haapamäki and C.B. Sandzén
Department of Surgical and Perioperative Sciences, Umeå University, Sweden

1. Introduction

The first cholecystectomy was performed by Langenbuch in 1882 (1), and the surgical approach changed very little in the next century. However, in the 1980s, reports began to appear that described the removal of the gallbladder through a 3-8 cm, muscle-sparing incision (small-incision cholecystectomy, or minicholecystectomy) (2-17). A few years later, laparoscopic cholecystectomy entered the scene (18, 19). These two minimally-invasive techniques have largely replaced the traditional open cholecystectomy, which used a 10 - 20 cm incision in elective gallbladder surgery (20). In 1993, a consensus conference at the National Institute of Health concluded that the experience of small-incision surgery or mini-laparotomy cholecystectomy was limited; and that laparoscopic cholecystectomy could be performed at a treatment cost that was equal to or slightly less than that of open cholecystectomy and offered substantial cost savings to the patient and society by reducing the time off work (21). The alternative to surgical removal of the gallbladder, lithotripsy combined with chemical dissolution of gallstones is restricted to single stone disease and runs a risk of stone recurrence (22, 23). However, it has been found to be associated with good long-term quality of life in selected patients (24).
The aim of this review is to discuss factors that influence the choice between cholecystectomy techniques, taking into account the applicability and cost of each technique.

2. Methods

We conducted a literature search, including a search of the Cochrane Library and PubMed (year 2010) with the keyword "cholecystectomy" and used the principles of evidence based medicine in the presentation of the findings (25-29).

3. Results and discussion

Cholelithiasis, the magnitude of the problem

The prevalence of cholelithiasis in European population is currently 10-15%, and it increases with age and female gender (30-33). Patients with cholelithiasis may be asymptomatic or symptomatic. Biliary colic is the only symptom specific to cholelithiasis (34). It is characterised by a high intensity, long duration pain located in the right upper abdominal quadrant; it can be referred, and often appears at night (35). Cholelithiasis may be complicated by acute cholecystitis, common bile duct stones (with pancreatitis or jaundice), or fistula (32). Gallstone disease is the most common among all abdominal diseases that lead to hospital care in the Western world (36); recently, an increase of hospital admissions for gallstone disease has been observed in England (37). This has made gallstone disease a health care problem with considerable economic consequences; moreover, this problem will most likely increase with increases in population age (38). The annual direct cost in the United States has been estimated to be approximately six billion USD (39, 40). No randomised controlled trials have favoured operative treatment of asymptomatic patients with cholelithiasis (41). A wait-and-see management approach may also be adopted for symptomatic patients with uncomplicated disease (42), particularly those with atypical symptoms (43). With the introduction of the laparoscopic technique, the cholecystectomy incidence increased substantially (15 - 80%) in Europe (38, 44, 45), Canada (46), the United States (47, 48), and Saudi-Arabia (49).

Comments on cholecystectomy techniques

Details of the laparoscopic technique (Figure 1) are readily available to any trainee and will not be discussed here. Essential equipment for small-incision cholecystectomy include

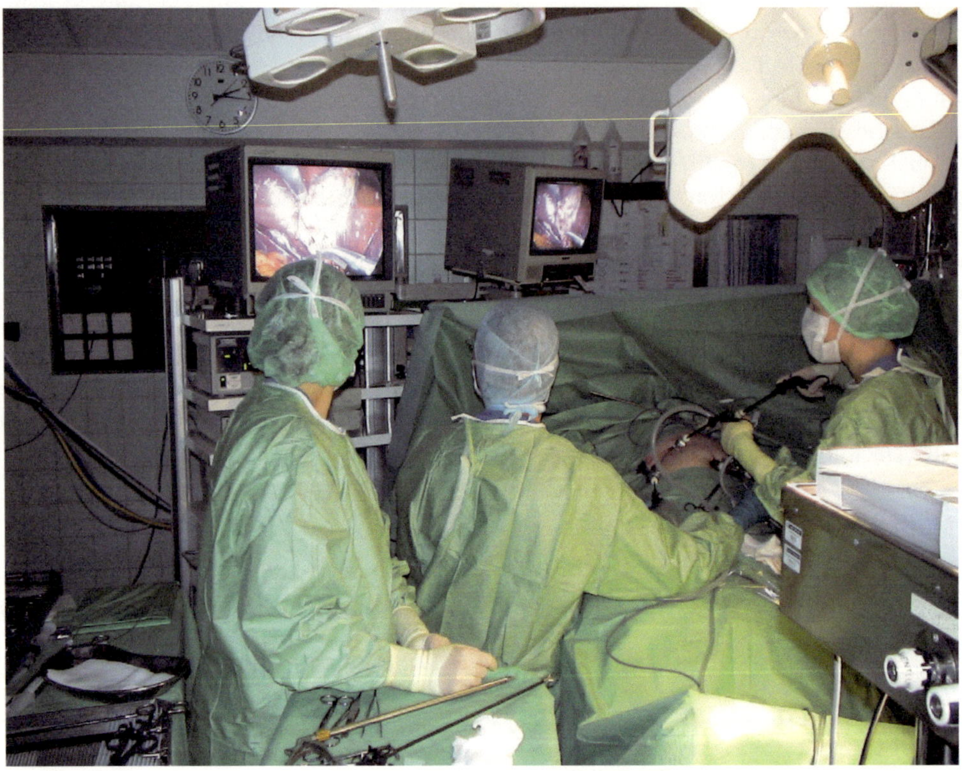

Fig. 1. Laparoscopic cholecystectomy with trainee (right). Consultant surgeon and nurse closely follow the operation.

Harrington-type retractors, headlamps, and magnification loops (Figure 2) (14). Briefly, the incision is performed over the right rectus muscle, two to three fingers below the xiphoid process (Figure 3) (10, 14). The anterior and the posterior rectus sheath are divided. The rectus muscle is left intact, but one or two cm may be divided medially. Intra-abdominal dissection is initiated at the triangle of Calot, although in patients with inflammation, a "fundus down" dissection may be advantageous. Before wound closure, a local anaesthetic agent is administered liberally in the rectus muscle compartment as well as subcutaneously. The rectus sheaths are sutured with non-absorbable suture and the subcutaneous layer with absorbable suture. When an extension of the incision must be performed in small-incision cholecystectomy, the incision is rarely extended lateral to the rectus muscle. Conversion from laparoscopic to open cholecystectomy typically requires a traditional 10 - 20 cm subcostal incision through the rectus muscle, the oblique muscles, and the transverse muscle, with the risk of causing denervation injury and subsequent incisional hernia.

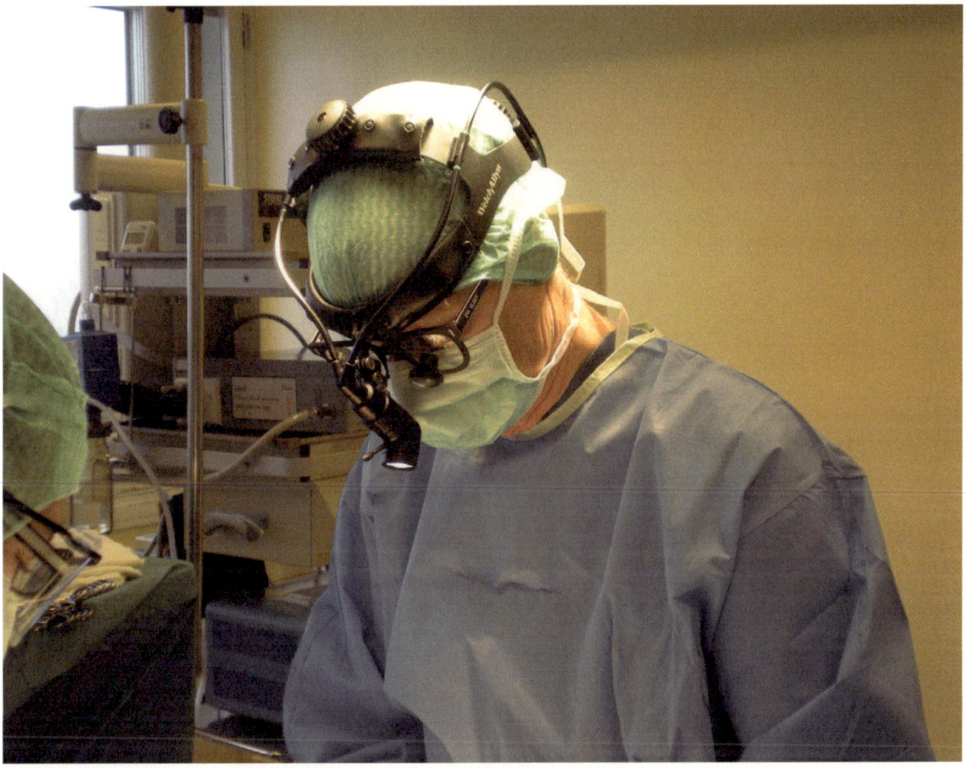

Fig. 2. Headlights and x2.5 magnification loops are necessary for performing a safe small-incision cholecystectomy.

Minimally-invasive techniques and day-case surgery

Both small-incision cholecystectomy (6, 7, 14, 17, 50-52) and laparoscopic cholecystectomy (50, 52-56) are compatible with ambulatory surgery. A Cochrane review has considered laparoscopic day-case surgery safe and effective for selected patients with symptomatic cholelithiasis (57).

Randomised controlled trials that compared open cholecystectomy, small-incision cholecystectomy, and laparoscopic cholecystectomy

Cochrane reviews demonstrate that small-incision and laparoscopic cholecystectomy should be considered equivalent with respect to complications and recovery, but the small-incision cholecystectomy requires a shorter operation time (58). However, trials with large numbers of patients are necessary to determine potential differences in serious adverse advents (59). Open cholecystectomy is associated with a longer hospital stay than the two minimally-invasive techniques (58). One randomised controlled trial concluded that small-incision cholecystectomy was also suitable for obese patients (17). Patient opinion of the cosmetic outcome of surgery did not differ significantly between small-incision and laparoscopic cholecystectomy one year after surgery (60). For both groups, the median value concerning patient views of the scar was 1 on a scale of 1 to 10, where 1= does not bother me at all, and 10=very disturbing. To judge the external validity of conclusions reached in randomised controlled trials, it is necessary to know outcomes for non-randomised patients treated at the units that participated in the trial. In one trial that compared the two minimally-invasive cholecystectomy techniques, the patients that received operations, but were excluded from the trials were older and tended to have more advanced disease (higher ASA-scores, more co-morbidities, more complications from gallstone disease) than the patients included in the trials (61).

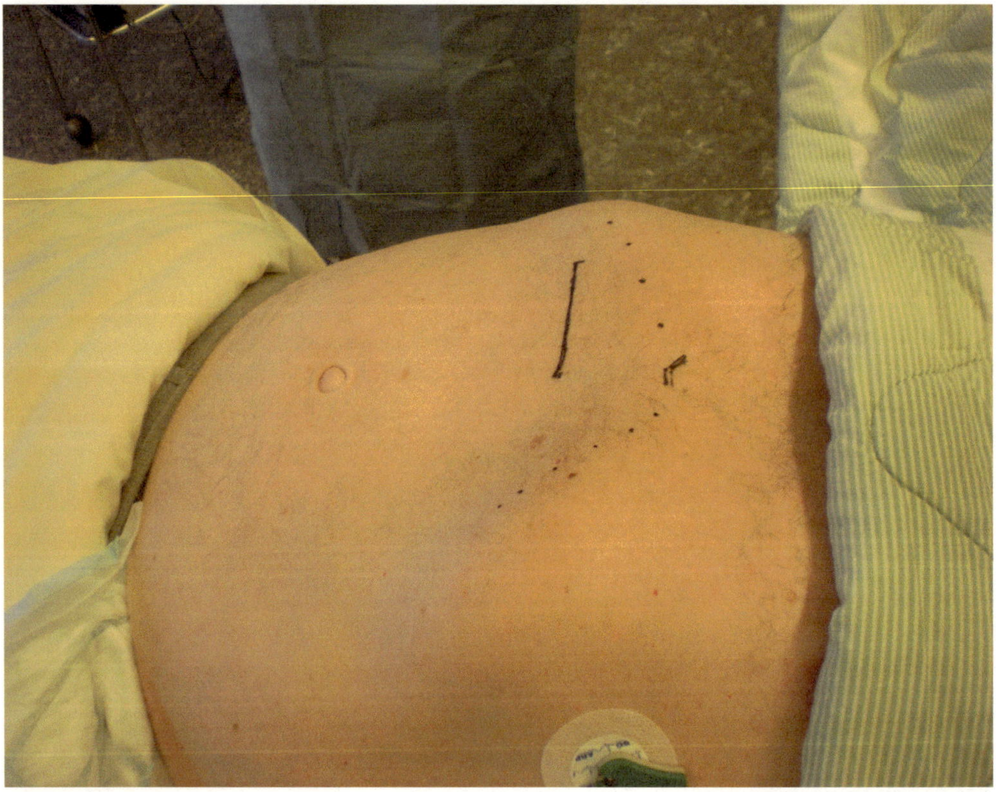

Fig. 3. Place for small-incision cholecystectomy. The incision is 6 -7 cm long, located over the right rectus muscle, 2 - 3 fingers below the xiphoid process (to the right). The costal margins are indicated by dots.

Cholecystectomy techniques from a population based perspective

In Sweden, laparoscopy has been the predominant cholecystectomy technique since 1993 (Sandzén et al, unpublished). From 2000 through 2003, 28% of patients who underwent cholecystectomy for benign, biliary diseases in Sweden had their operations completed as open procedures (62). Those patients showed a higher likelihood of having an acute admission and a complicated gallstone disease compared to patients that underwent laparoscopic cholecystectomy. They also had a higher mortality than expected, considering age and sex of the background population, both within 90 days of admission for cholecystectomy and 91-365 days postoperatively, indicating that these patients were sicker than the Swedish population in general. This suggested that efforts should be undertaken to reduce the surgical trauma in open biliary surgery (62). In the United States, 25% of all cholecystectomies were performed as open operations from 1998-2001, and 5-10% of laparoscopic cholecystectomies were converted to open operations (63). In Scotland, an audit reported that the open technique for gallbladder surgery was used in 11.4% of all cholecystectomies (4.0% primary and 7.4% converted laparoscopic) and concluded that also in the 2000s, open cholecystectomy is a common procedure with limited room in current trainee programs(64). Similar conclusions have been drawn from studies in the United States (65-67). Training programs for open cholecystectomy and common bile duct procedures have been considered necessary (68).

Population based studies have demonstrated that the incidence of bile duct injuries has increased after the introduction of laparoscopic cholecystectomy (69). In Sweden, there was a small to moderate long-term increase in the risk of bile duct injury after introduction of the laparoscopic technique compared to the prelaparoscopic era (70). This may be an underestimation of the real change, as the majority of bile duct injuries may be treated without reconstructive surgery today (71).

Cholecystectomy for complicated gallstone disease

The cholecystectomy technique should be chosen based on the particular type of gallstone complication in order to achieve smooth, early, definitive treatment. The complications include acute cholecystitis, common bile duct stones, and acute biliary pancreatitis.

For acute cholecystitis, an early randomised controlled trial showed that small-incision cholecystectomy was safe, reliable, and had advantages compared to traditional open cholecystectomy (72). Another randomised controlled trial found no clinically significant differences between traditional open cholecystectomy and laparoscopic cholecystectomy (73). Observational series have demonstrated that both small-incision (74) and laparoscopic cholecystectomy (75-79) are suitable for treating acute cholecystitis. According to meta-analyses, an early operation (open or laparoscopic) does not carry a higher risk of mortality or morbidity compared to delayed surgery, and therefore, should be the preferred treatment (80, 81). This is also applicable to older patients (81, 82). Laparoscopic cholecystectomy for acute cholecystitis, whether performed early or delayed, is associated with a higher conversion rate compared to elective cholecystectomy (81). In England, 40% of patients with acute gallbladder disease had an open operation (converted laparoscopic or traditional open cholecystectomy) (83). In Denmark, in 2004, 36% of cholecystectomies for acute cholecystitis were completed as open procedures (84). In Sweden, from 1995 through 1999, 68% of patients aged 70 years and older had open operations for acute cholecystitis (85).

Concomitant removal of common bile duct stones via choledochotomy can be successfully performed with open cholecystectomy (86), small-incision cholecystectomy (87), or laparoscopic cholecystectomy (88-90). According to a Cochrane review, choledochotomy is superior to endoscopic sphincterotomy for bile duct clearance in open gallbladder surgery. In contrast, laparoscopic choledochotomy and endoscopic sphincterotomy are equally effective in the short term, although the latter alternative requires an increased number of procedures (91). In laparoscopic surgery, endoscopic sphincterotomy is the method preferred by most surgeons for common bile duct clearance (37, 66, 92). However, laparoscopic choledochotomy and trancystic common bile duct exploration (93) with concomitant cholecystectomy are achievable, effective alternatives. Long-term observational studies have shown that, following endoscopic sphincterotomy, there is a risk of infection, gallstone formation, pancreatitis (94-98), and biliary carcinoma (96). After endoscopic retrograde cholangiopancreatography (ERCP), a prerequisite for sphincterotomy, there is an increased risk for cancer in bile ducts, liver, and pancreas compared to the background population (99). A Cochrane review indicated that patients with gallbladder *in situ* should be offered a cholecystectomy following common bile duct stone removal, provided they are fit for surgery (100). An observational study recommended a cholecystectomy within one week of sphincterotomy (101). Further randomised controlled trials are necessary to assess the benefits and risks of T-tube versus primary closure after both open (102) and laparoscopic common bile duct exploration (103, 104).

In acute pancreatitis, an early etiological diagnosis (<48 h after admission) is recommended, and in mild and moderate acute pancreatitis of biliary origin, an early cholecystectomy is recommended (105-109). In acute biliary pancreatitis without cholangitis, early ERCP does not lead to a significant reduction of complications or mortality (110). Deviations from these recommendations are common (111-117). However, a recent audit demonstrated that it is possible to follow the guidelines for acute biliary pancreatitis with a low associated mortality (118). According to one randomised trial (119) and other observational studies, in acute biliary pancreatitis, an early cholecystectomy can shorten the hospital stay (120, 121) and reduce the risk for recurrent pancreatitis (122) compared to a delayed operation.

Health care costs

An early randomised controlled trial concluded that hospital costs were higher for small-incision cholecystectomy than for laparoscopic cholecystectomy (123); in one trial no significant difference was found between the two methods (124). However, in all other randomised controlled trials, health care costs were found to be lower for small-incision compared to laparoscopic cholecystectomy also when re-usable laparoscopic instruments were used (125-129). In a cost-minimising analysis, small-incision cholecystectomy appeared to be more cost-effective than laparoscopic cholecystectomy, both from hospital and societal perspectives (130). To our knowledge, no formal systematic review has compared the costs of small-incision cholecystectomy and laparoscopic cholecystectomy. However, in a recent overview of Cochrane reviews, it was concluded that small-incision cholecystectomy "seems to be less costly" (58). Observational studies have supported that view (14-16). In laparoscopic surgery, endoscopic sphincterotomy is associated with a longer hospital stay (131) and is more costly than choledochotomy (132, 133). Health care costs are ultimately determined by more factors than the surgical technique used. Factors that modify the response to surgical trauma, including the use of steroids, use of ondansetron, or liberal administration of fluid (134-141), advice to patients concerning pain medication and postoperative activity may affect convalescence, return to work, and finally, the societal cost for cholecystectomy (142). Long-term costs for cholecystectomy should include costs for repair of abdominal wall hernias following large, subcostal incisions (Figure 4). Finally, overall costs for surgical training should take into account the costs for two learning curves for laparoscopic trainees (laparoscopic cholecystectomy and open cholecystectomy in case of conversion) versus one curve for minicholecystectomy trainees (small-incision cholecystectomy with extended incision when needed).

Medical ethics and cholecystectomy technique

Non-maleficence, beneficence, respect for autonomy, and justice are the cornerstones of principle-based medical ethics (143). Respect for autonomy involves providing evidence based information on the risks (including conversion/extended incision) and benefits of surgery in elective and emergency settings (144). Justice involves the fair distribution of resources among individuals in need of health care. External factors may affect the practice of justice (145). However, within the limits set by stakeholders, the health care system and the surgeon must always consider the cost-effectiveness of surgical care (146).

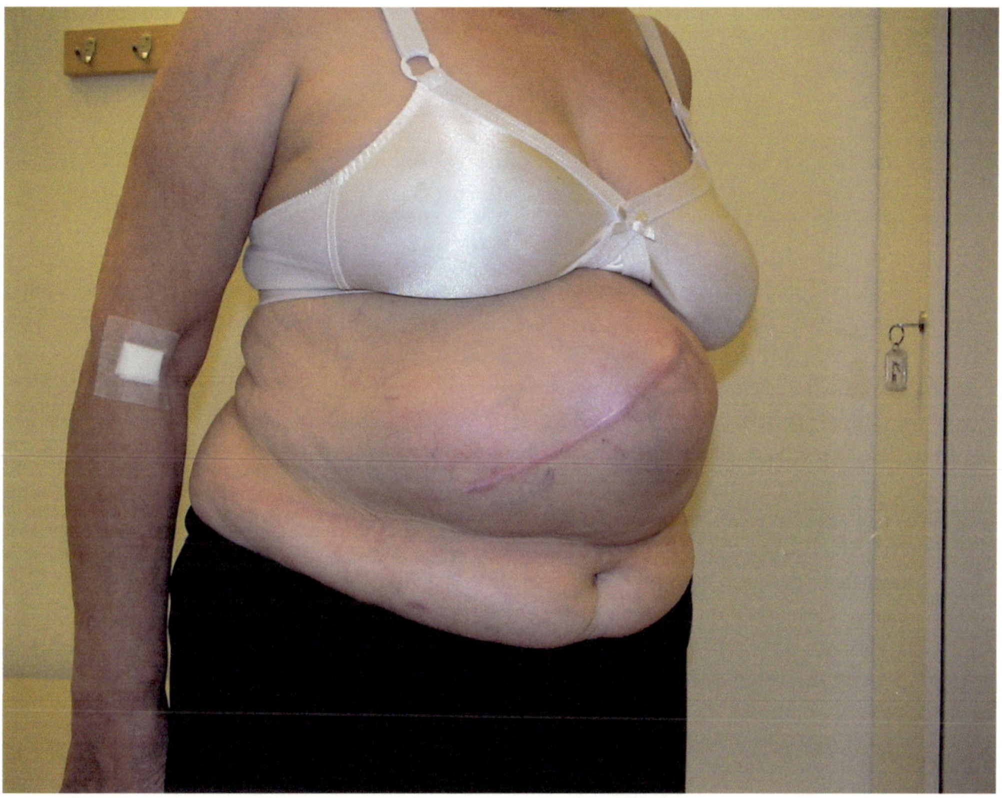

Fig. 4. Patient with a large abdominal wall hernia following subcostal incision in converted laparoscopic cholecystectomy.

4. Conclusions

Traditional open cholecystectomy is associated with a longer recovery than small-incision and laparoscopic cholecystectomy. To make a scientific evidence-based choice between small-incision cholecystectomy and laparoscopic cholecystectomy, surgeons and health care providers must scrutinize the evidence from randomised controlled trials and from defined populations, and they must consider the applicability of the techniques to their own setting. Conclusions reached may have a profound effect on costs and surgical training.

5. References

[1] Langenbuch C. Ein Fall von Extirpation der Gallenblase wegen chronischer Cholelithiasis: Heilung. Berliner Klin Wochenschr. 1882;19:725-7.
[2] Dubois F, Berthelot B. [Cholecystectomy through minimal incision (author's transl)]. La Nouvelle presse medicale. 1982 Apr 3;11(15):1139-41.
[3] Goco IR, Chambers LG. "Mini-cholecystectomy" and operative cholangiography. A means of cost containment. American Surgeon. 1983;49:143-5.
[4] Morton CE. Cost containment with the use of "mini-cholecystectomy" and intraoperative cholangiography. American Surgeon. 1985;51:168-9.
[5] Salembier Y. [Cholecystectomy through a short transverse incision]. Presse Med. 1986 Feb 8;15(5):210-1.
[6] Moss G. Discharge within 24 hours of elective cholecystectomy. The first 100 patients. Arch Surg. 1986 Oct;121(10):1159-61.
[7] Ledet WP, Jr. Ambulatory cholecystectomy without disability. Arch Surg. 1990 Nov;125(11):1434-5.
[8] Pelissier EP, Blum D, Meyer JM, Girard JF. Cholecystectomy by minilaparotomy without muscle section: a short-stay procedure. Hepatogastroenterology. 1992 Aug;39(4):294-5.
[9] Assalia A, Schein M, Kopelman D, Hashmonai M. Minicholecystectomy vs conventional cholecystectomy: a prospective randomized trial--implications in the laparoscopic era. World J Surg. 1993 Nov-Dec;17(6):755-9.
[10] Tyagi NS, Meredith MC, Lumb JC, Cacdac RG, Vanterpool CC, Rayls KR, et al. A new minimally invasive technique for cholecystectomy. Subxiphoid "minimal stress triangle": microceliotomy. Ann Surg. 1994 Nov;220(5):617-25.
[11] Belli G, Romano G, D'Agostino A, Iannelli A. Minilaparotomy with rectus muscle sparing: a personal technique for cholecystectomy. Giorn Chir. 1996;17(5):283-4.
[12] Daou R. [Cholecystectomy using a minilaparotomy]. Ann Chir. 1998;52(7):625-8.
[13] Sharma AK, Rangan HK, Choubey RP. Mini-lap cholecystectomy: a viable alternative to laparoscopic cholecystectomy for the Third World? The Australian and New Zealand journal of surgery. 1998 Nov;68(11):774-7.
[14] Seale AK, Ledet WP, Jr. Minicholecystectomy: a safe, cost-effective day surgery procedure. Arch Surg. 1999 Mar;134(3):308-10.
[15] Oyogoa SO, Komenaka IK, Ilkhani R, Wise L. Mini-laparotomy cholecystectomy in the era of laparoscopic cholecystectomy: a community-based hospital perspective. Am Surg. 2003 Jul;69(7):604-7.
[16] Syrakos T, Antonitsis P, Zacharakis E, Takis A, Manousari A, Bakogiannis K, et al. Small-incision (mini-laparotomy) versus laparoscopic cholecystectomy: a retrospective study in a university hospital. Langenbecks Arch Surg. 2004 Jun;389(3):172-7.
[17] Harju J, Juvonen P, Eskelinen M, Miettinen P, Paakkonen M. Minilaparotomy cholecystectomy versus laparoscopic cholecystectomy: a randomized study with special reference to obesity. Surg Endosc. 2006 Apr;20(4):583-6.
[18] Mühe E. Die erste Cholecystectomie durch das laparoskope. . Langenbecks Arch Chir. 1986;369.
[19] Dubois F, Berthelot G, Levard H. (Cholecystectomy by coelioscopy (see comments)]. Presse Med. 1989;18:980-2.

[20] Roslyn JJ, Binns GS, Hughes EF, Saunders-Kirkwood K, Zinner MJ, Cates JA. Open cholecystectomy. A contemporary analysis of 42,474 patients. Ann Surg. 1993 Aug;218(2):129-37.
[21] NIH Consensus conference. Gallstones and laparoscopic cholecystectomy. JAMA. 1993 Feb 24;269:1018-24.
[22] Plaisier PW, van der Hul RL, Nijs HG, den Toom R, Terpstra OT, Bruining HA. The course of biliary and gastrointestinal symptoms after treatment of uncomplicated symptomatic gallstones: results of a randomized study comparing extracorporeal shock wave lithotripsy with conventional cholecystectomy. Am J Gastroenterol. 1994 May;89(5):739-44.
[23] Plaisier PW, van der Hul RL, den Toom R, Nijs HG, Terpstra OT, Bruining HA. Gallstone lithotripsy: the Rotterdam experience. Hepatogastroenterology. 1994 Jun;41(3):260-2.
[24] Carrilho-Ribeiro L, Serra D, Pinto-Correia A, Velosa J, De Moura MC. Quality of life after cholecystectomy and after successful lithotripsy for gallbladder stones: a matched-pairs comparison. Eur J Gastroenterol Hepatol. 2002 Jul;14(7):741-4.
[25] www.cebm.net/index.aspx?o=1025. [11 Febraury 2011].
[26] Atkins D, Best D, Briss PA, Eccles M, Falck-Ytter Y, Flottorp S, et al. Grading quality of evidence and strength of recommendations. Bmj. 2004 Jun 19;328(7454):1490.
[27] Guyatt GH, Rennie D, Meade M, Cook D. Users' Guides to the Medical Literature: essentials of Evidence-Based Clinical Practice. 2nd ed: MGraw-Hill. Professional, 2008; 2008.
[28] Drummond MF, Sculpher MJ, Torrance GW, O'Brien BJ, Torrance GW. Methods for the economic evaluation of health care programmes. Oxford: Oxford University Press; 2005.
[29] Maier RV. What the surgeon of tomorrow needs to know about evidence-based surgery. Arch Surg. 2006 Mar;141(3):317-23.
[30] Jorgensen T. Prevalence of gallstones in a Danish population. Am J Epidemiol. 1987 Nov;126(5):912-21.
[31] Attili AF, Carulli N, Roda E, Barbara B, Capocaccia L, Menotti A, et al. Epidemiology of gallstone disease in Italy: prevalence data of the Multicenter Italian Study on Cholelithiasis (M.I.COL.). Am J Epidemiol. 1995 Jan 15;141(2):158-65.
[32] Jorgensen T. Treatment of gallstone patients. Copenhagen: National Institute of Public Health, Denmark, and Danish Institute for Health Technology Assessment; 2000.
[33] Portincasa P, Moschetta A, Palasciano G. Cholesterol gallstone disease. The Lancet. 2006;368.:230-9.
[34] Berger MY, van der Velden JJ, Lijmer JG, de Kort H, Prins A, Bohnen AM. Abdominal symptoms: do they predict gallstones? A systematic review. Scandinavian journal of gastroenterology. 2000 Jan;35(1):70-6.
[35] Berhane T, Vetrhus M, Hausken T, Olafsson S, Sondenaa K. Pain attacks in non-complicated and complicated gallstone disease have a characteristic pattern and are accompanied by dyspepsia in most patients: the results of a prospective study. Scandinavian journal of gastroenterology. 2006 Jan;41(1):93-101.
[36] Beckingham IJ, Krige JE. ABC of diseases of liver, pancreas, and biliary system: Liver and pancreatic trauma. BMJ. 2001 Mar 31;322(7289):783-5.

[37] Kang JY, Ellis C, Majeed A, Hoare J, Tinto A, Williamson RC, et al. Gallstones--an increasing problem: a study of hospital admissions in England between 1989/1990 and 1999/2000. Aliment Pharmacol Ther. 2003 Feb 15;17(4):561-9.

[38] Aerts R, Penninckx F. The burden of gallstone disease in Europe. Aliment Pharmacol Ther. 2003 Nov;18 Suppl 3:49-53.

[39] Sandler RS, Everhart JE, Donowitz M, Adams E, Cronin K, Goodman C, et al. The burden of selected digestive diseases in the United States. Gastroenterology. 2002 May;122(5):1500-11.

[40] Shaffer EA. Gallstone disease: Epidemiology of gallbladder stone disease. Best Pract Res Clin Gastroenterol. 2006;20(6):981-96.

[41] Gurusamy KS, Samraj K. Cholecystectomy versus no cholecystectomy in patients with silent gallstones. Cochrane Database Syst Rev. 2007(1):CD006230.

[42] Festi D, Reggiani ML, Attili AF, Loria P, Pazzi P, Scaioli E, et al. Natural history of gallstone disease: Expectant management or active treatment? Results from a population-based cohort study. Journal of gastroenterology and hepatology. 2010 Apr;25(4):719-24.

[43] Halldestam I, Kullman E, Borch K. Defined indications for elective cholecystectomy for gallstone disease. The British journal of surgery. 2008 May;95(5):620-6.

[44] Lam CM, Murray FE, Cuschieri A. Increased cholecystectomy rate after the introduction of laparoscopic cholecystectomy in Scotland. Gut. 1996;38:282-4.

[45] Mjåland O, Adamsen S, Hjelmqvist B, Ovaska J, Buanes T. Cholecystectomy rates, gallstone prevalence, and handling of bile duct injuries in Scandinavia. Surgical Endoscopy. 1998;12:1386-9.

[46] Cohen MM, Young W, Th,riault ME, Hernandez R. Has laparoscopic cholecystectomy changed patterns of practice and patient outcome in Ontario? Canadian Medical Association Journal. 1996;154(4):491-500.

[47] Steiner CA, Bass EB, Talamini MA, Pitt HA, Steinberg EP. Surgical rates and operative mortality for open and laparoscopic cholecystectomy in Maryland. The New England Journal of Medicine. 1994;330:403-8.

[48] Legorreta AP, Silber JH, Costantino GN, Kobylinski RW, Zatz SL. Increased cholecystectomy rate after the introduction of laparoscopic cholecystectomy. JAMA. 1993;270(12):1429-32.

[49] Al-Mulhim AA, Al-Ali AA, Albar AA, Bahnassy AA, Abdelhadi M, Wosornu L, et al. Increased rate of cholecystectomy after introduction of laparoscopic cholecystectomy in Saudi Arabia. World J Surg. 1999 May;23(5):458-62.

[50] Saltzstein EC, Mercer LC, Peacock JB, Daugherty SH. Outpatient open cholecystectomy. Surgery, Gynecology & Obstetrics. 1992;174:173-5.

[51] Amjad N, Fazal A. Mini cholecystectomy now a day stay surgery: anaesthetic management with multi modal analgesia. J Pak Med Ass. 2002;52:291-5.

[52] Harju J, Kokki H, Paakkonen M, Karjalainen K, Eskelinen M. Feasibility of minilaparotomy versus laparoscopic cholecystectomy for day surgery: a prospective randomised study. Scand J Surg. 2010;99(3):132-6.

[53] Arregui ME, Davis CJ, Arkush A, Nagan RF. In selected patients outpatient laparoscopic cholecystectomy is safe and significantly reduces hospitalization charges. Surg Laparoscop Endoscop. 1991;1:240-5.

[54] Richardson WS, Fuhrman GS, Burch E, Bolton JS, Bowen JC. Outpatient laparoscopic cholecystectomy. Outcomes of 847 planned procedures. Surg Endoscop. 2001; 15: 193-5.

[55] Vagenas K, Spyrakopoulos P, Karanikolas M, Sakelaropoulos G, Maroulis I, Karavias D. Mini-laparotomy cholecystectomy versus laparoscopic cholecystectomy: which way to go? Surg Laparosc Endosc Percutan Tech. 2006 Oct;16(5):321-4.

[56] Victorzon M, Tolonen P, Vuorialho T. Day-case laparoscopic cholecystectomy: treatment of choice for selected patients? Surg Endosc. 2007 Jan;21(1):70-3.

[57] Gurusamy KS, Junnarkar S, Farouk M, Davidson BR. Day-case versus overnight stay in laparoscopic cholecystectomy. Cochrane Database Syst Rev. 2008(1):CD006798.

[58] Keus F, Gooszen HG, van Laarhoven CJ. Open, small-incision, or laparoscopic cholecystectomy for patients with symptomatic cholecystolithiasis. An overview of Cochrane Hepato-Biliary Group reviews. Cochrane Database Syst Rev. 2010(1):CD008318.

[59] Keus F, Wetterslev J, Gluud C, Gooszen HG, van Laarhoven CJ. Trial sequential analyses of meta-analyses of complications in laparoscopic vs. small-incision cholecystectomy: more randomized patients are needed. J Clin Epidemiol. 2009 Dec 9.

[60] Ros A, Nilsson E. Abdominal pain and patient overall and cosmetic satisfaction one year after cholecystectomy: outcome of a randomized trial comparing laparoscopic and minilaparotomy cholecystectomy. Scandinavian journal of gastroenterology. 2004 Aug;39(8):773-7.

[61] Ros A, Carlsson P, Rahmqvist M, Backman K, Nilsson E. Non-randomised patients in a cholecystectomy trial: characteristics, procedures, and outcomes. BMC Surg. 2006;6:17.

[62] Rosenmuller M, Haapamaki MM, Nordin P, Stenlund H, Nilsson E. Cholecystectomy in Sweden 2000-2003: a nationwide study on procedures, patient characteristics, and mortality. BMC Gastroenterol. 2007;7:35.

[63] Livingston EH, Rege RV. A nationwide study of conversion from laparoscopic to open cholecystectomy. Am J Surg. 2004 Sep;188(3):205-11.

[64] Jenkins PJ, Paterson HM, Parks RW, Garden OJ. Open cholecystectomy in the laparoscopic era. The British journal of surgery. 2007 Nov;94(11):1382-5.

[65] Chung RS, Wojtasik L, Pham Q, Chari V, Chen P. The decline of training in open biliary surgery: effect on the residents' attitude toward bile duct surgery. Surg Endosc. 2003 Feb;17(2):338-40; discussion 41.

[66] Livingston EH, Rege RV. Technical complications are rising as common duct exploration is becoming rare. J Am Coll Surg. 2005 Sep;201(3):426-33.

[67] Chung RS, Ahmed N. The impact of minimally invasive surgery on residents' open operative experience: analysis of two decades of national data. Ann Surg. 2010 Feb;251(2):205-12.

[68] Schulman CI, Levi J, Sleeman D, Dunkin B, Irvin G, Levi D, et al. Are we training our residents to perform open gall bladder and common bile duct operations? The Journal of surgical research. 2007 Oct;142(2):246-9.

[69] Connor S, Garden OJ. Bile duct injury in the era of laparoscopic cholecystectomy. British Journal of Surgery. 2006;93:158-68.

[70] Waage A, Nilsson M. Iatrogenic bile duct injury: a population-based study of 152 776 cholecystectomies in the Swedish Inpatient Registry. Arch Surg. 2006 Dec;141(12):1207-13.
[71] de Reuver PR, Grossmann I, Busch OR, Obertop H, van Gulik TM, Gouma DJ. Referral pattern and timing of repair are risk factors for complications after reconstructive surgery for bile duct injury. Ann Surg. 2007 May; 245 (5):763-70.
[72] Assalia A, Kopelman D, Hashmonai M. Emergency minilaparotomy cholecystectomy for acute cholecystitis: prospective randomized trial--implications for the laparoscopic era. World J Surg. 1997 Jun;21(5):534-9.
[73] Johansson M, Thune A, Nelvin L, Stiernstam M, Westman B, Lundell L. Randomized clinical trial of open versus laparoscopic cholecystectomy in the treatment of acute cholecystitis. The British journal of surgery. 2005 Jan;92(1):44-9.
[74] Watanapa P. Mini-cholecystectomy: a personal series in acute and chronic cholecystitis. HPB (Oxford). 2003;5(4):231-4.
[75] Koo KP, Thirlby RC. Laparoscopic cholecystectomy in acute cholecystitis. What is the optimal timing for operation? Arch Surg. 1996 May;131(5):540-4; discussion 4-5.
[76] Peng WK, Sheikh Z, Nixon SJ, Paterson-Brown S. Role of laparoscopic cholecystectomy in the early management of acute gallbladder disease. The British journal of surgery. 2005 May;92(5):586-91.
[77] Wiseman JT, Sharuk MN, Singla A, Cahan M, Litwin DE, Tseng JF, et al. Surgical management of acute cholecystitis at a tertiary care center in the modern era. Arch Surg. 2010 May;145(5):439-44.
[78] Young AL, Cockbain AJ, White AW, Hood A, Menon KV, Toogood GJ. Index admission laparoscopic cholecystectomy for patients with acute biliary symptoms: results from a specialist centre. HPB (Oxford). 2010 May;12(4):270-6.
[79] Sanjay P, Moore J, Saffouri E, Ogston SA, Kulli C, Polignano FM, et al. Index laparoscopic cholecystectomy for acute admissions with cholelithiasis provides excellent training opportunities in emergency general surgery. Surgeon. 2010 Jun;8(3):127-31.
[80] Papi C, Catarci M, D'Ambrosio L, Gili L, Koch M, Grassi GB, et al. Timing of cholecystectomy for acute calculous cholecystitis: a meta-analysis. Am J Gastroenterol. 2004 Jan;99(1):147-55.
[81] Gurusamy K, Samraj K, Gluud C, Wilson E, Davidson BR. Meta-analysis of randomized controlled trials on the safety and effectiveness of early versus delayed laparoscopic cholecystectomy for acute cholecystitis. The British journal of surgery. 2010 Feb;97(2):141-50.
[82] Riall TS, Zhang D, Townsend CM, Jr., Kuo YF, Goodwin JS. Failure to perform cholecystectomy for acute cholecystitis in elderly patients is associated with increased morbidity, mortality, and cost. J Am Coll Surg. 2010 May;210(5):668-77, 77-9.
[83] David GG, Al-Sarira AA, Willmott S, Deakin M, Corless DJ, Slavin JP. Management of acute gallbladder disease in England. The British journal of surgery. 2008 Apr;95(4):472-6.
[84] Ainsworth AP, Adamsen S, Rosenberg J. Surgery for acute cholecystitis in Denmark. Scandinavian journal of gastroenterology. 2007 May;42(5):648-51.

[85] Nilsson E, Fored CM, Granath F, Blomqvist P. Cholecystectomy in Sweden 1987-99: a nationwide study of mortality and preoperative admissions. Scandinavian journal of gastroenterology. 2005 Dec;40(12):1478-85.
[86] Roukema JA, Carol EJ, Liem F, Jakimowicz JJ. A retrospective study of surgical common bile-duct exploration: ten years experience. Neth J Surg. 1986 Feb;38(1):11-4.
[87] Seale AK, Ledet WP, Jr. Primary common bile duct closure. Arch Surg. 1999 Jan;134(1):22-4.
[88] Martin IJ, Bailey IS, Rhodes M, O'Rourke N, Nathanson L, Fielding G. Towards T-tube free laparoscopic bile duct exploration: a methodologic evolution during 300 consecutive procedures. Ann Surg. 1998 Jul;228(1):29-34.
[89] Tokumura H, Umezawa A, Cao H, Sakamoto N, Imaoka Y, Ouchi A, et al. Laparoscopic management of common bile duct stones: transcystic approach and choledochotomy. J Hepatobiliary Pancreat Surg. 2002;9(2):206-12.
[90] Decker G, Borie F, Millat B, Berthou JC, Deleuze A, Drouard F, et al. One hundred laparoscopic choledochotomies with primary closure of the common bile duct. Surg Endosc. 2003 Jan;17(1):12-8.
[91] Martin DJ, Vernon DR, Toouli J. Surgical versus endoscopic treatment of bile duct stones. Cochrane Database Syst Rev. 2006(2):CD003327.
[92] Hüttl TP, Hrdina C, Geiger TK, Meyer G, Schildberg FW, Krämling HJ. Management of common bile duct stones - Results of a nationwide survey with analysis of 8 433 common bile duct explorations in Germany. Zentralblatt für Chirurgie. 2002;127:282-8.
[93] Paganini AM, Guerrieri M, Sarnari J, De Sanctis A, D'Ambrosio G, Lezoche G, et al. Thirteen years' experience with laparoscopic transcystic common bile duct exploration for stones. Effectiveness and long-term results. Surg Endosc. 2007 Jan;21(1):34-40.
[94] Bergman JJ, van der Mey S, Rauws EA, Tijssen JG, Gouma DJ, Tytgat GN, et al. Long-term follow-up after endoscopic sphincterotomy for bile duct stones in patients younger than 60 years of age. Gastrointest Endosc. 1996 Dec;44(6):643-9.
[95] Sugiyama M, Atomi Y. Follow-up of more than 10 years after endoscopic sphincterotomy for choledocholithiasis in young patients. The British journal of surgery. 1998 Jul;85(7):917-21.
[96] Tanaka M, Takahata S, Konomi H, Matsunaga H, Yokohata K, Takeda T, et al. Long-term consequence of endoscopic sphincterotomy for bile duct stones. Gastrointest Endosc. 1998 Nov;48(5):465-9.
[97] Rolny P, Andren-Sandberg A, Falk A. Recurrent pancreatitis as a late complication of endoscopic sphincterotomy for common bile duct stones: diagnosis and therapy. Endoscopy. 2003 Apr;35(4):356-9.
[98] Mandryka Y, Klimczak J, Duszewski M, Kondras M, Modzelewski B. [Bile duct infections as a late complication after endoscopic sphincterotomy]. Pol Merkur Lekarski. 2006 Dec;21(126):525-7.
[99] Stromberg C, Luo J, Enochsson L, Arnelo U, Nilsson M. Endoscopic sphincterotomy and risk of malignancy in the bile ducts, liver, and pancreas. Clin Gastroenterol Hepatol. 2008 Sep;6(9):1049-53.
[100] McAlister VC, Davenport E, Renouf E. Cholecystectomy deferral in patients with endoscopic sphincterotomy. Cochrane Database Syst Rev. 2007(4):CD006233.

[101] Schiphorst AH, Besselink MG, Boerma D, Timmer R, Wiezer MJ, van Erpecum KJ, et al. Timing of cholecystectomy after endoscopic sphincterotomy for common bile duct stones. Surg Endosc. 2008 Sep;22(9):2046-50.
[102] Gurusamy KS, Samraj K. Primary closure versus T-tube drainage after open common bile duct exploration. Cochrane Database Syst Rev. 2007(1):CD005640.
[103] Gurusamy KS, Samraj K. Primary closure versus T-tube drainage after laparoscopic common bile duct stone exploration. Cochrane Database Syst Rev. 2007(1):CD005641.
[104] Leida Z, Ping B, Shuguang W, Yu H. A randomized comparison of primary closure and T-tube drainage of the common bile duct after laparoscopic choledochotomy. Surg Endosc. 2008 Jul;22(7):1595-600.
[105] Uhl W, Warshaw A, Imrie C, Bassi C, McKay CJ, Lankisch PG, et al. IAP Guidelines for the Surgical Management of Acute Pancreatitis. Pancreatology. 2002;2(6):565-73.
[106] UK guidelines for the management of acute pancreatitis. Gut. 2005;54(Suppl 3):1-9.
[107] Banks PA, Freeman ML. Practice guidelines in acute pancreatitis. Am J Gastroenterol. 2006 Oct; 101(10):2379-400.
[108] Taylor E, Wong C. The optimal timing of laparoscopic cholecystectomy in mild gallstone pancreatitis. Am Surg. 2004 Nov;70(11):971-5.
[109] Kimura Y, Arata S, Takada T, Hirata K, Yoshida M, Mayumi T, et al. Gallstone-induced acute pancreatitis. J Hepatobiliary Pancreat Sci. 2010 Jan;17(1):60-9.
[110] Petrov MS, van Santvoort HC, Besselink MG, van der Heijden GJ, van Erpecum KJ, Gooszen HG. Early Endoscopic Retrograde Cholangiopancreatography Versus Conservative Management in Acute Biliary Pancreatitis Without Cholangitis: A Meta-Analysis of Randomized Trials. Ann Surg. 2008 Feb;247(2):250-7.
[111] Toh SK, Phillips S, Johnson CD. A prospective audit against national standards of the presentation and management of acute pancreatitis in the South of England. Gut. 2000 Feb;46(2):239-43.
[112] Hernandez V, Pascual I, Almela P, Anon R, Herreros B, Sanchiz V, et al. Recurrence of acute gallstone pancreatitis and relationship with cholecystectomy or endoscopic sphincterotomy. Am J Gastroenterol. 2004 Dec;99(12):2417-23.
[113] Lankisch PG, Weber-Dany B, Lerch MM. Clinical perspectives in pancreatology: compliance with acute pancreatitis guidelines in Germany. Pancreatology. 2005;5(6):591-3.
[114] Pezzilli R, Uomo G, Gabbrielli A, Zerbi A, Frulloni L, De Rai P, et al. A prospective multicentre survey on the treatment of acute pancreatitis in Italy. Dig Liver Dis. 2007 Sep;39(9):838-46.
[115] Al-Haddad M, Raimondo M. Management of acute pancreatitis in view of the published guidelines: are we compliant enough? Dig Liver Dis. 2007 Sep; 39 (9): 847-8.
[116] Sandzen B, Haapamaki MM, Nilsson E, Stenlund HC, Oman M. Cholecystectomy and sphincterotomy in patients with mild acute biliary pancreatitis in Sweden 1988 - 2003: a nationwide register study. BMC Gastroenterol. 2009;9:80.
[117] Nguyen GC, Boudreau H, Jagannath SB. Hospital volume as a predictor for undergoing cholecystectomy after admission for acute biliary pancreatitis. Pancreas. 2010 Jan;39(1):e42-7.

[118] Mofidi R, Madhavan KK, Garden OJ, Parks RW. An audit of the management of patients with acute pancreatitis against national standards of practice. The British journal of surgery. 2007 Jul;94(7):844-8.
[119] Aboulian A, Chan T, Yaghoubian A, Kaji AH, Putnam B, Neville A, et al. Early cholecystectomy safely decreases hospital stay in patients with mild gallstone pancreatitis: a randomized prospective study. Ann Surg. 2010 Apr;251(4):615-9.
[120] Alimoglu O, Ozkan OV, Sahin M, Akcakaya A, Eryilmaz R, Bas G. Timing of cholecystectomy for acute biliary pancreatitis: outcomes of cholecystectomy on first admission and after recurrent biliary pancreatitis. World J Surg. 2003 Mar;27(3): 256-9.
[121] Rosing DK, de Virgilio C, Yaghoubian A, Putnam BA, El Masry M, Kaji A, et al. Early cholecystectomy for mild to moderate gallstone pancreatitis shortens hospital stay. J Am Coll Surg. 2007 Dec;205(6):762-6.
[122] Nebiker CA, Frey DM, Hamel CT, Oertli D, Kettelhack C. Early versus delayed cholecystectomy in patients with biliary acute pancreatitis. Surgery. 2009 Mar;145(3):260-4.
[123] Barkun JS, Caro JJ, Barkun AN, Trindade E. Cost-effectiveness of laparoscopic and mini-cholecystectomy in a prospective randomized trial. Surg Endosc. 1995 Nov;9(11):1221-4.
[124] McGinn FP, Miles AJ, Uglow M, Ozmen M, Terzi C, Humby M. Randomized trial of laparoscopic cholecystectomy and mini-cholecystectomy. The British journal of surgery. 1995 Oct;82(10):1374-7.
[125] McMahon AJ, Russell IT, Baxter JN, Ross S, Anderson JR, Morran CG, et al. Laparoscopic versus minilaparotomy cholecystectomy: a randomised trial. Lancet. 1994 Jan 15;343(8890):135-8.
[126] Calvert NW, Troy GP, Johnson AG. Laparoscopic cholecystectomy: a good buy? A cost comparison with small-incision (mini) cholecystectomy. European Journal of Surgery. 2000;166:782-6.
[127] Srivastava A, Srinivas G, Misra MC, Pandav CS, Seenu V, Goyal A. Cost-effectiveness analysis of laparoscopic versus minilaparotomy cholecystectomy for gallstone disease. A randomized trial. Int J Technol Assess Health Care. 2001 Fall;17(4):497-502.
[128] Secco GB, Cataletti M, Bonfante P, Baldi E, Davini MD, Biasotti B, et al. [Laparoscopic versus mini-cholecystectomy: analysis of hospital costs and social costs in a prospective randomized study]. Chir Ital. 2002 Sep-Oct;54(5):685-92.
[129] Nilsson E, Ros A, Rahmqvist M, Backman K, Carlsson P. Cholecystectomy: costs and health-related quality of life: a comparison of two techniques. Int J Qual Health Care. 2004 Dec;16(6):473-82.
[130] Keus F, de Jonge T, Gooszen HG, Buskens E, van Laarhoven CJ. Cost-minimization analysis in a blind randomized trial on small-incision versus laparoscopic cholecystectomy from a societal perspective: sick leave outweighs efforts in hospital savings. Trials. 2009;10:80.
[131] Rogers SJ, Cello JP, Horn JK, Siperstein AE, Schecter WP, Campbell AR, et al. Prospective randomized trial of LC+LCBDE vs ERCP/S+LC for common bile duct stone disease. Arch Surg. 2010 Jan; 145(1):28-33.

[132] Schroeppel TJ, Lambert PJ, Mathiason MA, Kothari SN. An economic analysis of hospital charges for choledocholithiasis by different treatment strategies. Am Surg. 2007 May;73(5):472-7.
[133] Topal B, Vromman K, Aerts R, Verslype C, Van Steenbergen W, Penninckx F. Hospital cost categories of one-stage versus two-stage management of common bile duct stones. Surg Endosc. 2010 Feb;24(2):413-6.
[134] Holte K, Klarskov B, Christensen DS, Lund C, Nielsen KG, Bie P, et al. Liberal versus restrictive fluid administration to improve recovery after laparoscopic cholecystectomy: a randomized, double-blind study. Ann Surg. 2004 Nov; 240(5): 892-9.
[135] Liberman MA, Howe S, Lane M. Ondansetron versus placebo for prophylaxis of nausea and vomiting in patients undergoing ambulatory laparoscopic cholecystectomy. American Journal of Surgergy. 2000;179:60-2.
[136] Bisgaard T, Klarskov B, Kehlet H, Rosenberg J. Preoperative dexamethasone improves surgical outcome after laparoscopic cholecystectomy: a randomized double-blind placebo-controlled trial. Ann Surg. 2003 Nov;238(5):651-60.
[137] Feo CV, Sortini D, Ragazzi R, De Palma M, Liboni A. Randomized clinical trial of the effect of preoperative dexamethasone on nausea and vomiting after laparoscopic cholecystectomy. The British journal of surgery. 2006 Mar;93(3):295-9.
[138] Kehlet H, Wilmore DW. Evidence-based surgical care and the evolution of fast-track surgery. Ann Surg. 2008 Aug;248(2):189-98.
[139] Karanicolas PJ, Smith SE, Kanbur B, Davies E, Guyatt GH. The impact of prophylactic dexamethasone on nausea and vomiting after laparoscopic cholecystectomy: a systematic review and meta-analysis. Ann Surg. 2008 Nov;248(5):751-62.
[140] Fujii Y, Itakura M. Reduction of postoperative nausea, vomiting, and analgesic requirement with dexamethasone for patients undergoing laparoscopic cholecystectomy. Surg Endosc. 2010 Mar;24(3):692-6.
[141] Sanchez-Rodriguez PE, Fuentes-Orozco C, Gonzalez-Ojeda A. Effect of dexamethasone on postoperative symptoms in patients undergoing elective laparoscopic cholecystectomy: randomized clinical trial. World J Surg. 2010 May;34(5):895-900.
[142] Keus F, de Vries J, Gooszen HG, van Laarhoven CJ. Assessing factors influencing return back to work after cholecystectomy: a qualitative research. BMC Gastroenterol. 2010; 10:12.
[143] Beauchamp TL, Childress JF. Principles of biomedical ethics. 5 ed. Oxford: New York: Oxford University Press; 2001.
[144] Epstein RM, Alper BS, Quill TE. Communicating evidence for participatory decision making. JAMA. 2004 May 19;291(19):2359-66.
[145] Little M. Ethonomics: the ethics of the unaffordable. Arch Surg. 2000 Jan;135(1):17-21.
[146] Matthews JB. Cost containment: think globally, act locally. Arch Surg. 2010 Dec; 145(12):1136-7.

4

Laparoscopy-Assisted Distal Pancreatectomy

Masahiko Hirota et al.*
Department of Surgery,
Kumamoto Regional Medical Center, Kumamoto-city,
Japan

1. Introduction

The advantage of laparoscopic surgery is obvious and has been extended to pancreatic and splenic operations. Since 1994, various laparoscopic pancreatectomy, including pancreatoduodenectomy (Gagner & Pomp, 1994), enucleation (Gagner et al., 1996; Dexter et al., 1999), and distal pancreatectomy (Gagner et al. 1996; Sussman et al., 1996), have been performed. As for laparoscopic splenectomy, nowadays it can be conducted safely even for splenomegaly due to portal hypertension (Hama et al., 2008). Open pancreatic surgery requires a relatively large incision for a small lesion, and therefore the potential benefits of the laparoscopic approach are substantial. The most common indications for laparoscopic pancreatic resection were presumed benign pancreatic diseases, such as insulinoma or localized neuroendocrine neoplasms and branch type intraductal papillary mucinous neoplasms. The most common indication for laparoscopic pancreatic resection appears to be enucleations and distal pancreatectomy. Laparoscopic pancreatectomy, however, is still technically rather difficult because of the retroperitoneal position of the pancreas and the complex anatomical relationship between the pancreas and surrounding vessels. Thus, hand-assisted laparoscopic pancreatectomy is gaining recognition as a new and feasible technique that introduces a surgeon's hand into the abdominal cavity during laparoscopic surgery (Klingler et al., 1998; Shinchi et al., 2001; Kaneko et al., 2004). As a modification of hand-assisted laparoscopic pancreatectomy, we devised a method of spleen and gastrosplenic ligament preserving distal pancreatectomy, in which pancreatic resection is performed under direct vision extracorporeally (Hirota et al., 2009). Furthermore, laparoscopic assistance is also helpful in no-touch distal pancreatectomy for pancreatic cancer. For invasive pancreatic ductal cancers, the transection of the pancreas, splenic artery and vein, left gastroepiploic vessels, and short gastric vessels is performed at first to prevent the dissemination of cancer cells. Division of the pancreas, splenic artery, and splenic vein is done under direct vision through minilaparotomy at epigastrium. Division of the left gastroepiploic and short gastric vessels is done under laparoscope with left hand assistance. And then, retroperitoneal dissection is performed laparoscopically. In this way, the same no-touch distal pancreatectomy as open operation can be achieved.

---

*Daisuke Hashimoto, Kazuya Sakata, Hideyuki Kuroki, Youhei Tanaka, Takatoshi Ishiko,
Yu Motomura, Shinji Ishikawa, Yoshitaka Kiyota, Tetsumasa Arita, Atsushi Inayoshi and Yasushi Yagi
Department of Surgery, Kumamoto Regional Medical Center, Kumamoto-city, Japan

The three ways of laparoscopy-assisted distal pancreatectomy: 1) for benign lesions, 2) for low-grade malignant lesions, and 3) for invasive pancreatic ductal cancers, are presented in this chapter. Laparoscopic procedure is used for the retroperitoneal dissection under the left hand assistance in all types of lesions including cancers.

2. Laparoscopy-assisted distal pancreatectomy for benign lesions

In benign cases, such as insulinoma, branch type intraductal papillary mucinous neoplasm, spleen-preserving pancreatectomy is performed. An 8-cm minilaparotomy incision is made in the middle upper abdomen. For obese patients, 10-cm laparotomy is better. An abdominal wall disc for hand assistance is placed at the site of the minilaparotomy. Ultrasonography probe can be inserted through this site for intrapancreatic imaging. A total of the two trocars are then placed. After abdominal access is established, the gastrocolic omentum is divided, and the splenic flexure is mobilized. The short gastric and left gastroepiploic vessels are not divided to prevent splenic volvulus after the operation. Retrosplenic Gerota's fascia is transected on the surface of the left kidney (Figure 1a). Then, the posterior plane of Gerota's fascia is dissected from lateral to medial direction, allowing the distal pancreas and spleen detached from retroperitoneum.

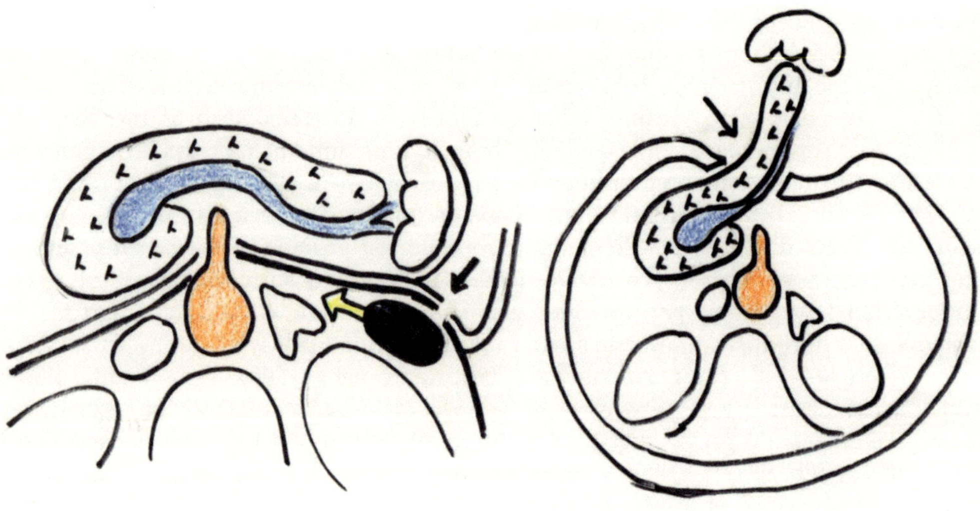

a b

Fig. 1. Procedures in laparoscopy assisted distal pancreatectomya) Retrosplenic Gerota's fascia is transected on the surface of the left kidney.Then, the posterior plane of Gerota's fascia is dissected from lateral to medial direction, allowing the distal pancreas and spleen detached from retroperitoneum. b)The distal pancreas and spleen are pulled out of the peritoneal cavity through the minilaparotomy for hand assistance at the epigastrium.

The distal pancreas, spleen, and left side of stomack are then pulled out of the peritoneal cavity through the minilaparotomy for hand assistance at the epigastrium (Figure 1b).

Spleen and gastrosplenic ligament preserving pancreatectomy is performed under direct vision (Figure 2). The advantage of extracorporeal procedure is the safety and certainty in dissection of the splenic vessels and preparation of the pancreatic stump. The transected main pancreatic duct is doubly ligated, and the transected pancreatic stump is sewn manually. The preserved spleen, stomach and splenic vessels are placed back in the peritoneal cavity after resection.

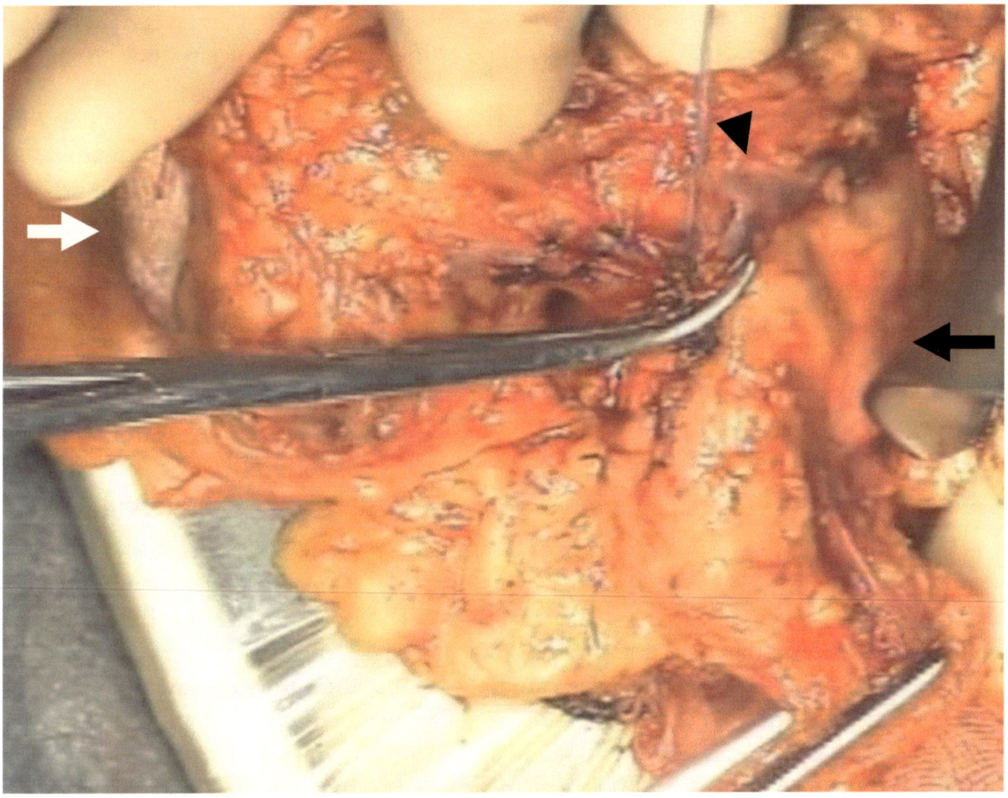

Fig. 2. Dissection of the distal pancreas. The distal pancreas (black arrow) is dissected from the surrounding tissues (spleen, splenic artery, splenic vein, stomach) under direct vision extracorporeally. White arrow: spleen, black arrow head: splenic vessels.

Distal pancreatectomy with preservation of the spleen was first reported in 1988 (Warshow, 1988). The advantage of preserving the spleen is obvious; it reduces the risk of postoperative severe inflammation and peripheral blood count aberration. Preserving the spleen has been a major procedure in distal pancreatectomy. Warshow reported a case of splenic abscess that occurred after sacrificing the splenic artery and vein (Warshow, 1988). Kimura et al. reported five patients successfully treated with splenic vessel-preserving distal pancreatectomy to maintain the blood supply to the spleen and to avoid splenic necrosis and abscess (Kimura et al., 1996; Kimura et al., 2010). Spleen-preserving pancreatectomy has recently been shown to have comparable risk of complication to standard pancreatectomy where the spleen is removed. Nevertheless, spleen-preserving pancreatectomy remains an uncommon and technically demanding operation, due to the difficulty in dissecting the distal pancreas from the splenic vessels. Another advantage of our procedure is the safety in dissecting the distal pancreas from the splenic vessels. The displacement of the spleen with the inherent risk of torsion or hemorrhage is another disadvantage of spleen-preserving pancreatectomy. If spleen-preserving pancreatectomy is performed, the spleen is often free in the abdomen, where it is prone to torsion or trauma. Various techniques have been described to reposition the spleen (splenopexy). Appu et al. report a novel technique for splenic repositioning and fixation, using peritoneal pocket (Appu et al., 2005). We experienced one case of splenic bleeding due to venous congestion after spleen-preserving pancreatic tail resection using Appu's splenopexy. After that experience we are preserving the gastrosplenic ligament.

This approach is suitable for the very distal lesion of the pancreas. However, if the posterior plane of Gerota's fascia is dissected, this method could be applied to more proximal lesion. For obese patients, because the pulling out through the small laparotomy is difficult, 10 cm incision is preferable. This procedure is applicable only for lesions in the pancreatic body and tail. For the benign head lesions, another approach should be conducted (Hirota et al., 2007).

Preservation of gastrosplenic ligament and extracorporeal preparation of transected pancreatic stump and splenic vessels under direct vision are useful measures for troubles in spleen-preserving distal pancreatectomy under minimal incision approach assisted by laparotomy.

3. Laparoscopy-assisted distal pancreatectomy for low grade malignant lesions

In low-grade malignant cases, such as mutinous cystic neoplasm, solid pseudopapillary neoplasm, medium-sized neuroendocrine neoplasm, the procedure is almost the same as in benign cases except the resection of the spleen and splenic vessels for lymph node dissection. The distal pancreas and spleen are pulled out of the peritoneal cavity through the minilaparotomy at the epigastrium (Figure 3). Pancreatic resection and closure of the residual pancreatic stump is performed safely under direct vision extracorporeally.

The successful management of the pancreatic stump remains the challenge of this procedure. In some laparoscopic enucleation series, the rate for low volume pancreatic fistula is reported to be high (Mabrut et al., 2005). This complication does not create an important problem as long as the main duct is not injured. Even though self-limiting, the pancreatic fistula formation rate remains high after either laparoscopic enucleation or resection. Pancreatic fistula after distal pancreatectomy has been a topic of decades, even in the era of laparoscopic pancreatectomy. Patterson et al. collected data from the literature on morbidity after open and laparoscopic pancreatic resections, and found that the rate of pancreatic fistula ranged from 20% to 33% after laparoscopic pancreatectomy and from 5% to 23% after open pancreatectomy (Patterson et al., 2001). The way in which the surgeon approaches the pancreatic transection seems to be important. Ninety-seven percent of the patients underwent laparoscopic transection of the pancreas by use of a stapling technique (Mabrut et al., 2005). Closing the pancreatic stump with interrupted mattress sutures and selectively ligating the pancreatic duct, the usual practice in open surgery, are more difficult to replicate laparoscopically. This factor could explain the high rate of pancreas-related complications. Hand-sewn parenchymal closure and duct ligation are an advantage of this extracorporeal pancreatic resection, to prevent pancreatic juice leakage, compared with the procedure done by laparoscopy only. We could safely and securely handle the pancreatic duct and fine branches of the splenic vessels under the direct vision.

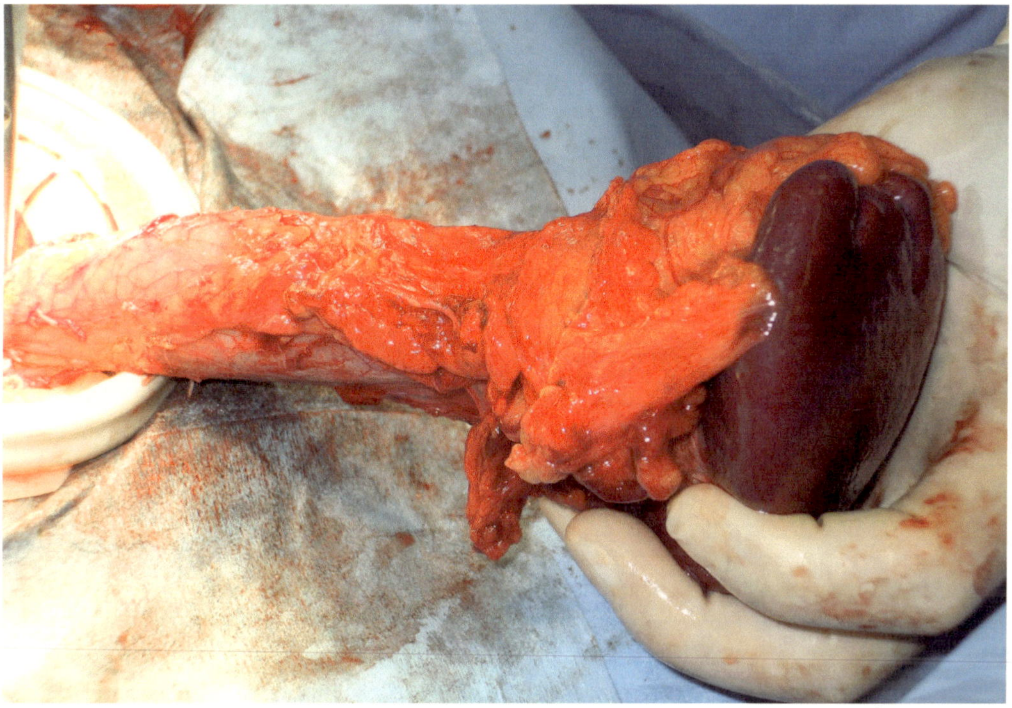

Fig. 3. Dissected distal pancreas and spleen. The distal pancreas and spleen are pulled out of the peritoneal cavity through the minilaparotomy at the epigastrium. Pancreatic resection and closure of the residual pancreatic stump is performed under direct vision.

4. Laparoscopy-assisted distal pancreatectomy for invasive pancreatic ductal cancers

Laparoscopic assistance is also helpful in no-touch distal pancreatectomy for pancreatic cancer. The aim of no-touch distal pancreatectomy is to decrease the shedding of cancer cells, and to achieve negative transection margins. All drainage vessels from the pancreatic body and tail have been ligated and divided during the early phase of the operation. Squeezing and handling the tumor prior to ligation of the surrounding vessels during pancreatectomy may increase the risk of shedding cancer cells into the portal vein, retroperitoneum and/or peritoneal cavity. Although the no-touch isolation technique has not been shown to increase cancer survival or decrease recurrence, it is theoretically promising (Hirota et al., 2005; Hirota et al., 2010).

Another aim is to resect cancers by wrapping them within Gerota's fascia. Perirenal tissue beyond Gerota's fascia is often protected from the autodigestion in severe acute pancreatitis.

Because cancer cell invasion is dependent on protease activity, Gerota's fascia may function as a barrier against protease-mediated invasion of cancer cells.
Division of the pancreas, splenic artery, and splenic vein is done under direct vision through minilaparotomy at epigastrium. Following the division of the gastrocolic ligament, the posterior surface of the pancreatic neck is tunneled by blunt dissection. The pancreas is transected after ligating the left side of the pancreas. The splenic artery and vein are ligated and divided at the origin and at the confluence with the superior mesenteric vein, respectively. As mentioned by Fagniez and Munoz-Bongrand, early division of the pancreatic neck provides superior access to control the splenic vessels (Fagniez & Munoz-Bongrand, 1999). Then, division of the left gastroepiploic and short gastric vessels is done under laparoscope with left hand assistance. At this point, all drainage vessels from the pancreatic body and tail have been ligated and divided. Lastly, retroperitoneal dissection behind the Gerota's fascia is performed lateral to medial direction laparoscopically.

5. Conclusion

Laparoscopic assistance is useful in distal pancreatectomy. This technique can be applied to both benign and malignant lesions. For benign lesions, preservation of gastrosplenic ligament and extracorporeal preparation of transected pancreatic stump under direct vision are useful measures to prevent post-operative complications.

6. References

Appu, S.; Young, A.B. & Lawrentschuk, N. (2005). Peritoneal "pillowcase" for the displaced spleen post-distal pancreatectomy. Journal of Hepatobiliary Pancreatic Surgery, Vol.12, pp. 470-473.

Dexter, S.P.; Martin, I.G.; Leindler, L.; Fowler, R. & McMahon, M.J. (1999).Laparoscopic enucleation of a solitary pancreatic insulinoma. Surgical Endoscopy, Vol.13, pp. 406-408.

Fagniez, P.L. & Munoz-Bongrand, N. (1999), Vascular control during left splenopancreatectomy in cancer. Annales de Chirurgie, Vol.53:, pp. 632-634, (in French with English abstract).

Gagner, M. & Pomp, A. (1994), Laparoscopic pylorus-preserving pancreatoduodenectomy. Surgical Endoscopy, Vol.8, pp. 408-410.

Gagner, M.; Pomp, A. & Herrera, M.F. (1996), Early experience with laparoscopic resections of islet cell tumors. Surgery, Vol.120, pp. 1051-1054.

Hama, T.; Takifuji, K.; Uchiyama, K.; Tani, M.; Kawai, M. & Yamaue, H. (2008), Laparoscopic splenectomy is a safe and effective procedure for patients with splenomegaly due to portal hypertension. Journal of Hepatobiliary Pancreatic Surgery, Vol.15, pp. 304-309.

Hirota, M.; Shimada, S.; Yamamoto, K.; Tanaka, E.; Sugita, H.; Egami, H. & Ogawa, M. (2005), Pancreatectomy using the no-touch isolation technique followed by extensive intraoperative peritoneal lavage to prevent cancer cell dissemination: a pilot study. JOP, Vol.6, pp. 143-151.

Hirota, M.; Kanemitsu, K.; Takamori, H.; Chikamoto, A.; Ohkuma, T.; Komori, H.;

Miyanari, N.; Ishiko, T. & Baba, H. (2007), Local pancreatic resection with preoperative endoscopic transpapillary stenting. American Journal of Surgery, Vol.194, pp. 308-310.

Hirota, M.; Ichihara, A.; Furuhashi, S.; Tanaka, H.; Takamori, H. & Baba, H. (2009), Spleen and gastrosplenic ligament preserving distal pancreatectomy under a minimum incision approach assisted by laparotomy. Journal of Hepatobiliary Pancreatic Surgery, Vol.16, pp. 792-795.

Hirota, M.; Kanemitsu, K.; Takamori, H.; Chikamoto, A.; Tanaka, H.; Sugita, H.; Sand, J., Nordback, I. & Baba, H. (2010), Pancreatoduodenectomy using a no-touch isolation technique. American Journal of Surgery, Vol.199, pp. e65-e68.

Kaneko, H.; Takagi, S.; Joubara, N.; Yamazaki, K.; Kubota, Y.; Tsuchiya, M.; Otsuka, Y. & Shiba, T. (2004), Laparoscopy-assisted spleen-preserving distal pancreatectomy with conservation of the splenic artery and vein. Journal of Hepatobiliary Pancreatic Surgery, Vol.11, pp. 397-401.

Kimura, W.; Inoue, T.; Futakawa, N.; Shinkai, H.; Han, I. & Muto, T. (1996), Spleen-preserving pancreatectomy with conservation of the splenic artery and vein. Surgery, Vol.120, pp. 885-890.

Kimura, W.; Yano, M.; Sugawara, S.; Okazaki, S.; Sato, T.; Moriya, T.; Watanabe, T.; Fujimoto, H.; Tszuka, K.; Takeshita, A. & Hirai, I. (2010). Spleen-preserving distal pancreatectomy with conservation of the splenic artery and vein: techniques and its significance. Journal of Hepatobiliary Pancreatic Sciences, Vol. 17, pp. 813-823.

Klingler, P.J.; Hinder, R.A.; Menke, D.M. & Smith, S.L. (1998), Hand-assisted laparoscopic distal pancreatectomy for pancreatic cystadenoma. Surgical Laparoscopy & Endoscopy, Vol.8, pp. 180-184.

Mabrut, J.Y.; Fernandez-Cruz, L.; Azagra, J.S.; Bassi, C.; Delvaux, G.; Weerts, J.; Fabre, J.M.; Boulez, J.; Baulieux, J.; Peix, J.L.; Gigot, J.F.; Hepatobiliary and Pancreatic Section of the Royal Belgian Society of Surgery; Belgian Group for Endoscopic Surgery; & Club Coelio. (2005), Laparoscopic pancreatic resection: results of a multicenter European study of 127 patients. Surgery, Vol.137, pp. 597-605.

Patterson, E.J.; Gagner, M.; Salky, B.; Inabnet, W.B.; Brower. S.; Edye, M.; Gurland, B.; Reiner, M & Pertsemlides, D. (2001), Laparoscopic pancreatic resection: single-institution experience of 19 patients. Journal of the American College of Surgeons, Vol.193, pp. 281-287.

Shinchi, H.; Takao, S.; Noma, H.; Mataki, Y.; Iino, S. & Aikou, T. (2001), Hand-assisted laparoscopic distal pancreatectomy with minilaparotomy for distal pancreatic cystadenoma. Surgical Laparoscopy Endoscopy & Percutaneous Techniques, Vol.11, pp. 139-143.

Sussman, L.A.; Christie, R. & Whittle, D.E. (1996), Laparoscopic excision of distal pancreas including insulinoma. Australian & New Zealand Journal of Surgery, Vol.66, pp. 414-416.

Warshow, A.L. (1988), Conservation of the spleen with distal pancreatectomy. Archives of Surgery, Vol.123, pp. 550-553.

Part 2

Laparoscopic Liver Surgery

5

Laparoscopic Liver Resection

Robert M. Cannon[1] and Joseph F. Buell[2]
[1]*University of Louisville Dept of Surgery,*
[2]*Tulane University Dept of Surgery*
United States of America

1. Introduction

Since the introduction of the laparoscopic cholecystectomy, there has been explosive growth in the field of minimally invasive surgery. Commonly accepted laparoscopic procedures have now come to include bariatric and anti reflux procedures, distal pancreatectomy, splenectomy, hernia repair, and colon resection. The adoption of laparoscopy to the field of liver surgery; however, has been slower to take off. Initial concerns included inadequate exposure and ability to attain hemostasis, fear of gas embolism, and doubts over the oncologic adequacy of the less invasive procedure. The earliest reports of laparoscopic liver surgery were limited to wedge resections for staging or isolated metastases(Lefor, AT & Flowers, JL 1994). Laparoscopic liver resection finally started to gain serious widespread attention after publication of Cherqui's initial thirty patient experience(Cherqui, D et al 2000). Since that time, the field has seen explosive growth, with over 2,804 cases now described in the world literature(Nguyen, KT et al 2009). Despite its widespread acceptance, laparoscopic liver resection remains a daunting technical challenge suited to a relatively small number of centers that have taken the time and effort to develop concurrent expertise in both open hepatic surgery and laparoscopy. Once these hurdles are overcome; however, laparoscopic liver resection is a safe and highly effective procedure offering numerous patient benefits. In this chapter, we will describe the indications for laparoscopic liver resection, and outline the steps that should be taken by fledgling groups wishing to embark upon creating a laparoscopic liver resection program.

2. Benign disease

Benign liver tumors represent a diagnostic and therapeutic challenge. Traditionally, a highly conservative approach to benign hepatic tumors has been favored, owing to the historically high morbidity and mortality associated with open liver surgery. As operative and anesthetic techniques have improved, these hurdles have come down. Despite the increased safety of hepatic surgery, the indications for resection of benign hepatic tumors have changed little: symptomatic lesions, asymptomatic lesions at high risk of rupture or malignant degeneration, and inability to exclude malignancy nonoperatively. Because of concerns over oncologic adequacy, benign lesions represent the ideal starting point for a laparoscopic liver surgery program. Despite the attractiveness of minimally invasive surgery; however, surgeons should be cautioned that the ability to perform a laparoscopic resection should not change the indications for operation.

2.1 Hemangioma

2.1.1 Epidemiology and presentation

Hemangioma represents the most common benign liver tumor, accounting for 5-20% of liver lesions(Buell, JF et al 2010). These tumors typically occur in females in the third through fifth decades. Symptoms typically do not occur until the tumors grow relatively large (>5cm), and typically consist of abdominal pain resulting from stretching of Glisson's capsule. There have been reports of spontaneous, traumatic, or iatrogenic rupture. A rare consequence of hemangioma is a consumptive coagulopathy resulting from sequestration of platelets and clotting factors within the tumor vasculature known as the Kasabach-Merritt syndrome. There is no potential for malignant degeneration with hepatic hemangioma.

2.1.2 Diagnostic evaluation

Hemangiomas demonstrate a typical pattern of enhancement on triple phase contrast enhanced CT. The lesion appears as a well circumscribed hypodense mass with peripheral enhancement in the arterial phase that will progress toward the center of the lesion. This pattern is typically known as centripetal enhancement. Sensitivity of triple phase CT has been reported from 75-85% with specificity of 75-100%(Trotter, JF & Everson, GT 2001). Even better results have been reported with the use of magnetic resonance imaging, with reported sensitivity and specificity of up to 95% and 100%, respectively (Semelka, RC et al 2001). Because of the highly vascular nature of these tumors, percutaneous biopsy of suspected hemangiomas is contraindicated.

2.1.3 Indications for surgical resection

As there is no malignant potential, symptomatic disease is the only generally accepted indication for surgical resection of hemangiomas. It should again be stressed that the availability of laparoscopy should not extend the indications for operation to asymptomatic patients. If pain is the indication for surgery, a thorough diagnostic workup is imperative to rule out other sources before attributing the symptoms to the hemangioma. The indication for surgery is more clear cut for large ruptured hemangioma, with patients often presenting in shock. Because of the dire consequences of rupture of large hemangioma, some surgeons would advocate the prophylactic resection of large lesions in patients with high risk occupations in areas remote from medical care. This opinion is controversial and should not be broadly applied.

2.2 Focal nodular hyperplasia

Focal nodular hyperplasia (FNH) is generally thought to arise as a hyperplastic proliferation of cells arising from an arterial malformation. This malformation may be congenital in nature such as telangiectasia or arteriovenous malformation, or may result from vascular injury (Paradis, V 2010; Wanless, IR et al 1985). Hyperplasia is thought to be a polyclonal process resulting from the hyperperfusion resulting from increased arterial flow (Gaffey, MJ et al 1996). The polyclonal nature of these lesions has significant impact on the radiographic evaluation of FNH, as it is the only common benign lesion that appears hot on Technetium sulfur colloid scan. This is from increased uptake of tracer in Kuppfer cells present within the lesion.

2.2.1 Epidemiology, radiographic evaluation, and presentation

FNH is typically an incidentally discovered lesion in women of late child bearing age, presenting most commonly from age 30 to 50. The female to male ratio has been reported at up to 8:1 (Mortele, KJ & Ros, PR 2002). Unlike hepatocellular adenoma, FNH is not influenced by oral contraceptive use. The radiographic appearance of focal nodular hyperplasia is typically diagnostic. On triple phase computed tomography, FNH will show transient enhancement on arterial phase. On delayed imaging, the characteristic central scar then becomes hyperenhancing. This central scar represents the vascular pedicle of the lesion and is pathognomonic. The most common diagnostic difficulty is distinguishing FNH from adenoma, which may best be achieved by contrast enhanced MRI. In this setting, sensitivity and specificity can reach 97% and 100%, respectively (Terkivatan, T et al 2006).

On histologic examination, FHN consists of benign hepatocytes arranged in a nodular pattern that are separated by fibrous septae originating in the central scar. Steatosis within the lesion may be evident (Paradis, V 2010). FNH is asymptomatic in upwards of 80% of cases (Buell, JF et al 2010). In very rare instances, these lesions may present with hemorrhage. There are no reported cases of malignant degeneration of FNH thus far. Because of this, there is no indication for resection of asymptomatic lesions, regardless of the size and number of lesions. Surgical resection is reserved for the rare cases in which the lesion is symptomatic or when the diagnosis is not secure.

2.3 Hepatocellular adenoma

Hepatic adenoma is a less common benign hepatic neoplasm, arising most commonly in women of child bearing age. There is a strong association between development of these lesions and oral contraceptive or androgenic steroid use. While the incidence is 0.1 per year per 100,000 patients who don't use oral contraceptives, there is a marked increase to up to 4 per 100,000 oral contraceptive users (Paradis, V 2010). The introduction of modern contraceptives with lower estrogen content has led to a decrease in incidence (Rooks, JB et al 1979). Less common risk factors for the development of hepatocellular adenoma include glycogen storage disease type I and type III (Micchelli, ST et al 2008)

2.3.1 Radiographic features

Though typically presenting as solitary lesions, adenoma may also be present as multiple lesions. Hepatic adenomas can grow quite large, with tumors of up to 30cm reported in the literature. Ultrasonography typically lacks diagnostic utility for adenomas, which can range from hypo to hyper-echoic. Reported sensitivity of ultrasound is only around 30%(Di, SM et al 1996). The CT appearance is that of a discrete, hypodense lesion showing enhancement on arterial phase followed by washout on later images. T1 weighted MRI will show a hypo- to hyperintense lesion, while T2 images will show a lesion that is more isointense. Enhancement with gadolinium contrast is typically present on the arterial phase, with rapid washout in the venous phase. The fat content of these lesions creates a typical decrease in intensity on fat-suppressed MRI images (Motohara, T et al 2002).

2.3.2 Clinical presentation

Patients with hepatocellular adenoma are more likely to present with symptomatic disease than those with FNH. Epigastric or right upper quadrant pain is present in 25-50% of patients (Buell, JF et al 2010). Spontaneous hemorrhage is also relatively common with these lesions, occurring in over 20% of patients. These complications are more likely to occur in men and with lesions greater than 5cm in diameter (Dokmak, S et al 2009). Perhaps the most feared complication of hepatocellular adenoma is malignant degeneration. The risk has been reported in the range of 8-10%(Dokmak, S et al 2009; Paradis, V 2010). Although 5cm is the generally accepted size at which malignant degeneration becomes a concern, cases have been reported in lesions as small as 4cm (Micchelli, ST et al 2008). There is also a greater risk of malignant degeneration in males and in patients with the metabolic syndrome. Malignancy within adenomas is typically discovered only after surgical resection.

2.3.3 Management

In the case of small adenomas in the setting of oral contraceptive use, a period of observation following the cessation of contraception is warranted. Surgical resection in this setting is then reserved for lesions which fail to regress or continue to grow after stopping the offending medication. As with other benign lesions, symptomatology that can clearly be attributed to the adenoma is also an indication for surgical resection. The presence of multiple adenomas, or adenomatosis, is an arbitrary distinction rather than a distinct pathologic subtype, thus indications for resection are the same as for solitary adenoma. Because of the well defined risk of malignant degeneration, there are also cases where resection of asymptomatic lesions is warranted. Generally accepted criteria include adenomas greater than 5cm in size, or any adenoma in a male, regardless of size (Dokmak, S et al 2009).

2.4 Other benign lesions

2.4.1 Angiomyolipoma

Angiomyolipoma is a rare benign tumor of mesenchymal origin. They most commonly occur in women and are discovered as incidental findings. Histologically, angiomyolipoma is composed of fat cells, blood vessels, and smooth muscle. CT imaging will show early enhancement that remains throughout the more delayed phases. Positive staining with HMB-45, with negative staining for cytokeratins 18 and 19, help to secure the diagnosis (Ding, GH et al 2011; Sturtz, CL & Dabbs, DJ 1994). Malignant degeneration is very rare, as is rupture, with three cases reported in the world literature. Because of the rare nature of serious complications, an initially conservative management strategy of imaging follow up is recommended when the diagnosis is established. Recently proposed guidelines for surgical resection of angiomyolipoma are as follows: symptomatic disease, tumors greater than 6cm, tumors which grow on repeated imaging, tumors showing extrahepatic growth with risk of rupture, and inability to make a definitive diagnosis on imaging or biopsy (Ding, GH et al 2011).

2.4.2 Nodular regenerative hyperplasia

Nodular regenerative hyperplasia (NRH) is characterized by diffuse involvement of the liver by multiple regenerative nodules in the absence of significant fibrosis. The incidence of NRH in a large autopsy series has been reported at 2.6% (Wanless, IR 1990). The disease typically manifests in the setting of systemic disorders such as Felty's syndrome or with the use of chemotherapeutic agents, of which azathioprine is the most common (Reshamwala, PA et al 2006). Complications are rare, as demonstrated by Wanless' series in which only 1 of 64 patients suffered any form of complication from NRH. Specific treatment for NRH is not needed. Diagnosis is made on liver biopsy, with reticulin staining being particularly helpful in identifying the changes of hyperplasia. Therapy, instead, is directed at treating the underlying disorder or withdrawing the offending medication.

2.4.3 Inflammatory pseudotumor

Inflammatory pseudotumor of the liver is a benign reactive process, the pathogenesis of which is unclear. In the majority of cases in the literature, an infectious agent was found to be the causative agent. Symptoms, when present, are generally nonspecific including body pain, fever, weight loss, leukocytosis, and elevated transaminases. CT findings are generally not specific for the diagnosis, although spontaneous regression on followup imaging in 4-6 weeks is commonly reported to occur (Seki, S et al 2004). Histological features include replacement of liver parenchyma by densely hylanized collagenous tissue and chronic inflammatory infiltrates. These features are missed on FNA, making core needle biopsy critical for accurate diagnosis (Tsou, YK et al 2007). In a review of eight cases, Tsou et al have suggested that inflammatory pseudotumor may best be thought of as a variant of a healing liver abscess. Thus, treatment consists of antibiotic therapy and nonsteroidal anti-inflammatory drugs. With appropriate therapy, the lesion can be expected to spontaneously regress. Surgical therapy is thus reserved for cases with severe symptoms or when malignancy is unable to be reliably excluded.

2.5 Technical considerations for resection

The majority of benign liver lesions are asymptomatic, leaving surgical resection as an appropriate therapy only in cases of symptomatic disease that is clearly attributable to the lesion, or when the diagnosis remains in doubt following appropriate workup. The exception is for hepatocellular adenoma, where the risk of malignant degeneration mandates resection for lesions larger than 5cm or cases occurring in men.

2.5.1 Patient positioning

There are three commonly used patient positions employed in laparoscopic liver resection: supine, lateral decubitus, and the so-called French position in which the patient is supine with the legs in stirrups and the surgeon is positioned between the patient's legs. The appropriate position is determined based on the location of the tumor, and the surgical technique to be employed. The French position has the advantage of allowing the surgeon to operate with both hands while assistants can retract from either side of the table. The supine position is best employed when approaching lesions on the left lobe or right anterior sector of the liver. The lateral decubitus position places the patient recumbent on their left side at an angle of sixty degrees. This position allows access to the posterior segments of the right liver, as the left side down positioning prevents the liver from falling dependently into the operative field. When a hand port is to be employed, it is generally placed in the right upper quadrant as dictated by the position of the tumor being resected.

2.5.2 Anesthesia and intraoperative care

The use of low CVP anesthesia has been a critical factor in the improved safety of modern hepatic surgery. This technique mandates the use of central venous catheters and arterial lines for patient monitoring. During the parenchymal transection phase, central venous pressure is lowered to between 2 and 4 mmHg with the use of nitrates, nitrous oxide, and dieresis. Combined with the tamponade effect of pneumoperitoneum, this technique minimizes blood loss from venous parenchymal bleeding (Tranchart, H et al 2010). Concern has been raised over the possibility of carbon dioxide embolism during laparoscopic liver surgery; however, extensive use of CO2 as an intravenous contrast agent in interventional radiology procedures shows that these fears are probably overstated (Hawkins, IF & Caridi, JG 1998). Argon embolism, on the other hand, is a legitimate fear, and we advocate against the use of the argon beam coagulator on hepatic parenchymal veins. Furthermore, it is prudent to lower insufflations pressures during use of the argon beam.

Minimization of blood product usage is another key component of intraoperative care. The use of intraoperative thromboelastography (TEG) allows for near real time assessment of the coagulation cascade with replacement of coagulation factors as appropriate. The cell saver is well accepted as a means of minimizing blood transfusion requirements during operation for benign indications. Cell saver use in the setting of malignancy is more controversial; however, the employment of adjunctive measures such as leukocyte depletion filters may minimize the burden of tumor cells in salvaged blood (Liang, TB et al 2008).

2.5.3 Parenchymal transection techniques

A number of parenchymal transection techniques have been described in the literature, with none of them showing clear superiority over the others. Which technique is ultimately chosen thus becomes dependent upon the individual surgeon's comfort level with a given technique. Here we describe two of the more common strategies: electrosurgical dissection and stapler hepatectomy.

Electrosurgical transection techniques rely upon the surgeon's ability to operate two devices simultaneously. The surgeon should use a device such as the Harmonic Scalpel or Enseal (Ethicon Endosurgery, Cincinnatti, OH) in the dominant hand. This device is used to incise Glisson's capsule and for the majority of parenchymal transection. The device should not be fully introduced into the parenchyma to prevent tearing of large vessels. When active bleeding is encountered, it is immediately controlled with bipolar cautery forceps which are held in the surgeon's other hand. Larger vessels require the use of laparoscopic clips. The simultaneous use both devices is facilitated by sitting on a tall stool, which allows the surgeon to operate the foot pedals independently.

Our group has favored the use of stapler hepatectomy. This technique provides the advantage of more rapid parenchymal transection, without the need for prior control of individual hepatic vessels. The first centimeter of parenchyma is relatively devoid of major vessels, and is incised with electrosurgical devices as described above. The dissection then proceeds using the thin blade of the stapler as a dissector. Care must be taken to avoid inadvertent manipulation of the stapler during firing, which can lead to tearing of major vessels and subsequent hemorrhage. The use of hand assistance is helpful in stabilizing the stapler to prevent such complications. We have preferred the use of a 25 mm vascular staple load for parenchymal transection.

When intraoperative hemorrhage is encountered, the presence of a hand in the abdomen is highly beneficial in allowing digital control of bleeding vessels prior to attaining definitive hemostasis. The "quick stitch" as described by Koffron has proven highly useful in laparoscopic control of bleeding vessels. The quick stitch is a precut 10cm suture with two vascular clips placed on the tail of the suture. After the suture is placed and hemostasis is obtained, the closure is secured by additional clips place on the proximal end. Should conversion be necessary during a pure laparoscopic procedure, it should initially be to a hand assist method rather than to full laparotomy. In all cases, conversion should not be viewed as a failure or complication, but rather as a measure of prudent judgment (Buell, JF et al 2009a).

3. Laparoscopic liver surgery for malignancy

After becoming comfortable with resection of benign lesions, the logical progression in the development of a laparoscopic liver program is the resection of malignant lesions. These lesions require an increased degree of skill on the part of the surgeons in order to attain adequate margins and maintain oncologic adequacy. The presence of cirrhosis in the setting of HCC or steatohepatitis following neoadjuvant chemotherapy for colorectal metastasis make proper patient selection and timing of operation critical. The consideration of adjunctive techniques such as transarterial chemoemboliztion for preoperative downstaging also becomes important. Here, we will discuss laparoscopic management of the two most common malignant hepatic tumors: colorectal metastases and hepatocellular carcinoma.

3.1 Colorectal metastases

Colorectal metastases are the most common malignant hepatic tumor. Results following open resection of these lesions have been excellent, with 5 year survival rates exceeding 50% in many centers (House, MG et al 2010). Such outcomes have set a high standard by which laparoscopic resection must be measured. The adoption of laparoscopy to this field has been hindered by concerns of tumor seeding at port sates and the possibility of missing extrahepatic lesions by inadequate inspection of the peritoneal cavity(Hsu, TC 2008; Johnstone, PA et al 1996). These hurdles have slowly been brought down, and laparoscopic resection is now a standard part of the therapeutic arsenal for hepatic malignancy.

3.1.2 Patient selection

Patient selection criteria for laparoscopic resection of colorectal metastases are similar to those applied for open resection. Initial evaluation requires precise definition of tumor anatomy and exclusion of extrahepatic disease. We favor triple phase CT as the initial radiographic evaluation. When combined with digital arterial reconstruction, evaluation of aberrant vascular anatomy, which can be present in nearly half of all patients, is afforded. Evaluation of baseline liver function is performed with evaluation of bilirubin, INR, and albumin. A thorough history and physical exam is necessary to assess general fitness for major abdominal surgery. Tumor resectability is defined by the SSAT as an expected negative margin resection with preservation of at least 2 contiguous hepatic segments with adequate inflow, outflow, and biliary drainage and a future liver remnant of more than 20% for normal parenchyma(Charnsangavej, C et al 2006).

3.1.3 Neoadjuvant therapy

The use of chemotherapy and chemoradiation for metastatic colon and rectal cancer has become a mainstay of therapy. Modern chemotherapeutic regimens generally consist of 5-fluorouracil combined with either oxaliplatin (FOLFOX) or irinotecan (FOLFIRI) have produced excellent response rates, and have been able to render 10-30% of previously unresectable disease amenable to surgical therapy. Agents such as cetuximab and bevacizumab have shown even better response rates. This efficacy is not without a price, however. Bevacizumab has a black box warning for spontaneous intestinal perforation. Traditional chemotherapeutic combinations are hepatotoxic, leading to the phenomenon of chemotherapy associated steatohepatitis (CASH). These considerations are important, as patients are often referred for hepatic surgery after neoadjuvant therapy has been initiated.

3.1.4 Operative considerations and oncologic adequacy

The most critical factor to producing positive outcomes is the attainment of negative operative margins (R0 resection). Facility with laparoscopic intraoperative ultrasound is a must for surgeons approaching malignant liver lesions, allowing for precise definition of tumor anatomy and planning of resection planes. As long as negative microscopic margins are obtained, there does not appear to be a minimum necessary margin width (Pawlik, TM et al 2005).

The approach to synchronous disease has received considerable attention, as it will be present in up to 25% of patients with colorectal liver metastases (Martin, RC et al 2009). There are three possible surgical strategies in this setting: the classic approach of colorectal resection followed by hepatectomy, a simultaneous resection of colorectal and hepatic disease, and a reverse strategy of metastasectomy followed by primary tumor resection. The drawback of the classic strategy is the delay in metastasectomy while patients receive adjuvant therapy. The combined strategy eliminates this delay, at the cost of greater surgical insult with possibly higher morbidity. The reverse strategy was described to eliminate the delay in metastasectomy while avoiding the surgical insult of the combined approach. With appropriate patient selection, groups from MD Anderson and the University of Louisville have demonstrated that the combined approach can be undertaken without increased morbidity and mortality. Brouquet's analysis of all three strategies found similar morbidity, mortality, and survival across groups, showing that no approach is clearly superior for all patients (Brouquet, A et al 2010).

With increasing worldwide experience of laparoscopic resection of colorectal metastases, the oncologic integrity of laparoscopy compared with open techniques has been shown to be comparable. Nguyen's review of the world literature found only one case of port site recurrence, which occurred in a case of metastatic renal cell carcinoma that ruptured prior to resection (Nguyen, KT et al 2009). Castaing's comparison of 60 patients undergoing laparoscopic resection and 60 patients undergoing open resection provided the first evidence of long term efficacy of laparoscopic resection for colorectal metastases. Five year survival in the laparoscopic group in this series was 62%, which was comparable to the 56% five year survival in the open group. There was no difference in width of resection margins between groups, while the laparoscopic group included a greater percentage of patients undergoing combined hepatic and colorectal resection (Castaing, D et al 2009). Such results confirm that laparoscopic resection is a safe and effective alternative to open surgery for hepatic colorectal metastases.

3.2 Hepatocellular carcinoma

Hepatocellular carcinoma (HCC) is the sixth most common malignancy and the third most common cause of cancer death worldwide (Parkin, DM et al 2005). In the United States, where chronic hepatitis C infection is the main risk factor, there has been an increase in the incidence of HCC over the past several decades (El-Serag, HB & Mason, AC 1999). Most patients present with relatively advanced disease, making curative treatment such as resection and liver transplantation applicable in only 30-40% of patients in Western centers

(Bruix, J & Llovet, JM 2002). One of the major limiting factors in preventing resectability is impaired hepatic function, with the vast majority of cases in Western patients developing in the background of cirrhosis. Thus, appropriate patient selection becomes paramount in achieving successful outcomes. Because of these limitations, the role of laparoscopic liver resection has remained more limited than for other disease states.

3.2.1 Patient selection

Much of the patient selection process for resection of HCC centers around assessment of the underlying liver parenchyma. The Child-Pugh classification system provides a rough framework from which to base the selection process. In generally, Child A patients are able to tolerate limited forms of resection, while Child B and C patients are typically referred for more palliative procedures such as systemic therapy or transarterial chemoembolization. In the West, assessment is directed at determining the presence of significant portal hypertension. Generally, patients with hepatic-venous pressure gradient of less than 10, esophageal varices of no greater than grade 1, and platelet counts of over 100,000 are considered acceptable risk. In addition, bilirubin levels must be normal.

A common technique in Eastern centers is the assessment of indocyanine green clearance rate (ICG). This technique involves the injection of an organic dye which is then measured in the peripheral blood after a 15 minute interval. Clearance of the dye is used as a surrogate for hepatic metabolic function. ICG retention of no more than 10-20% is considered to be acceptable. Using this technique in 1056 consecutive patients with normal bilirubin and no ascites, Imamura has been able to achieve hepatic resection with zero operative mortality (Imamura, H et al 2003).

Advances in imaging technology have lead to the increasing use of systemic liver volumetry as a preoperative risk assessment tool. A future liver remnant to standard liver volume ratio of greater than 20% is considered safe in patients with healthy liver parenchyma, while ratios of 30-40% are considered necessary for patients with compensated cirrhosis. An insufficient future liver remnant may be addressed with the use of adjunctive techniques such as portal vein embolization, which will be discussed in greater detail in the section on resection in cirrhotics.

Tumor related factors that preclude surgical resection include extrahepatic disease and invasion of the main portal vein, vena cava, and common hepatic artery. Multinodular disease that can't be resected with an adequate future liver remnant is also a relative contraindication to resection, although there is a role for resection of the dominant lesion with radiofrequency ablation of the remaining disease in highly selected cases. Although size alone is not a criteria for resectability, there is a practical limit to the size of lesion that can be safely approached laparoscopically. The recent international position statement for laparoscopic liver surgery recommends limitation of the laparoscopic approach to tumors <5cm in diameter for all but the most experienced of centers (Buell, JF et al 2009a).

3.2.2 Technical considerations and oncologic adequacy

Unlike the case of hepatic colorectal metastases, there does appear to be a benefit to wider surgical margins in patients with HCC. For patients with solitary HCC lacking vascular invasion, a margin of at least 2cm has proven beneficial in a randomized controlled trial setting. Furthermore, the tendency of HCC to spread via the portal venous system favors the use of planned anatomic resection in patients with adequate hepatic reserve. The inability to perform anatomic resection should not be considered a contraindication, however, as more

limited resection as been shown to be beneficial in the setting of cirrhosis (Rahbari, NN et al 2011).
Despite the limitations imposed by the greater difficulties in technical resection and patient selection, laparoscopic resection has proven to be a safe and effective alternative to open surgery in appropriately selected patients. Lai has demonstrated 5 year survival of 50%, with disease free survival of 36%, while Dagher has shown 5 year overall and disease free survival of 64.9% and 32.2%, respectively (Dagher, I et al 2010; Lai, EC et al 2009). Others have shown laparoscopic resection to be associated with lower morbidity and postoperative ascites compared to open resection (Belli, G et al 2009b). Although hepatocellular carcinoma in the setting of cirrhosis represents the most difficult of diseases to approach via laparoscopy, these results show that the technique is safe and effective when performed in centers that have acquired the appropriate experience.

4. Laparoscopic resection in cirrhotics

As noted above, the cirrhotic patient represents a unique challenge to the laparoscopic liver surgeon. The possibility of postoperative liver failure resulting from inadequate remnant liver function is a dreaded complication to be avoided at all costs. One technique that can potentially prevent this problem is the use of preoperative portal vein embolization (PVE). The effectiveness of PVE is based on the remarkable regenerative capacity of the liver. The technique involves occlusion of the tumor bearing segments of the liver, which induces hypertrophy in the remaining hepatic segments. Generally, reimaging 6 weeks after PVE is performed to assess the adequacy of hypertrophy to provide an adequate future liver remnant. Failure to achieve adequate hypertrophy indicates a severely diseased liver that is not amenable to resection.
A meta-analysis of PVE has been found that the procedure is safe and able to induce adequate hypertrophy to reduce post resection liver failure in a considerable proportion of patients (Abulkhir, A et al 2008). Preoperative PVE is currently recommended in cirrhotic patients with predicted future liver remnant of less than 40%. For centers using ICG retention, values of 10-19% with a FLR of 40-60% also represents an indication for portal vein embolization (Rahbari, NN et al 2011).
For cirrhotic patients able to undergo liver resection, laparoscopy provides a number of unique benefits. The smaller incisions cause less disruption of the abdominal wall collateral circulation. As complete evacuation of ascites is not necessary for a laparoscopic procedure, intraoperative fluid shifts are lessened. This contributes to the reduction in postoperative ascites seen with laparoscopy compared to open hepatectomy (Dagher, I et al 2009; Gigot, JF et al 2002). Another unique benefit is the reduced adhesion formation following laparoscopic surgery. For patients undergoing resection of HCC, salvage transplantation remains an important option for recurrences that are within the Milan criteria. Laurent found that liver transplants following laparoscopic compared to open resection were performed in less time, with less blood loss and transfusion requirement (Laurent, A et al 2009). Similarly, Belli has found repeat hepatectomy following initial laparoscopic resection to be faster and safer, with less blood loss and risk of visceral injury (Belli, G et al 2009a).

5. Development of a laparoscopic liver resection program

The recent international consensus conference on laparoscopic liver surgery has developed guidelines for the establishment and credentialing of a laparoscopic liver surgery program

(Buell, JF et al 2009b). Prior to embarking upon beginning a program in laparoscopic liver surgery, it is necessary to acquire experience with both advanced laparoscopy and open hepatic surgery. These requirements have made the widespread adoption of laparoscopic liver surgery appropriately slow. As advanced laparoscopy becomes an increasingly important part of general surgery training programs, these prerequisites will become less of a hurdle, with the expected more rapid acceptance of laparoscopic liver surgery.

After establishing the necessary expertise in laparoscopy and open hepatic surgery, the ideal starting point is small, benign lesions in the periphery of the liver. Extensive use of hand assistance is also critical in reducing the learning curve. Koffron has described the hybrid technique, in which mobilization of the liver is performed laparoscopically, and parenchymal transection is then performed in an open fashion through the hand port incision (Koffron, AJ et al 2007). He has termed this approach "laparoscopic liver surgery for everyone," and we agree that this approach represents an ideal starting point for a laparoscopic liver program.

Once comfortable with performing more limited resections, the next step in development is the performance of major, anatomic resections. In this setting, the left lateral segmentectomy is the ideal starting point. Although much attention is given to the parenchymal transection phase, it should be noted that the greatest risk for vascular injury and subsequent conversion to an open procedure is actually during the mobilization phase. The most commonly injured vessel in this setting is the phrenic vein, which must be carefully identified and avoided. Conversion, as we have emphasized previously, should not be viewed as a failure or complication. Instead, the decision to convert to an open or hand assisted procedure rather than continue with a potentially unsafe situation laparoscopically is a mark of good surgical judgment.

Experience with resection of lesions located in the peripheral segments of the liver provides a foundation of skills, including mobilization, transection, hemostasis, and laparoscopic ultrasound. Once this fundamental skill set has been developed thoroughly, the surgeon is then able to proceed to more difficult lesions. At this point, malignant and/or large lesions located in the right and posterior segments of the liver can then be approached in the culmination of programmatic development. We have found that facility with minor resections can be achieved in 30 to 50 cases. More difficult resections such as formal lobectomy and right posterior resection require an additional 60 to 80 cases to master. Thus, the road to development of a laparoscopic liver resection program is long and often arduous, but is highly rewarding to both the surgeon and the patient when properly travelled.

6. Conclusion

Nearly 15 years after first being described, laparoscopic liver resection has been gradually gaining acceptance in a number of centers worldwide. As the necessary skills in advanced laparoscopy and hepatic surgery become more widespread, we anticipate that the further adoption of laparoscopic liver resection will increase more rapidly. The maturation of long term series have proven the oncologic adequacy of the laparoscopic approach in a variety of settings. With the development of a greater number of surgeons who are proficient in laparoscopic liver surgery, many more patients will benefit from decreased blood loss, less postoperative pain, and shorter lengths of stay. From being a novel procedure practiced in only a handful of centers worldwide, laparoscopic liver resection is now established as a safe and effective technique in the therapeutic decision tree for patients with surgical disease of the liver. We believe that this acceptance will continue to grow to the point that the laparoscopic approach will, as has been seen with colon resection, eventually be adopted as the standard of care in appropriately selected patients.

7. References

Abulkhir, A et al Preoperative portal vein embolization for major liver resection: a meta-analysis Ann.Surg.2008;247(1):49-57

Belli, G et al Laparoscopic redo surgery for recurrent hepatocellular carcinoma in cirrhotic patients: feasibility, safety, and results Surg.Endosc.2009a;23(8):1807-1811

Belli, G et al Laparoscopic and open treatment of hepatocellular carcinoma in patients with cirrhosis Br.J.Surg.2009b;96(9):1041-1048

Brouquet, A et al Surgical strategies for synchronous colorectal liver metastases in 156 consecutive patients: classic, combined or reverse strategy? J.Am.Coll.Surg.2010; 210(6):934-941

Bruix, J & Llovet, JM Prognostic prediction and treatment strategy in hepatocellular carcinoma Hepatology2002;35(3):519-524

Buell, JF et al The international position on laparoscopic liver surgery: The Louisville Statement, 2008 Ann.Surg.2009a;250(5):825-830

Buell, JF et al The international position on laparoscopic liver surgery: The Louisville Statement, 2008 Ann.Surg.2009b;250(5):825-830

Buell, JF et al Management of benign hepatic tumors Surg.Clin.North Am.2010;90(4):719-735

Castaing, D et al Oncologic results of laparoscopic versus open hepatectomy for colorectal liver metastases in two specialized centers Ann.Surg.2009;250(5):849-855

Charnsangavej, C et al Selection of patients for resection of hepatic colorectal metastases: expert consensus statement Ann.Surg.Oncol.2006;13(10):1261-1268

Cherqui, D et al Laparoscopic liver resections: a feasibility study in 30 patients Ann.Surg.2000;232(6):753-762

Dagher, I et al Laparoscopic hepatectomy for hepatocellular carcinoma: a European experience J.Am.Coll.Surg.2010;211(1):16-23

Dagher, I et al Laparoscopic versus open right hepatectomy: a comparative study Am.J.Surg.2009;198(2):173-177

Di, SM et al Natural history of focal nodular hyperplasia of the liver: an ultrasound study J.Clin.Ultrasound1996;24(7):345-350

Ding, GH et al Diagnosis and treatment of hepatic angiomyolipoma J.Surg.Oncol.2011

Dokmak, S et al A single-center surgical experience of 122 patients with single and multiple hepatocellular adenomas Gastroenterology2009;137(5):1698-1705

El-Serag, HB & Mason, AC Rising incidence of hepatocellular carcinoma in the United States N.Engl.J.Med.1999;340(10):745-750

Gaffey, MJ et al Clonal analysis of focal nodular hyperplasia of the liver Am.J.Pathol.1996;148(4):1089-1096

Gigot, JF et al Laparoscopic liver resection for malignant liver tumors: preliminary results of a multicenter European study Ann.Surg.2002;236(1):90-97

Hawkins, IF & Caridi, JG Carbon dioxide (CO2) digital subtraction angiography: 26-year experience at the University of Florida Eur.Radiol.1998;8(3):391-402

House, MG et al Survival after hepatic resection for metastatic colorectal cancer: trends in outcomes for 1,600 patients during two decades at a single institution J.Am.Coll.Surg.2010; 210(5):744-745

Hsu, TC Intra-abdominal lesions could be missed by inadequate laparoscopy Am.Surg.2008;74(9):824-826

Imamura, H et al One thousand fifty-six hepatectomies without mortality in 8 years Arch.Surg.2003;138(11):1198-1206

Johnstone, PA et al Port site recurrences after laparoscopic and thoracoscopic procedures in malignancy J.Clin.Oncol.1996;14(6):1950-1956

Koffron, AJ et al Laparoscopic liver surgery for everyone: the hybrid method Surgery2007; 142(4):463-468

Lai, EC et al Minimally invasive surgical treatment of hepatocellular carcinoma: long-term outcome World J.Surg.2009;33(10):2150-2154

Laurent, A et al Laparoscopic liver resection facilitates salvage liver transplantation for hepatocellular carcinoma J.Hepatobiliary.Pancreat.Surg.2009;16(3):310-314

Lefor, AT & Flowers, JL Laparoscopic wedge biopsy of the liver J.Am.Coll.Surg.1994; 178(3):307-308

Liang, TB et al Intraoperative blood salvage during liver transplantation in patients with hepatocellular carcinoma: efficiency of leukocyte depletion filters in the removal of tumor cells Transplantation2008;85(6):863-869

Martin, RC et al Simultaneous versus staged resection for synchronous colorectal cancer liver metastases J.Am.Coll.Surg.2009;208(5):842-850

Micchelli, ST et al Malignant transformation of hepatic adenomas Mod.Pathol.2008; 21(4):491-497

Mortele, KJ & Ros, PR Benign liver neoplasms Clin.Liver Dis.2002;6(1):119-145

Motohara, T et al MR imaging of benign hepatic tumors Magn Reson.Imaging Clin.N.Am.2002;10(1):1-14

Nguyen, KT et al World review of laparoscopic liver resection-2,804 patients Ann.Surg.2009; 250(5):831-841

Paradis, V Benign liver tumors: an update Clin.Liver Dis.2010;14(4):719-729

Parkin, DM et al Global cancer statistics, 2002 CA Cancer J.Clin.2005;55(2):74-108

Pawlik, TM et al Effect of surgical margin status on survival and site of recurrence after hepatic resection for colorectal metastases Ann.Surg.2005;241(5):715-22, discussion

Rahbari, NN et al Hepatocellular carcinoma: current management and perspectives for the future Ann.Surg.2011;253(3):453-469

Reshamwala, PA et al Nodular regenerative hyperplasia: not all nodules are created equal Hepatology2006;44(1):7-14

Rooks, JB et al Epidemiology of hepatocellular adenoma. The role of oral contraceptive use JAMA1979;242(7):644-648

Seki, S et al A clinicopathological study of inflammatory pseudotumors of the liver with special reference to vessels Hepatogastroenterology2004;51(58):1140-1143

Semelka, RC et al Focal liver lesions: comparison of dual-phase CT and multisequence multiplanar MR imaging including dynamic gadolinium enhancement J.Magn Reson.Imaging2001;13(3):397-401

Sturtz, CL & Dabbs, DJ Angiomyolipomas: the nature and expression of the HMB45 antigen Mod.Pathol.1994;7(8):842-845

Terkivatan, T et al Focal nodular hyperplasia: lesion characteristics on state-of-the-art MRI including dynamic gadolinium-enhanced and superparamagnetic iron-oxide-uptake sequences in a prospective study J.Magn Reson.Imaging2006;24(4):864-872

Tranchart, H et al Laparoscopic resection for hepatocellular carcinoma: a matched-pair comparative study Surg.Endosc.2010;24(5):1170-1176

Trotter, JF & Everson, GT Benign focal lesions of the liver Clin.Liver Dis.2001;5(1):17-42, v

Tsou, YK et al Inflammatory pseudotumor of the liver: report of eight cases, including three unusual cases, and a literature review J.Gastroenterol.Hepatol.2007; 22(12):2143-2147

Wanless, IR Micronodular transformation (nodular regenerative hyperplasia) of the liver: a report of 64 cases among 2,500 autopsies and a new classification of benign hepatocellular nodules Hepatology1990;11(5):787-797

Wanless, IR et al On the pathogenesis of focal nodular hyperplasia of the liver Hepatology1985; 5(6):1194-1200

6

Hilar Glissonean Access in Laparoscopic Liver Resection

Akihiro Cho

Division of Gastroenterological Surgery, Chiba Cancer Center Hospital
Japan

1. Introduction

Laparoscopy for liver resection is a highly specialized field, as laparoscopic liver surgery presents severe technical difficulties. However, the recent rapid development of technological innovations, improvements in surgical skills and the accumulation of extensive experience by surgeons have improved the feasibility and safety of a laparoscopic approach for properly selected patients [1]. Since the first report of laparoscopic anatomical left lateral sectionectomy in 1996 [2], increasing numbers of laparoscopic anatomical liver resections have been reported [3-6]. However, laparoscopic anatomical resection has not been widely accepted because major technical difficulties remain, such as hilar dissection and pedicle control. During open anatomical liver resections, each Glissonean pedicle is often ligated and divided en bloc extrahepatically [7, 8]. Using the same concept, we describe herein a novel technique by which each Glissonean pedicle can be easily and safely encircled and divided en bloc extrahepatically during laparoscopic anatomical liver resection.

2. Surgical technique

Laparoscopic encircling of the hepatoduodenal ligament is usually performed using an Endo Retract Maxi (Fig. 1) or Endo Mini-Retract (Covidien Japan, Tokyo, Japan) to be used as a tourniquet for complete interruption of blood inflow to the liver only if necessary [9].

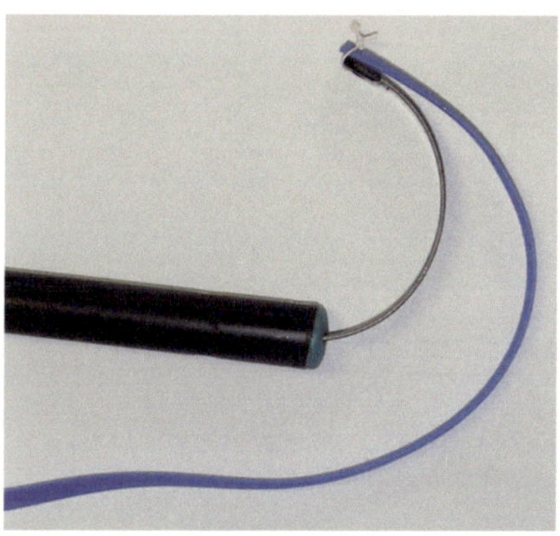

Fig. 1. Endo Retract Maxi in activated position. Vessel tape is preliminarily fixed to the tip of the metallic arch.

2.1 Encircling right-sided Glissonean pedicles, including the right, anterior, and posterior pedicles

After dividing the cystic artery and duct and dissecting the gallbladder neck, the peritoneum of the hepatoduodenal ligament is dissected at the hepatic hilum (Fig. 2). Retracting the round ligament and gallbladder allows a good operative field of view, facilitating the encircling of each Glissonean pedicle. The metallic arch of an Endo Retract Maxi or Endo Mini-Retract is then meticulously extended between the hepatic parenchyma and the bifurcation of the right and left Glissonean pedicles, so the tip of the metallic arch is visualized (Fig. 3). Although the metallic arch is blindly deployed behind the Glissonean bifurcation, the tip can be safely delivered into the dorsal side of the hepatoduodenal ligament because the blade is blunt. The right Glisonean pedicle is encircled extrahepatically (Fig. 4). In the same way, the metallic arch of Endo Mini-Retract is meticulously extended between the hepatic parenchyma and the bifurcation of the anterior and posterior Glissonean pedicles, then the anterior or posterior Glisonean pedicle is extrahepatically encircled (Fig. 5) [10, 11]. Hepatic parenchymal dissection along the Cantle line facilitates inserting an endocopic stapler and dividing the right anterior and posterior Glissonean pedicles respectively (Fig. 6).

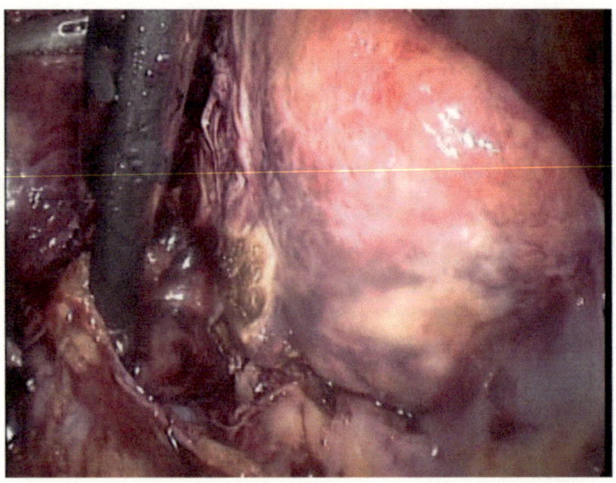

A

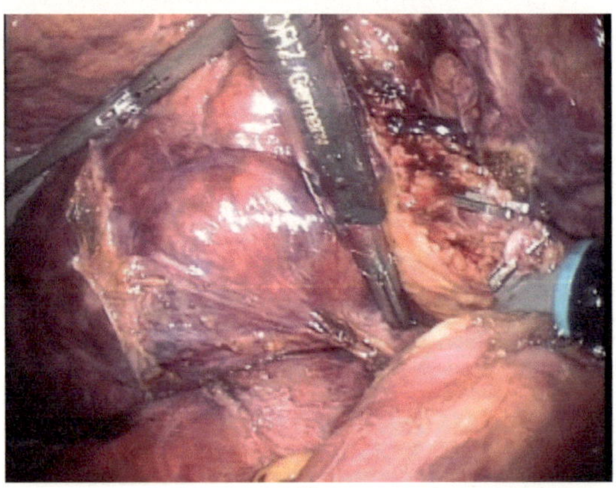

B

Fig. 2. Dissection between the hepatic parenchyma and the Glissonean bifurcation is performed from the ventral side (A) and dorsal side (B).

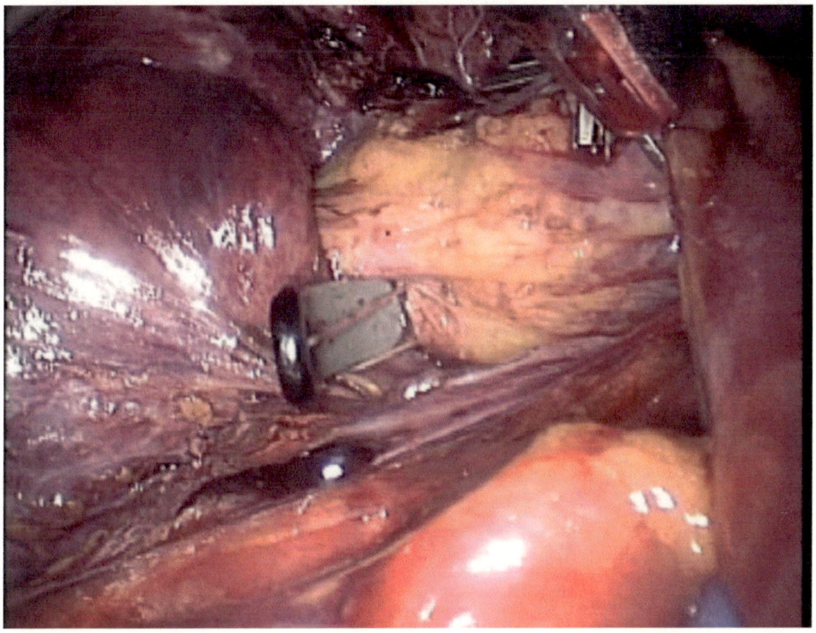

A

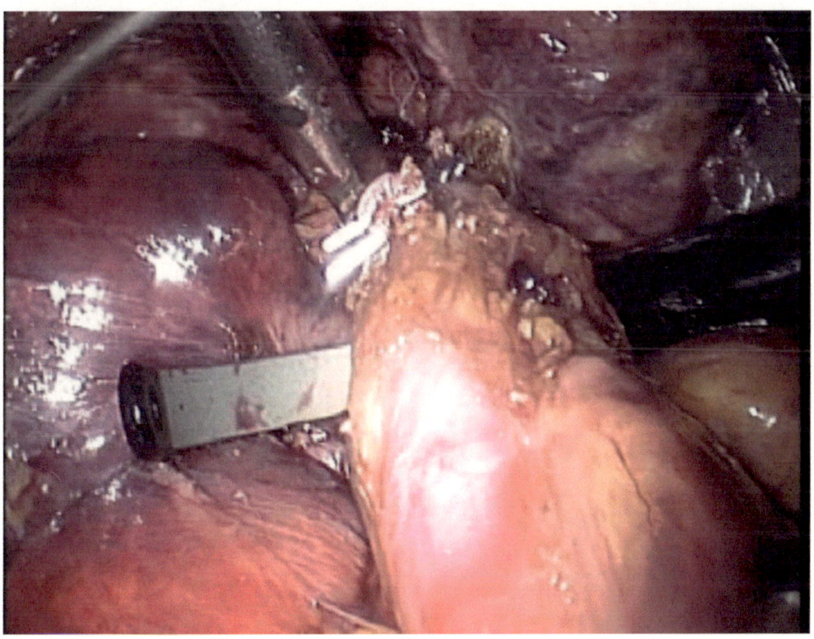

B

Fig. 3. An Endo Retract Maxi is introduced between the hepatic parenchyma and the bifurcation of the right and left Glissonean pedicles, so the tip of the metallic arch is visualized (A). The metallic arch is then meticulously extended (B).

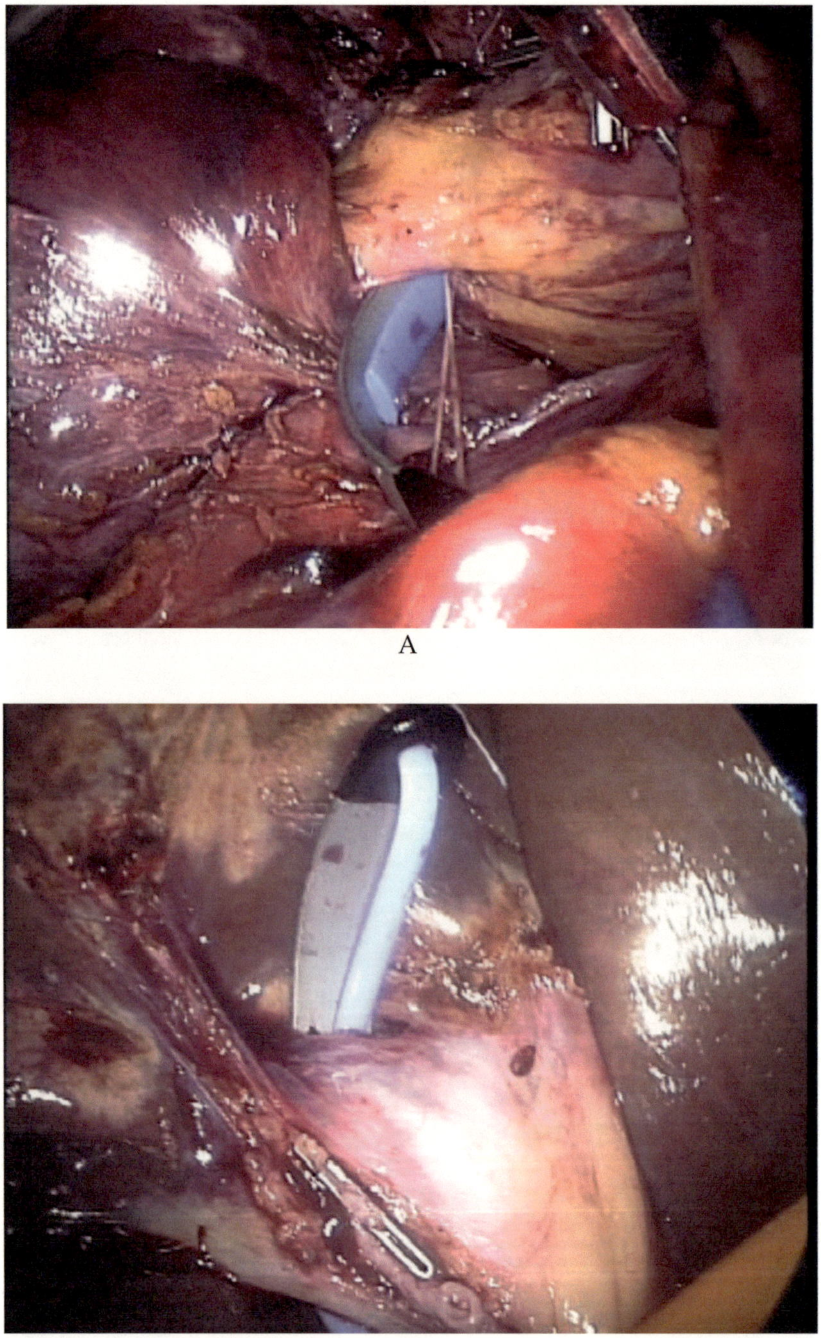

A

B

Fig. 4. The right Glissonean pedicle is encircled with an Endo Retract Maxi from the ventral side (A) and dorsal side (B).

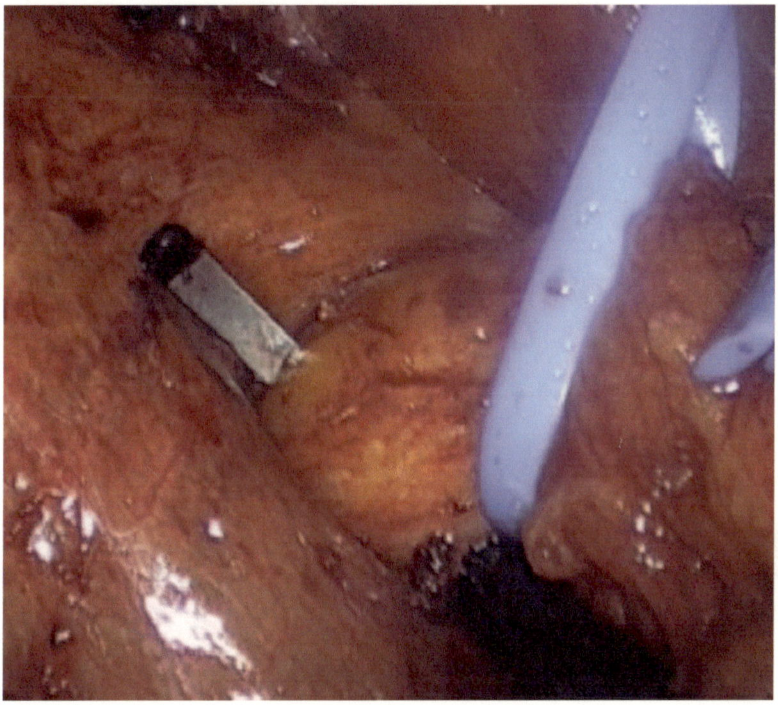

A

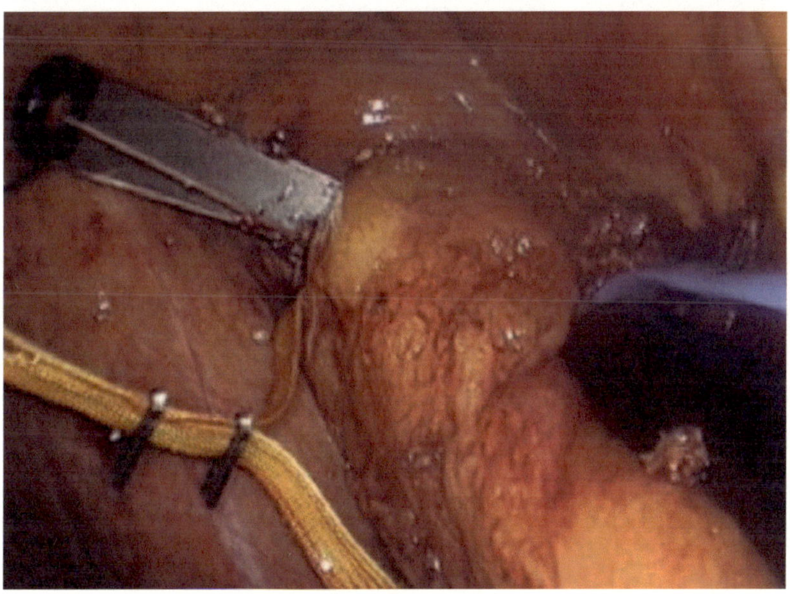

B

Fig. 5. The metallic arch of Endo Mini-Retract is extended between the hepatic parenchyma and the bifurcation of the anterior and posterior Glissonean pedicles, then the posterior (A) or anterior (B) Glisonean pedicle is extrahepatically encircled.

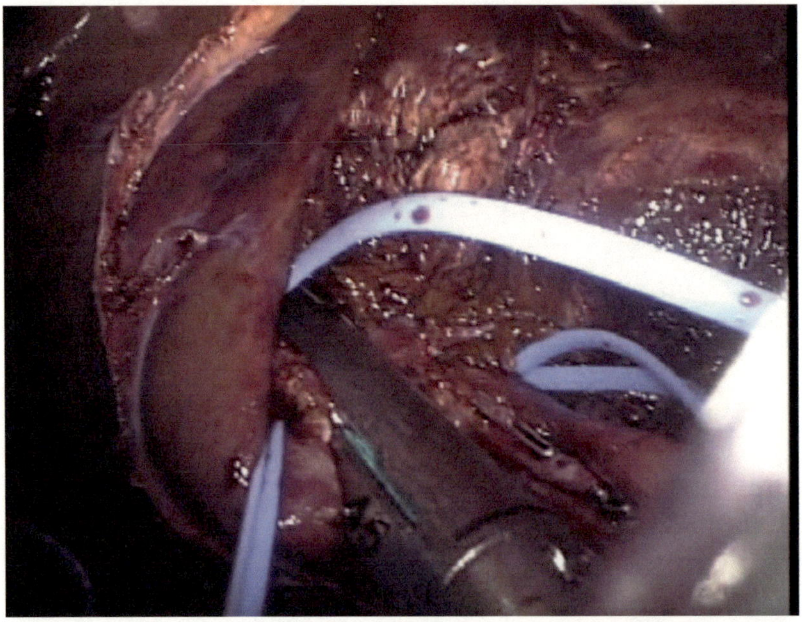

A

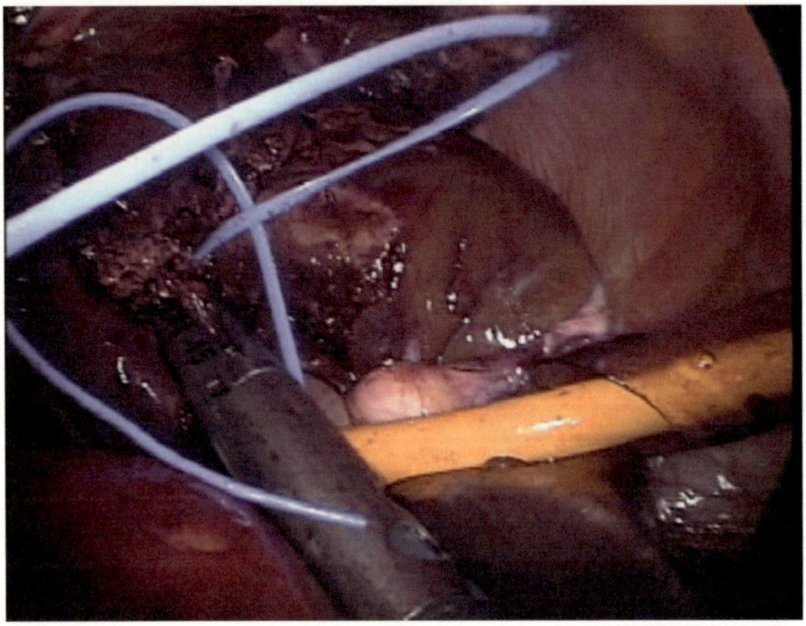

B

Fig. 6. The posterior (A) and anterior (B) Glisonean pedicles are divided respectively using an endocopic stapler.

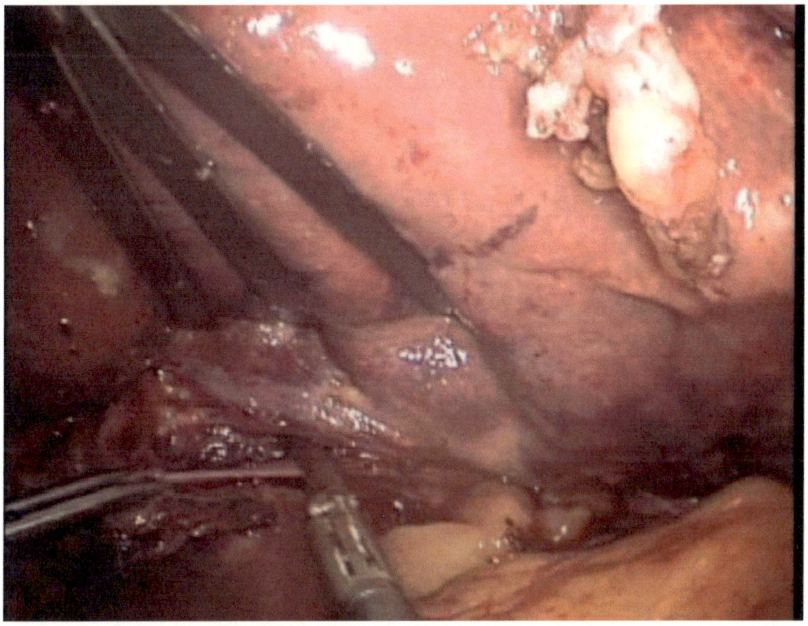

Fig. 7. The ligamentum venosum is divided.

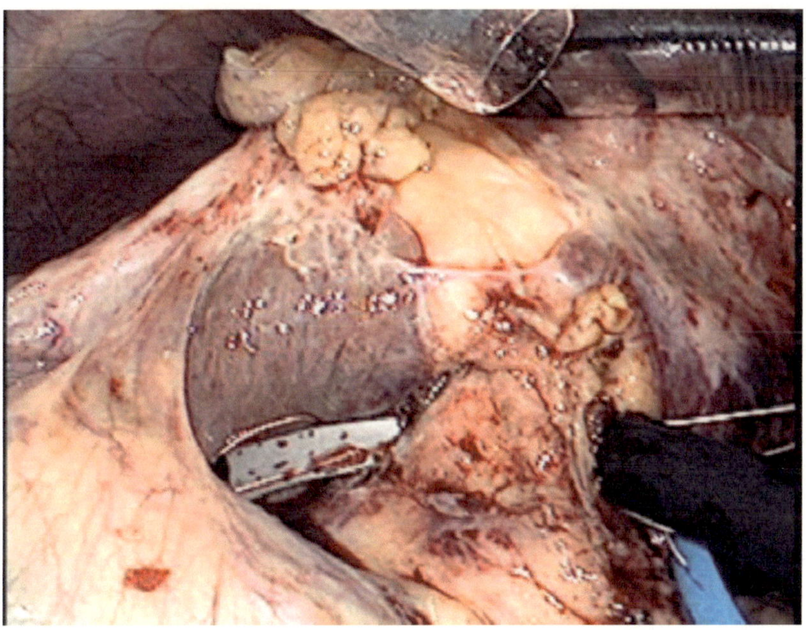

Fig. 8. The metallic arch of an Endo Retract Maxi is meticulously extended behind the umbilical plate, so the left Glisonean pedicle is encircled extrahepatically.

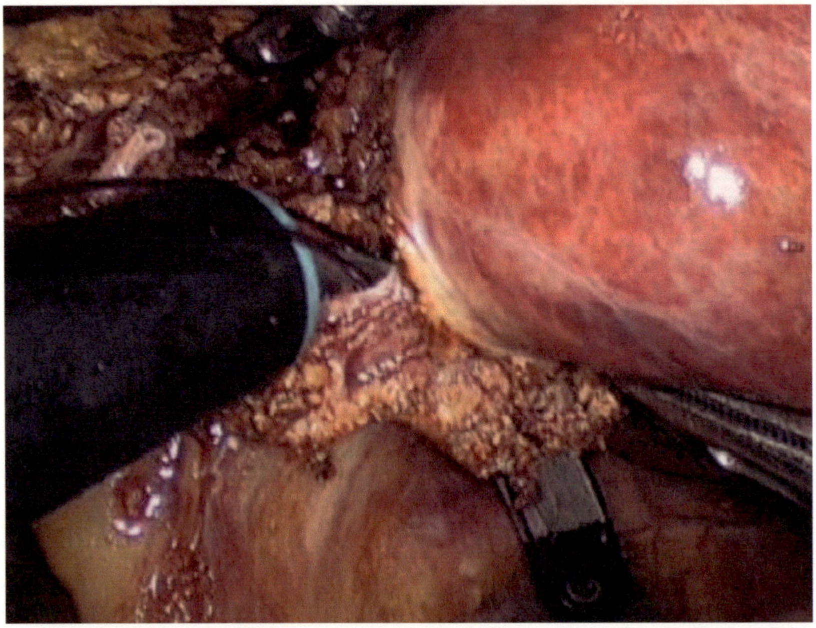

Fig. 9. The medial Glissonean pedicle is encircled with an Endo Mini Retract.

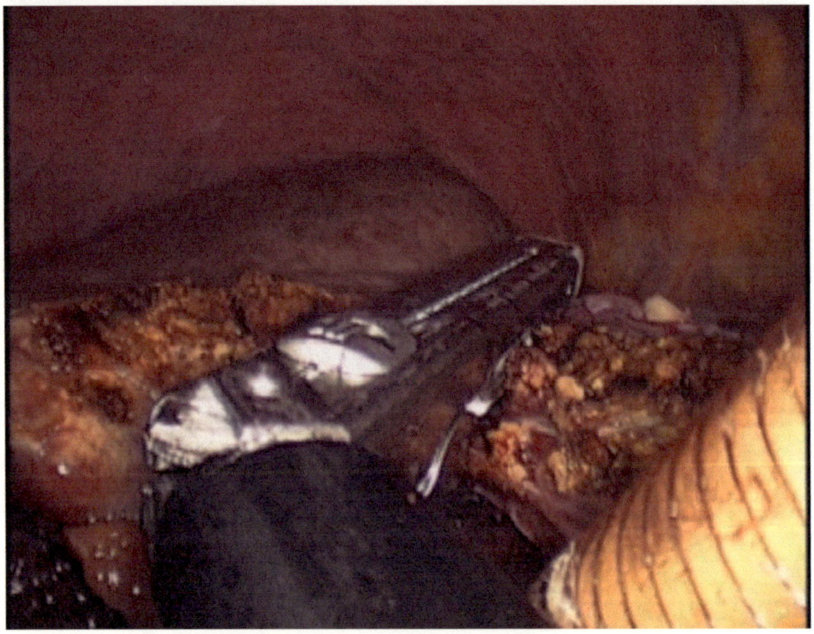

Fig. 10. The medial Glissonean pedicle is divided using an endocopic stapler.

2.2 Encircling left-sided Glissonean pedicles, including the left, medial, and lateral pedicles

Dividing the ligamentum venosum (Fig. 7) and retracting the round ligament upward extends the umbilical portion, facilitating isolation of its root. A parenchymal bridge is divided if present. Dissection between the hepatic parenchyma and umbilical plate is performed. The metallic arch of an Endo Retract Maxi or Endo Mini-Retract is meticulously extended behind the umbilical plate, so the left Glisonean pedicle is encircled extrahepatically (Fig. 8). Hepatic parenchyma is divided along the main portal fissure, which facilitates dividing the left Glissonean pedicle using an endoscopic stapler. A little dissection of the hepatic parenchyma along the umbilical fissure facilitates isolation of the root of the medial Glissonean pedicle (G4) or lateral Glissonean pedicles (G2, G3). Dissection between the hepatic parenchyma and umbilical plate is performed, and G2, G3, or G4 is extrahepatically encircled using Endo Mini-Retract (Fig. 9) and divided using an endoscopic stapler based on resection type (Fig. 10).

3. Comments

Laparoscopic anatomical segmental resection has not been widely accepted due to technical difficulties in controlling each Glissonean pedicle laparoscopically. Previous reports relating to laparoscopic hemihepatectomy have described separate dissection and division of each of the hepatic artery, duct and portal vein [3-6], or an intrahepatic Glissonean approach [12, 13]. The entire length of primary branches of the Glissonean pedicle and the origin of secondary branches are located outside the liver and the trunks of the secondary and more peripheral branches run inside the liver [8]. Therefore, the right, left, anterior, posterior, medial, or lateral Glissonean pedicle can be encircled and divided en bloc extrahepatically. Using an Endo Retract Maxi or Endo Mini-Retract, an extrahepatic Glissonean approach can be safe and feasible. However, each Glissonean pedicles should be divided as distally as possible to avoid biliary injury. The right Glissonean pedicle should not be transacted en bloc but the right anterior and posterior Glissonean branches should be divided respectively. The left Glissonean pedicle should be divided at the root of the umbilical portion to avoid injury of the right hepatic duct. Therefore, the pedicle should be encircled left to the Spiegel branch. In addition, each pedicles show shorter extrahepatic courses, and thus are better divided after some amount of parenchymal dissection.

4. References

[1] Buell JF, Cherqui D, Geller DA, O'Rourke N, Iannitti D, Dagher I, Koffron AJ, Thomas M, Gayet B, Han HS, Wakabayashi G, Belli G, Kaneko H, Ker CG, Scatton O, Laurent A, Abdalla EK, Chaudhury P, Dutson E, Gamblin C, D'Angelica M, Nagorney D, Testa G, Labow D, Manas D, Poon RT, Nelson H, Martin R, Clary B, Pinson WC, Martinie J, Vauthey JN, Goldstein R, Roayaie S, Barlet D, Espat J, Abecassis M, Rees M, Fong Y, McMasters KM, Broelsch C, Busuttil R, Belghiti J, Strasberg S, Chari RS; World Consensus Conference on Laparoscopic Surgery: The international position on laparoscopic liver surgery: The Louisville Statement, 2008. Ann Surg 2009; 250: 825-380.

[2] Azagra JS, Goergen M, Gilbart E, Jacobs D: Laparoscopic anatomical (hepatic) left lateral segmentectomy-technical aspects. Surg Endosc.1996; 10: 758-761.

[3] O'Rourke N, Fielding G: Laparoscopic right hepatectomy: surgical technique. J Gastrointest Surg2004; 8: 213-216.
[4] Dagher I, Di Giuro G, Lainas P, Franco D: Laparoscopic right hepatectomy with selective vascular exclusion. J Gastrointest Surg2009; 13: 148-149.
[5] Han HS, Cho JY, Yoon YS: Techniques for performing laparoscopic liver resection in various hepatic locations. J Hepatobiliary Pancreat Surg2009; 16: 427-432.
[6] Gayet B, Cavaliere D, Vibert E, Perniceni T, Levard H, Denet C, Christidis C, Blain A, Mal F: Totally laparoscopic right hepatectomy. Am J Surg2007; 194: 685-689.
[7] Takasaki K, Kobayashi S, Tanaka S, Saito A, Yamamoto M, Hanyu F: Highly anatomically systematized hepatic resection with Glissonean sheath code transection at the hepatic hilus. Int Surg1990; 75: 73-77.
[8] Takasaki K: Glissonean pedicle transection method for hepatic resection: a new concept of liver segmentation. J Hepatobiliary Pancreat Surg1998; 5: 286-291.
[9] Cho A, Yamamoto H, Nagata M, Takiguchi N, Shimada H, Kainuma O, Souda H, Gunji H, Miyazaki A, Ikeda A, Matsumoto I: Safe and feasible inflow occlusion in laparoscopic liver resection. Surg Endosc2009; 23: 906-908.
[10] Cho A, Asano T, Yamamoto H, Nagata M, Takiguchi N, Kainuma O, Souda H, Gunji H, Miyazaki A, Nojima H, Ikeda A, Matsumoto I, Ryu M, Makino H, Okazumi S: Laparoscopy-assisted hepatic lobectomy using hilar Glissonean pedicle transection. Surg Endosc2007; 21: 1466-1468.
[11] Cho A, Yamamoto H, Kainuma O, Souda H, Ikeda A, Takiguchi N, Nagata M: Safe and feasible extrahepatic Glissonean access in laparoscopic anatomical liver resection. Surg Endosc2011; 25: 1333-1336.
[12] Machado MA, Makdissi FF, Galvão FH, Machado MC: Intrahepatic Glissonian approach for laparoscopic right segmental liver resections. Am J Surg 2008; 196: 38-42.
[13] Topal B, Aerts R, Penninckx F: Laparoscopic intrahepatic Glissonian approach for right hepatectomy is safe, simple, and reproducible. Surg Endosc 2007; 21: 2111.

7

Laparoscopic Liver Surgery

Steven A. White, Rajesh Y. Satchidanand and Derek M. Manas
Department of Hepatobiliary and Transplant Surgery,
The Freeman Hospital, Newcastle upon Tyne, Tyne and Wear,
England

1. Introduction

Recent improvements in cross sectional imaging, chemotherapy and advances in the techniques of liver resection have resulted in rates of 5 year survival approaching 60% for patients with colorectal liver metastasis. Historically liver resection was perceived as a formidable operation but now liver resection is safe and specialist centres should expect low mortality rates in the region of 1-2%[1,2]. Consequently, many more patients are now referred for liver resection and its indications are continually being revised and expanded.

At the same time there have been many advances in minimally invasive laparoscopic surgical techniques so much so that laparoscopic liver resection (LLR) is becoming an increasingly popular option amongst laparoscopic enthusiasts. Indeed the first laparoscopic liver resection was described nearly 20 years ago for focal nodular hyperplasia[3]. In a recent review by Nguyen and colleagues [4,5] over 3,000 laparoscopic liver resections have now been reported in various series and meta-analyses [6 7 8]. Despite this enthusiasm doubts still remain over its more widespread application because of the risks of complications and whether there is any patient benefit [9-11]. The latter is still very difficult to demonstrate in the absence of any well designed randomized controlled trials. Like laparoscopic cholecystectomy that came before, it is now very unlikely that any well designed Randomised controlled trials (RCT) will ever be performed. Perhaps the most important RCT that should have been done is outcome after laparoscopic left lateral resection versus open resection. Yet for laparoscopic enthusiasts the advantages are so obvious they would now be very reluctant to offer open resection in a trial setting. The situation is very different for major resections e.g. right hepatectomy where any advantage is still very difficult to demonstrate. In this situation a RCT would be difficult to design as few centres regularly perform this operation and large numbers would be needed because of high rates of conversion and recruiting patients with tumours distributed in such away that they can be resected laparoscopically.

2. Indications and contra-indications

2.1 International consensus - The Louisville statement

In 2008 a consensus meeting was convened in Louisville to discuss the position of LLR amongst some of the worlds leading hepatobiliary surgeons. This was a very important development and the following guidelines were suggested as follows[11]:

1. LLR can be performed safely in specialized centres with results comparable to those achieved after open resection

2. The main indications are for both symptomatic benign and malignant tumours the latter being predominantly Hepatocellular carcinoma (HCC) and liver metastasis (colorectal-CRLM) and in determinant liver lesions.
3. It is important that the indications for resection of benign liver tumours are not expanded (e.g. asymptomatic tumours where there is no diagnostic doubt)
4. Harvested grafts for living donation should only be performed in very specialised centres and should be scrutinized in a world registry [12 13-15].

Other areas of discussion focused on patient safety and contraindications with the following guidelines being suggested

1. The contraindications for LLR should be the same as those for open resection.
2. Other contraindications include;
3. The presence of dense adhesions and failing to progress after prolonged dissection
4. Tumour adjacent to a major vascular structure
5. Tumour too large to manipulate
6. The need for a portal lymphadenectomy.

2.2 Benign liver tumours

Paired comparisons between laparoscopic and open resection for benign tumours have not been frequently reported [16 17 18]. A few series are dedicated to LLR for benign tumours only but these can be subdivided into solid or cystic [19 20]. Most studies report outcomes in series mixed for both benign and malignant tumours [21]. The largest series of LLR for benign tumours have been reported by Koffron et al. (n=177) [22]. Forty seven were hepatic adenomas the others being made up of haemangiomas (n=37), FNH (n=23) and liver cysts (n=70). It is not clear in this article what the indications for resection were. Most centres report predominantly resection of malignant tumours. From the Newcastle series of 69 patients; 28% constitute benign lesions and 72% malignant. The most common benign lesions include hepatic adenoma **(Figure 1)**, symptomatic FNH (or where there was diagnostic doubt), biliary cysts, angiomyolipoma, haemangioma, biliary haematoma and polycystic liver disease. In our experience most of these lesions were resected in patients with a known diagnosis of colorectal carcinoma where there was diagnostic doubt regarding a liver lesion despite cross sectional imaging by CT and MRI and in some cases contrast enhanced ultrasound. It is important not to expand the indications for resection just because it can be done laparoscopically. In general for benign tumours most report less morbidity (including incisional hernias), shorter hospital stay and faster time to oral intake [19].

2.3 Malignant liver tumours

Although there have been many reports of LLR for malignant tumours being resected including hilar cholangiocarcinoma [23] and neuroendocrine/carcinoid tumours, for the purposes of this chapter discussion will concentrate on the most commonly resected malignant tumours e.g. CRLM and HCC.

2.4 Colorectal

One of the disadvantages of LLR for CRLM is that all patients have had previous surgery and initial dissection can be tedious because of adhesions. Especially when patients have had a previous right hemicolectomy or cholecystectomy. Indeed in one patient in the authors series LLR was abandoned after 3 hours of dissection and failure to progress.

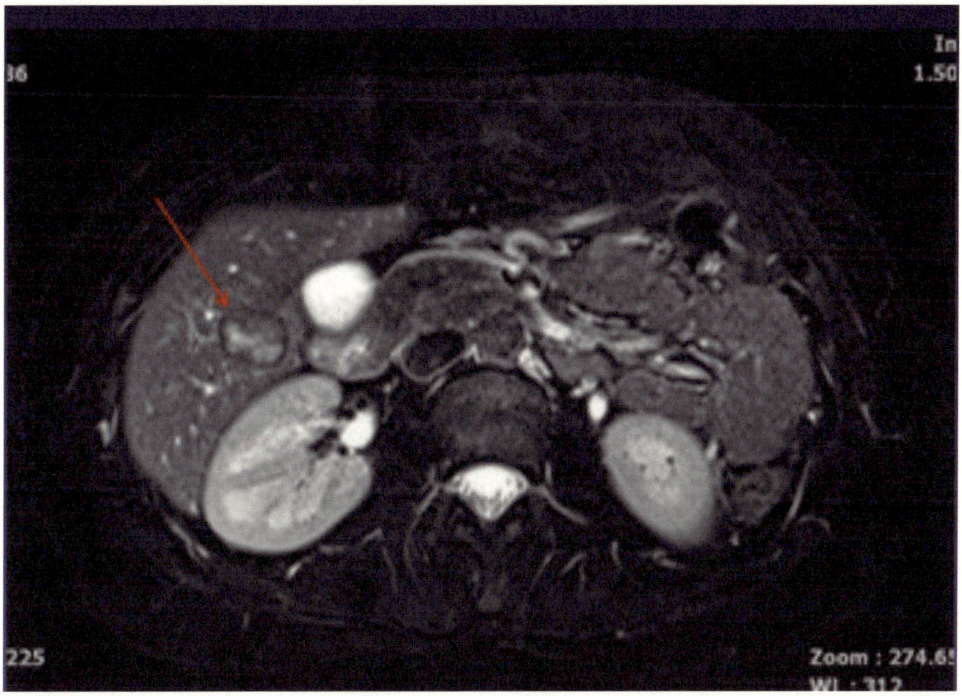

Fig. 1. Hepatic Adenoma ideally placed for Laparoscopic resection

Surgery for LLR should be divided in two broad categories, a) Those patients with metastasis confined to liver and b) those patients with concomitant extra-hepatic disease. Essentially all patients with CRLM who have had radical treatment for their primary CRC should be considered resectable and falls into one of the following groups;

A. Those patients with metastasis confined to liver

i. Unilobar or bilobar disease
ii. Single or multiple metastases
iii. Remnant liver is approximately 20-30%. Total liver volume (TLV) dependent on remnant function or equivalent to at least two liver segments

B. Those patients with concomitant extra-hepatic disease

i. CRLM in the presence of resectable or ablatable pulmonary disease
ii. CRLM in the presence of resectable isolated extra-hepatic disease e.g. spleen, adrenal or resectable local recurrence
iii. CRLM in the presence of resectable invasion of adjacent structures (e.g. diaphragm, adrenal).

With respect to extra-hepatic disease. Elias et al. have reported overall 5-year crude survival rates of 28% when hepatic and extra-hepatic disease are both resected in a curative manner, however in this situation it must be accepted that an R0 resection will not be possible in 50% of patients [24]. More importantly, the presence of extra hepatic disease does not appear to influence outcome when resection is complete along with the liver metastases [25] . Nevertheless it cannot be denied that there are few long term survivors in the presence of peritoneal disease [26]. Certainly these types of patients should be carefully evaluated by open surgery and not by LLR. The easiest patients to consider for LLR are those with disease confined to a single segment who ideally have a solitary metastasis in the anterior segments (IVb, V and in some cases VI) **(Figure 2.)** or in the left lateral segment (group Ai or Aii). Laparoscopic posterior sectionectomy has been described but they are significantly more challenging [27-29].

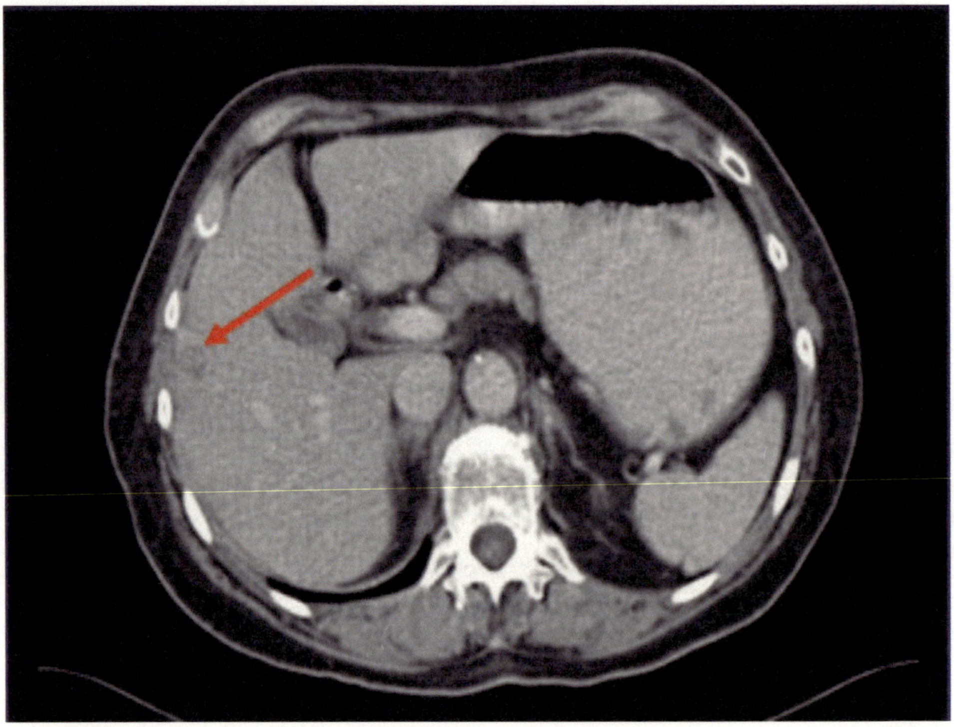

Fig. 2. Colorectal metastasis in segment VI for laparoscopic resection

Patients with extra-hepatic disease (group B) fall into a very difficult group as resection of extra-heptic disease may require more advanced laparoscopic skills which could be more easily dealt with by open surgery. The temptation to laparoscopically resect a single lesion and then perhaps laparoscopically ablate a more difficult lesion should be avoided and open surgery performed.

With respect to nodal disease, regional metastasis to peri-hepatic lymph nodes deposits should not be regarded as a contraindication to open resection but does reduce long-term outcome. Recent studies suggest up to 20% of patients will have hepatic nodal involvement at the time of resection [30]. It is very difficult to evaluate this laparoscopically. Resection of nodes involving second tier nodes (i.e.celiac nodes) is far more controversial and offers no survival benefit. Another problem highlighted by the MSKCC group is the ability to identify which lymph nodes are involved during open surgery. Routine sampling of lymph node stations and lymphadenectomy is unnecessary and time consuming, without any evidence of benefit. The best approach is selective sampling based on intra-operative assessment and pre-operative imaging [31]. Again performing this laparoscopically would not be advisable.

One of the main advantages of LLR, in our experience, has been its use with synchronous tumours **(Figure 3).** LLR can be performed at the same time with a laparoscopic colorectal specialist who removes the primary in one sitting. Up to 25% of patients may present in this way [32]. Nonetheless there are no significant publications with any reasonable numbers to draw on any useful conclusions as to whether there is any benefit with combined laparoscopic procedures [33 34]. Minimally invasive techniques have obvious advantages over two major laparotomies in a short space of time. With advances in chemotherapy more patients are now becoming operable with their primary still in situ as there liver disease can be controlled. This cohort is becoming increasingly more common and challenging [35 36]. Generally these patients have either laparoscopic right hemicoloectomy or laparoscopic anterior resection with excision of either a solitary or unilobar metastasis. A further group includes those patients who have major colonic resection with clearing of a single lobe and then further downstaging chemotherapy prior to definitive resection by a second open liver resection. Recent reports have suggested no significant differences in post-operative morbidity or mortality or 5 year survival rates in those patients with synchronous disease who need a minor hepatectomy with colonic resection [37 38] . In patients who require a major hepatectomy, a test of time, to enable an assessment of the biological behaviour of the disease and to provide adjuvant treatment, is still sensible. Although simultaneous laparoscopic major liver resection e.g. right hepatectomy along with major colonic resection e.g. anterior resection have been successfully described [39 40] the authors would not recommend this without a careful assessment of the patients fitness because of the need for prolonged anaesthesia beyond 5 hours.

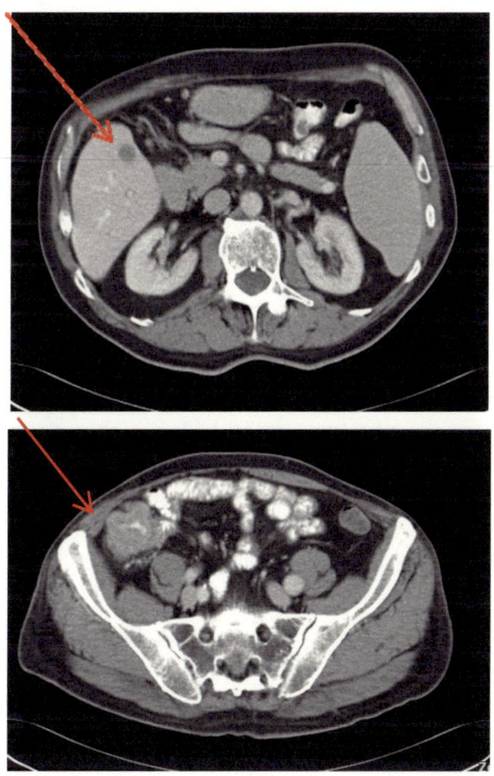

Fig. 3. Colorectal metastasis with the primary colonic tumour still in situ ideal for simultaneous laparoscopic

Two-thirds of patients undergoing liver resection for CRLM will develop recurrence of their disease within 2 years [32]. One third will manifest with liver only disease and a small proportion of them will be suitable for repeat liver resection [41]. Technically repeat liver resections are demanding. However long-term survival is similar to those following initial liver resections for open resections [42 43] . In a series of 60 third hepatectomies [43] complication rates were similar to those having first and second hepatectomies with no obvious survival disadvantage. Five year survival rates of 32% have been reported after open resection. Multivariate analysis suggests a curative resection (R0) as the most important predictor of improved survival after open resection. There are no studies reporting repeat LLR but these are likely to be technically more challenging. Further studies are needed to evaluate repeat LLR in terms of survival rates and complications.

2.5 Hepatocellular carcinoma

The treatment of HCC covers a broad spectrum including surgical (Resection, Ablation or Liver Transplant-LT) and non-surgical treatments (Sphere therapy, TACE, Sorafenib). Mortality after liver resection in large series of non cirrhotics are now around 3%. Yet in large volume centres in the east, mortality after resection for HCC in cirrhotics is now approaching zero. Substantial refinements in the surgical techniques have played an important role including the development of liver "hardware" such as ultrasonic dissectors, low CVP anaesthesia, hepatoduodenal compression (Pringle's manoeuvre) and vascular staplers have all contributed to reducing blood loss, post-op morbidity and mortality [44].

There is no doubt that the results of LT for primary HCC have improved dramatically in the last decade following the publication of the Milan criteria by Mazzaferro et al. in 1996 [45]. Consequently more patients with HCC are being referred for consideration of LT and the management of these patients on the ever expanding waiting list present an interesting cohort of patients to discuss. With this in mind bridging treatments such as resection, chemo-embolisation or ablation by RFA are becoming increasingly important The clinical characteristics after such treatments are also important in terms of predicting overall prognosis.

One of the disadvantages of resection is tumour recurrence as some suggest that this can hinder subsequent LT [46] yet this has not been substantiated by others and in terms of technical difficulty is no different to re-transplantation for other indications [47]. To avoid this problem there is a niche for the development of LLR which can reduce morbidity and have an impact on curative intent as a potential bridging treatment. Resection can be useful as a bridging treatment if patients are Childs A with a low MELD score, have a small tumour <3cm without any obvious macroscopic tumour thrombus [44]. Overall 3 year survival rates in patients with Child's A cirrhosis can be as high as 93% [48] for segmental resections. Segmental resections are best performed given the risks of recurrence with non segmental resections due to microscopic satellite nodules that are not easily visualised by intra-operative ultrasound. Comparisons of LLR with open resection for HCC in cirrhotic patients are favourable [49 50 51 52] but the main advantage of LLR is a shorter hospital stay and less blood loss. LLR is also less likely to lead to problematic adhesions if LT is required at a later date. Numerous single centre [49 50 53 54] and multi-centre series [55] have published their series of LLR in patients with HCC and cirrhosis confirming it is safe and reproducible without oncological compromise or survival.

3. Imaging

3.1 Computed tomography

This modality is the work-horse of all imaging techniques in the pre-operative planning phase for LLR. Present generation triple phase multi-detector CT scanning technology enables image acquisition during a single-breath hold, of the entire chest and abdomen and pelvis. The improved resolution results in excellent detection of lesions in solid organs and enables better local, regional and distant staging. The other advantage of CT scanning is the high incidence of detection of lesions in the lung, liver and pelvis, when intravenous contrast is used with arterial or venous phase scanning. Slice thickness or maximum collimation should be 3- 5mm. The sensitivity for detecting a metastatic lesion approaches 80%, which increases to 90% when CT angiography is used, however lesions less than 1 cm in size are liable to be missed [56]. Contrast enhanced helical CT is the investigation of choice in the initial evaluation of liver tumours assessing response to chemotherapeutic agents and for post-operative surveillance for tumour recurrence.

3.2 Magnetic resonance imaging

Magnetic resonance imaging has an extremely high sensitivity in identifying and characterizing small lesions within the liver. In addition patients are not exposed to radiation but the procedure is far more expensive and labour intensive. One of its limitations is the identification of extra hepatic disease. The technique is very sensitive to respiratory artefact and this can limit its resolution in certain patients who are unable to hold their breath for a sufficient length of time. Contrast agents such as gadolinium and the liver specific super magnetic iron oxide result in very high sensitivities in diagnosing small (less than 1 cm) liver metastases [57] and differentiating between potentially malignant and benign liver lesions (e.g. FNH, adenoma etc). Usually MR imaging is utilised just prior to resection, in order to identify small lesions not visualised by conventional CT scanning but this is not universally routine.

3.3 Intra-operative ultrasound

Intra-operative ultrasound (IOUS) is an essential pre-requisite for assessment of the liver prior to commencement of liver resection. IOUS allows for mapping of the major vascular and ductal structures in relation to the metastasis and aids in planning the final approach to resection. It also serves as a guide in confirming the accuracy of the plane of dissection. However following chemotherapy, when fatty change supervenes and in the presence of cirrhosis, identification of small iso-echoic masses becomes poor, decreasing the sensitivity of IOUS. IOUS must be used before, during and at the end of resection in order to keep R1 resection rates as low as possible. It is also important to leave an adequate margin around the tumour and to mark the margins prior to commencing parenchymal transaction. This is also useful to avoid coning as it is very difficult to estimate the depth of a tumour without measuring the dimensions.

4. Anaesthesia

One of the overlooked contra-indications for LLR is the patients inability to withstand a prolonged pneumoperitoneum especially with major resections e.g. right hepatectomy. Results of left lateral liver resection suggest that resection time can be comparable to open.

The median duration in the literature is around 2-3 hours [58] . In the authors experience laparoscopic left lateral resection can be performed as quick laparoscopically as open once the learning curve has been overcome. Transection time can be less than 1 hour as reported in a recent meta-analysis [59]. For major hepatectomy operative times are prolonged and the duration of anaesthesia can be in excess of 5 hours compared to 3 hours for open surgery [60] [61]. This can be reduced by performing a hybrid resection or, using a hand-port as it is generally the parenchymal transection and dealing with the right hepatic vein that causes the prolonged pneumoperitoneum. In the UK most centres use epidural anaesthesia for post-operative pain relief but for LLR the duration of anaesthesia can be significantly reduced as an epidural and central venous pressure line are no longer required.
Few studies have reported the consequences of the prolonged peritoneum. There is no doubt that increased intra-abdominal pressure reduces liver, renal lower limb and mesenteric blood flow. It also increases cardiac output and arterial pressures . The presence of obesity exacerbates these problems further. Careful consideration therefore needs to be given to those patients with significant renal and cardiac disease. There is also experimental evidence that prolonged peritoneum can impair post-operative liver regeneration, oxidative stress and hepatocellular damage[62]. Sometimes the pneumoperitoneum can have advantages in that during bleeding a careful increase in intra-abdominal pressure can reduce bleeding and allow parenchymal transection without portal clamping. However prolonged pneumoperitoneum with portal clamping can cause a significant reduction in hepatic oxygen tensions, tissue hypoxia, with higher transaminase and increased tissue necrosis [63]. Gas embolism is also thought to be of concern in that it can cause haemodynamic disturbance in 50% of episodes but usually has no clinical consequences as the solubility of carbon dioxide is greater than nitrogen. It is important to avoid high intra-abdominal pressures when dissecting the major venous structures in an effort to avoid this problem [64]. By controlling the differential pressures between the pneumoperitoneum and central venous pressure the risk of air embolism can be reduced significantly.

5. Techniques of laparoscopic liver resection

Definitions of laparoscopic liver surgery have been standardised. There are 3 techniques, totally laparoscopic, hand assisted and hybrid [11]. Hand assisted can be used either at the start of the operation or introduced at any time to aid dissection. This is most often performed during right hepatectomy or major resection and to control bleeding. Hybrid procedures comprise either totally laparoscopic converted to hand assisted and then the operation is completed through a small incision usually this is for parenchymal transection or to aid mobilisation of the right or left lobe after hilar dissection.

5.1 Patient positioning

During resection of the left lateral segment, and tumours within the anterior segments e.g. IVb, V, VI the patient is positioned in the supine position with split legs with the surgeon standing in between them and the assistants on each side **(Figure 4).** For tumours placed in the posterior segments (VI and VII), patients are positioned in the left lateral decubitus position. For those patients positioned supine with split legs, five ports (ENDO PATH Xcel ™, Ethicon Endosurgery, LLC, USA) are positioned; three 12 mm ports: the first at the umbilicus (sometimes higher if distance between the xiphoid and umbilicus is greater than 15 cm), the second and third working ports in the right and left mid clavicular line; and two

5 mm ports in the right and left anterior axilliary line **(Figure 5).** For tumours positioned in segments IVa and VIII, high up towards the dome of the right diaphragm a further 10mm port is placed at the xiphisternum to allow for CUSA parenchymal division (Integra, Saint Priest, France, USA)

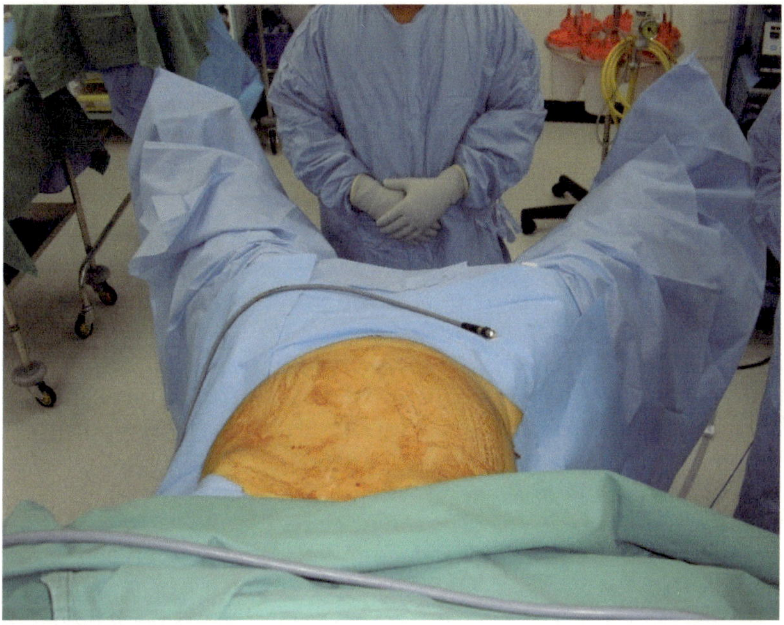

Fig. 4. The surgeons preferred position for lap resection

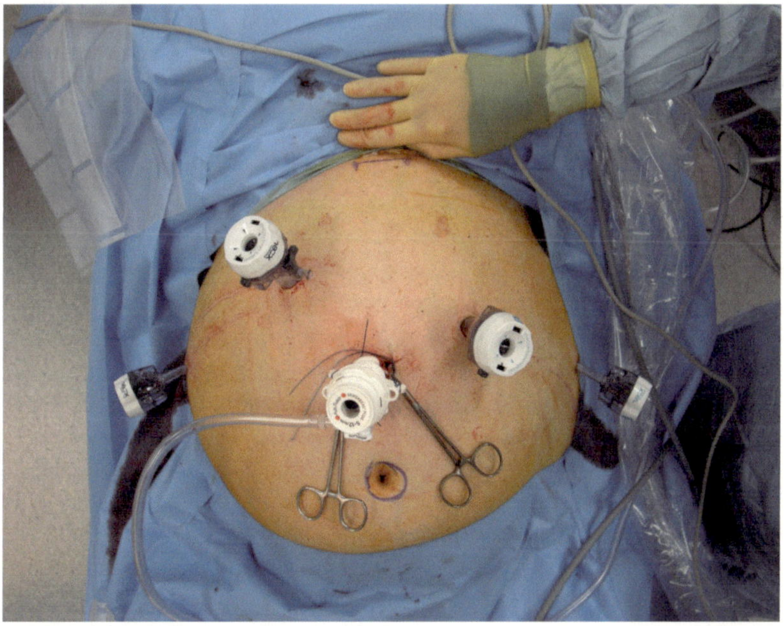

Fig. 5. Port position for lap left lateral resection

Left hepatectomy can usually be performed using similar port positions to left lateral resection. For right hepatectomy the surgeon stands between the patients legs with two assistants on either side. The right side and right shoulder are slightly elevated. Ports are shifted to the right and are placed as far across as the mid axillary line **(Figures 7a and 7b).** A hand port, if required, is usually placed in the right iliac fossa **(Figure 8).** If it is placed too high the hand will be over the liver, if it placed too low the surgeon has to stoop for prolonged periods which can become uncomfortable. A laparoscopic port can also be placed through the hand port to assist with totally laparoscopic dissection. Right hepatectomy hepatectomy should only be performed if the tumour is located away from the hilum or the RHV or IVC so as to give an oncologically sound resection.

5.2 Pringle's manoeuvre

A staging laparoscopy is performed first to rule out the presence of significant extra-hepatic disease although this is often limited due to dense pelvic adhesions. Laparoscopic ultrasound (7.5 MHz, Aloka Co. Ltd, Tokyo, Japan) of the liver is then performed to define the vascular anatomy and to confirm the location of metastases. The liver can be lifted by two methods; early in our series a Nathanson hook was placed at the xiphisternum as described for Nissen's Fundiplication. This elevates the left lateral segment and the hepato-duodenal ligament off the inferior vena cava thus ensuring good access through the foramen of Winslow and giving fixed retraction for all hilar dissection. Now either a hand retractor (fan), diamond flex or goldfinger retractor can be placed through a 5mm port to elevate the LLS. The xiphisternal Nathanson Hook can then be replaced with a 5mm port after hilar dissection to assist with tumours high on the dome of VIII.

An alternative method is to retract the falciform ligament towards the shoulder but this uses an instrument through a 5 mm port. A better approach is to divide the falciform ligament and then place an Endoloop ™ (Autosuture, Tyco Healthcare UK Ltd) around the free edge of the ligamentum teres. This can be retracted superiorly by bringing this through the anterior abdominal wall using an 'Endo Close™' (Autosuture, Tyco Healthcare UK Ltd) device. The suture is then held in a haemostat thus holding the ligament against the anterior abdominal wall. The gallbladder can also be used for retraction but some patients may have already had this removed. Calot's triangle should be dissected first and the cystic duct and cystic artery divided.. Sometimes it is necessary to partially dissect the infundibulum of the gallbladder prior to retraction over the liver. This elevates the liver and also assists with access to the posterior surface of V and VI.

Once the liver has been retracted and the hepato-duodenal ligament has been lifted a tape can then be placed. The pars lucida is opened, care being taken to look for an accessory left hepatic artery. To place a tourniquet around the hepato-duodenal ligament a 'Gold finger' (Gold finger ™, Blunt Dissector and Suture Retrieval System, Ethicon Endo Surgery, Johnson & Johnson, USA) is used. This is an endoscopic dissector previously developed for laparoscopic bariatric surgery. The Gold finger is a long instrument with a versatile tip which is used to help position laparoscopic gastric bands and creation of a retro-gastric tunnel. The tip is blunt and includes a slot to snare and pull a pre-tied suture, and a keyhole for multiple gastric bands. The tip can be set at varying degrees between the neutral position and 90 degrees. It has multi-positional flexibility, is malleable and provides precise articulation. The Gold finger has a one-handed, ergonomic operation which enables precise dissection and controlled grasping and snaring. It is also disposable and ensures sterility and consistent performance.

A nylon tape is passed through the snare in the tip of a Gold finger ™ (Ethicon Endo Surgery, Johnson & Johnson, USA). As the tip of the Gold finger is blunt and atraumatic, it can safely be introduced through a 10 mm working port in the right upper quadrant. It is best to do this through the right sided port as the natural curvature of the liver from this side avoids placing the tip into the caudate lobe and porta-hepatis if done from the left side. The hepato-duodenal ligament is then cradled by the 'Gold finger ™' (Ethicon Endo Surgery, Johnson & Johnson, USA). The Gold finger is then advanced beyond the porta-hepatis until the tip with the nylon tape can be visualised on the left side of the hepato-duodenal ligament. As the tip of the Gold finger is atraumatic, it can be safely deployed the tip is then flexed and articulated to 90 degrees. The tape can then be grasped through the port placed in the left upper quadrant in the mid-clavicular line **(Figure 6).** The two ends are positioned through the port onto the anterior abdominal wall and placed through a 'snugger' using tubing (Suction tubing 10 cm, 7 mm, Pennine Healthcare Ltd, UK). The port is removed and replaced with the tape lying adjacent to the side of the port.
Portal triad clamping (Pringle's manoeuvre) is one of the methods used to reduce bleeding from the hepatic transection plane. This manoeuvre of encircling the hepato-duodenal ligament with a nylon tape is widely used and is easily performed during conventional open surgery. However, this step can be difficult and technically challenging during laparoscopic liver surgery and not all surgeons place a tape laparoscopically for fear of injury to the IVC and structures within the porta hepatitis. For major laparoscopic resection it is a vital adjunct to reduce haemorrhage. This is as a result of the two dimensional view during laparoscopy and the ergonomics of most laparoscopic instruments make this manipulation blind with the potential of injury to vital structures. Most of the literature on totally laparoscopic liver resection mentions the placement of a tape or vascular sling around the portal triad in the hepato-duodenal ligament in case a Pringle's manoeuvre is necessary during parenchymal division [21] although opinions differ [65] [14] [66] and once experience has been gained for minor resections is often not necessary at all, even in some cirrhotic patients [67] Nonetheless it is our policy to always place a tape around the hepatoduodenal ligament for training purposes.
Some surgeons use a tape around the hepato-duodenal ligament with intra-peritoneal clamping. However, this uses up an extra port as an instrument clamps it on the inside. Moreover laparoscopic instruments are not robust enough to give a satisfactory clamp. The technique of using the Gold finger to facilitate placement of a tape around the hepato-duodenal ligament for the Pringle manoeuvre is an easy, safe and efficient technique. This manoeuvre is performed easily in a few minutes. Although this technique has evolved in a small series we believe this to be a simplified technique that is much easier and safer for laparoscopic liver resection.

6. Parenchymal transection and haemostasis

6.1 Hilar dissection

There are many preferences for hilar dissection for major resection e.g. right trisectionetomy, right hepatectomy or left hepatectomy. Intra-hepatic [68] or extra-hepatic [69] (conventional or anterior approach) division of major structures have both been described. It is the authors practice to divide all major structures extra-hepatically with the exception of the hepatic bile duct. This is divided last of all, within the liver parenchyma, using a suitable stapling device. Fortunately the use of vascular staplers with roticulators has overcome most of the problems relating to the management of major pedicles and vessels, these can be either 45 or 60mm varieties. When the bile duct is divided within the liver there is less risk of damaging the remnant hepatic duct.

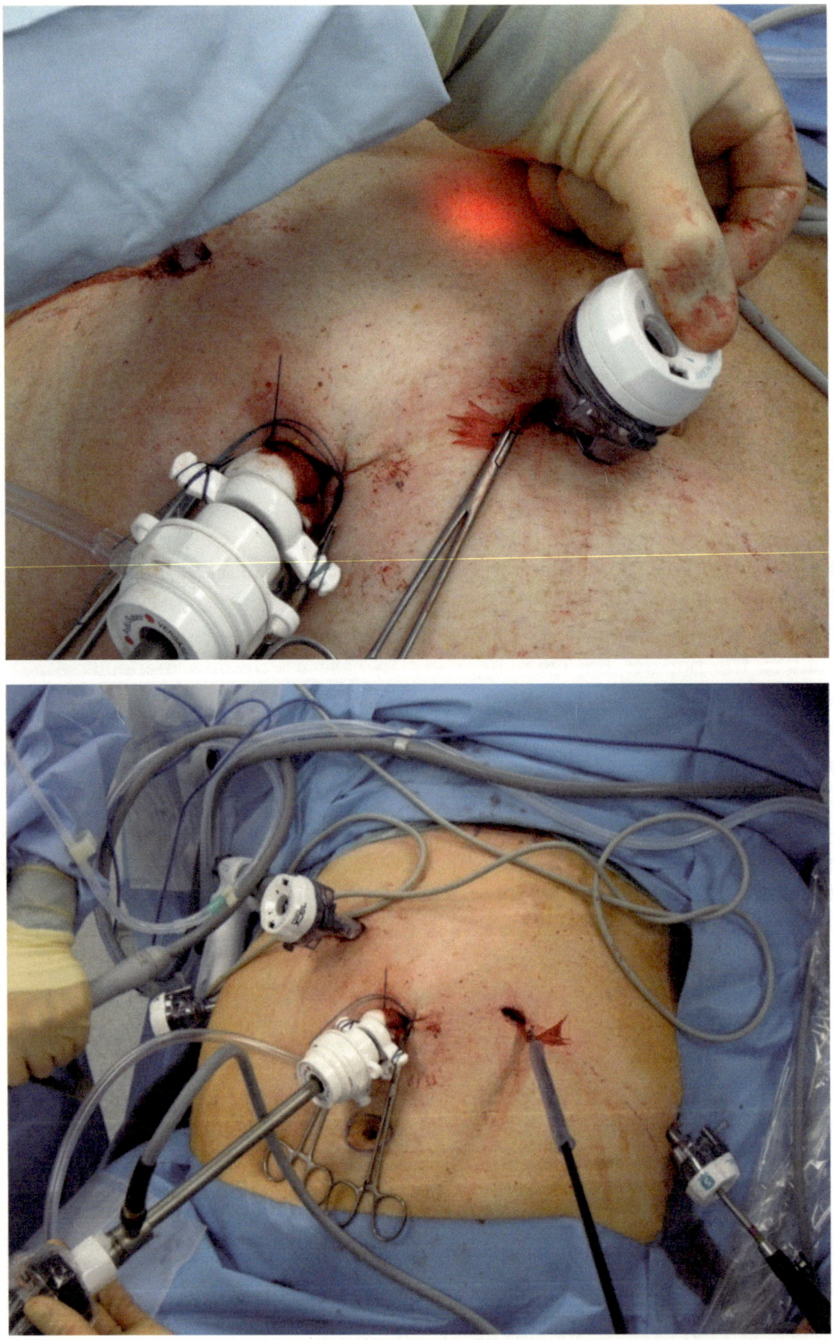

Fig. 6. Hepatoduodenal tape positioned lateral to the port for a Pringle manoeuvre

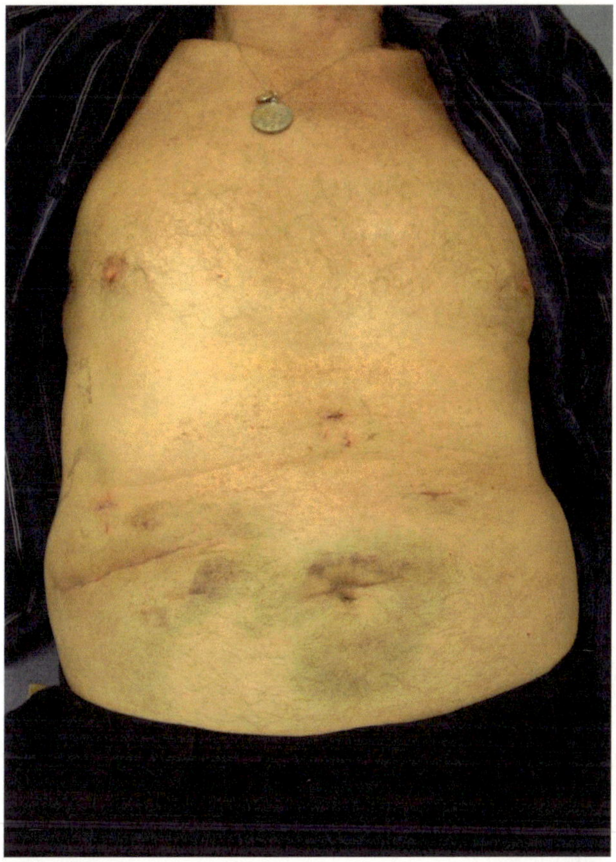

Fig. 7a. Port position for laporoscopic right hepatectomy with RIF incision

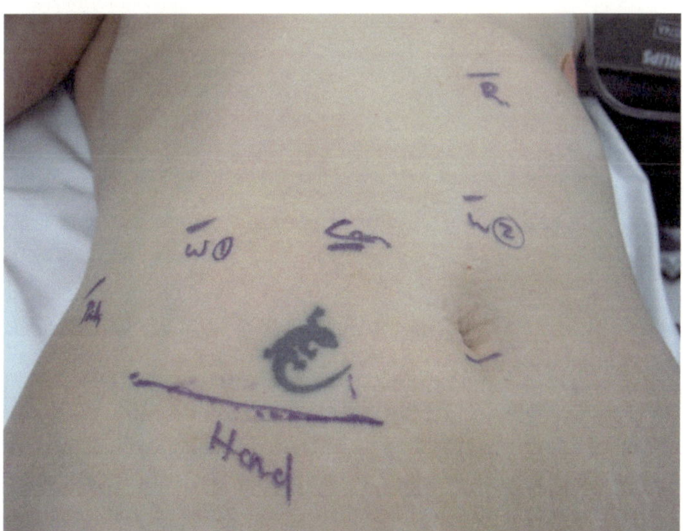

Fig. 7b. Pre-operative marking for hand assisted right hepatectomy

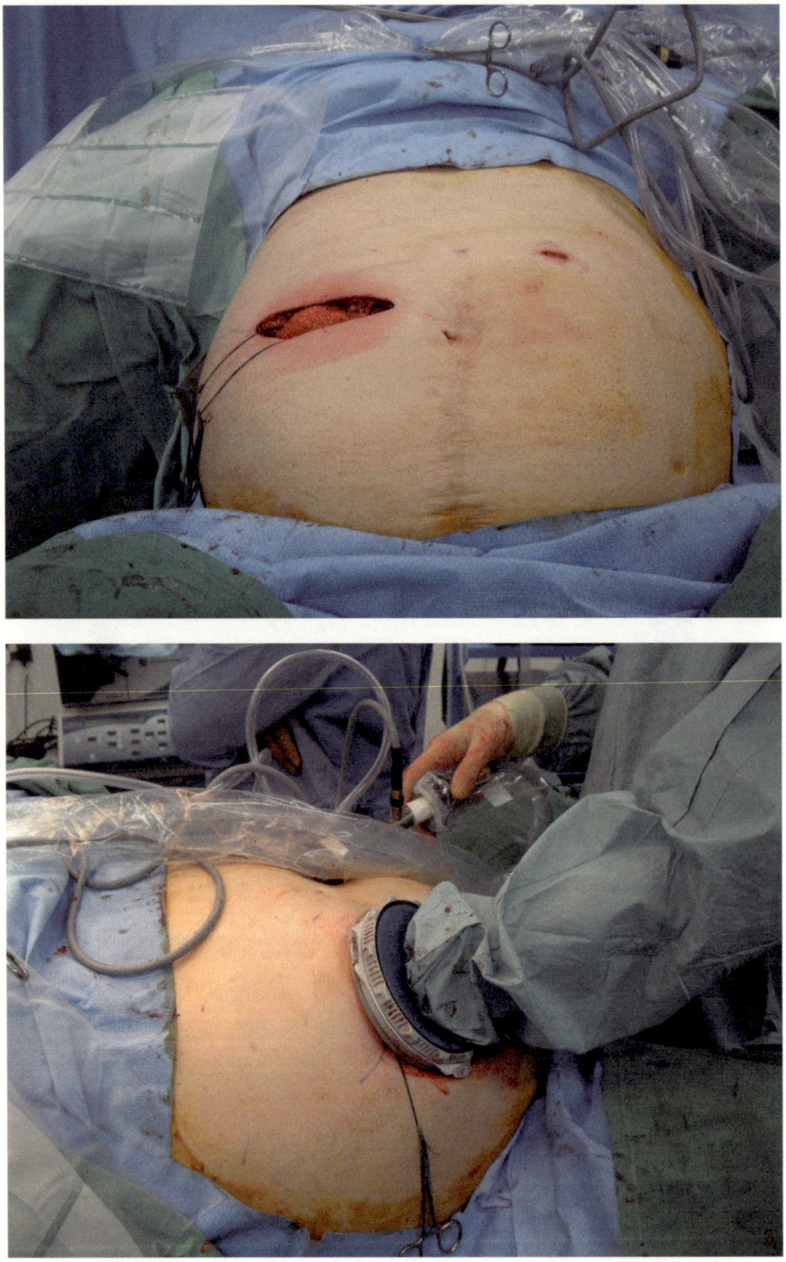

Fig. 8. Hand assisted liver resection

Hilar dissection can be tedious and difficult especially when there are extensive adhesions. Major structures can be inadvertently injured and troublesome bleeding can be difficult to deal with for the inexperienced surgeon. Extensive dissection in the hepatoduodenal ligament is never necessary and can lead to devascularisation of the common hepatic duct or remnant hepatic duct. For a right hepatectomy identification of major structures such as the right hepatic artery (RHA), and right portal vein (RPV) can be approached either anteriorly or laterally, posterior to the hepatic duct.. The author's preference is to use locking clips such as Weck Clips. The portal vein can be approached differently. This can be divided using either a vascular stapler or Weck clips. However, care needs to be taken when achieving vascular control as bleeding at the portal confluence can be difficult to stop. Dividing the caudate process prior to this assists this manoeuvre by allowing more room. Tiny venous tributaries supplying the true caudate lobe and caudate process may also be encountered.

The posterior or Glissonian approach described by Launois and Jamieson [70] avoids hilar dissection within the hepatoduodenal ligament. The basic concept is that the major right sided structures such as RHA, RPV and RHD are enveloped in a tough fibrous Glissonian sheath. This is more common for hand assisted procedures [71]. Keeping very close, posterior to the sheath a finger is used to encircle the right pedicle. If inflow to the remnant is confirmed the whole pedicle is ligated using a vascular stapling device. There is certainly no doubt that the posterior approach is the quickest way for inflow division [72,73].

Another technique for right hepatectomy is the anterior approach [68]. This avoids the potential hazard of major injury to the RHV with injudicious mobilization of liver and the potential for hepatic ischaemia. Another problem that is avoided is IVC obstruction when the liver is continually rotated to the left. It also has a theoretical advantage of less propagation of tumour cells during the mobilisation phase as the liver is only mobilised once the RHV has been disconnected. The anterior approach involves hilar dissection and inflow control, complete parenchymal transection and division of the RHV only then is liver mobilised. Survival appears to be better for the anterior approach 'open procedures', when compared to the conventional mobilisation technique for patients with HCC[74].

6.2 Parenchymal transection

Haemorrhage can be exsanguinating and unpredictable particularly after sustained use of chemotherapy. However it is the constant steady bleeding sustained in the phase of parenchymal transection that contributes most to the overall blood loss. A variety of techniques and surgical adjuncts can be used to aid parenchymal transection. Most experience is with the Cavitational ultrasonic aspirator (CUSA ™), bipolar sealing device Tissue Link, The Habib x4 ™ radiofrequency device or the Harmonic Scalpel ultrasonically activated shears (now Harmonic ACE ™). The Harmonic Scalpel ® cuts and coagulates by using ultrasound. Vessels are coapted (tamponaded) and sealed by a protein coagulum. Coagulation occurs by means of protein denaturation when the blade, vibrating at 55,000 Hz, couples with protein, denaturing it to form a coagulum that seals small coapted vessels. The newer Harmonic ACE version appears to be more effective in that it is faster and seals vessels up to 5mm in diameter and seals up to twice systolic pressure. However after a 15 second application heat can be 140 °C 1cm away from the tip causing significant lateral thermal damage away from the tissues being sealed [75]. Their powerful compression forces are directed at the tip of the device as well [76].

Newer generation devices include the LOTUS Torsion ™, which uses torsional ultrasound, transfers less energy to adjacent structures. The torsional waveform is thought to be safer as there are only weak frictional forces at the tip of the active blade and reduces' distal drilling' and tissue charring. The Ligasure ™ device which utilises low voltage bi-polar radiofrequency energy seals vessels up to 7mm in diameter up to 3 times systolic pressure and monitors changes in tissue impedance and adjusts the energy output accordingly causing less collateral tissue damage to within 1.5mm of the grasping jaws [77]. Tissuelink (Aquamantys TM) works using transcollation (transforming collagen) technology sealing small biliary radicals, no charringand gives a bloodless operating field. This device delivers radiofrequency energy and saline simultaneously to achieve temperatures of 100°C [78]. The major disadvantage is that is can be slower and is more expensive. A cheap and effective time honoured method is bipolar diathermy giving good haemostasis on the liver parenchyma using a power of up to 80 watts. There have been concerns regarding Argon Beam Coagulation (ABC) and gas embolism[79] because of the stream of argon gas when the instrument is activated particularly on the liver bed when there are large open vessels. It is strongly advisable not to use ABC in this situation.

There are no well designed controlled studies comparing different haemostatic techniques during LLR but these have been reviewed in detail elsewhere [80] [81]. Attention to detail regarding securing the bile ducts, identifying and ligating the medium and larger vascular structures are important in ensuring minimal blood loss, bile leaks and achieving an oncologically sound surgical procedure. To realize this, various techniques might be needed at different stages of the operation and therefore a working knowledge of all available techniques is useful.

7. Laparoscopic versus open liver resection - The evidence

7.1 The learning curve/patient benefit

Most studies reporting laparoscopic liver resection report a learning curve. How long that learning curve is depends on the type of resection. Small resections less than 2cm require little additional skill to that needed for a complex laparoscopic cholecystectomy when positioned in the anterior segments V, IVb or left lateral segment on the proviso the surgeon has completed a recognised training program in HPB surgery. For more major resections e.g. right heptectomy, left hepatectomy the bar is significantly raised and should only be attempted by surgeons who regularly perform complex laparoscopic procedures. The main limiting factor is technical difficulty and access. Some would suggest that increasing size of tumour is not a limiting factor [60] but this is not what has been recommended in the Louisville guidelines [11].

It cannot be denied that not everyone is suitable for a laparoscopic liver resection. Most centres suggest that up to 30% [68] [29] are suitable although those centres performing more major resections regularly report higher rates up to 80% but also report higher rates with hand assisted techniques [82] [4]. One study suggests a learning curve of 60 cases is adequate to demonstrate quicker operating times and a lower conversion rate [83]. Indeed during our 4 year experience the conversion rate has decreased from 14% to 3%. The commonest reason for conversion is usually technical or due to bleeding.

Most studies doing detailed analysis report reduced operating time when different era's are evaluated[68]. For example, laparoscopic left lateral resection can become significantly quicker[84] [58] as in our experience, yet for major resection (e.g. right hepatectomy) there is still some progress to be made to reduce operating times compared to open (5 hours versus 3 hours) [61,68] even procedures up to 10 hours have been reported [60]. Also anatomical resections are generally quicker than non anatomical wedge resections [68]. Nonetheless the learning curve is difficult to assess as it depends on the definition of success which to most would be disease free survival which is rarely discussed. One study has addressed this in detail in a non randomized study comparing 120 patients. There does not appear to be any difference in overall 5 year survival in those having either LLR or open resection in terms of disease free survival [85]. Most studies report no difference in rates of R0 resection and no increased risk of positive margins after LLR as reviewed elsewhere [10]. Although a recent meta-analysis suggests the risk of an R0 resection (<1cm) is twice as high after LLR than for open resection[86]. Indeed R1 resection rates of up to 43% have been reported [18] and non segmental resections may have the highest risk [87].

For left lateral resections and segmental resections blood loss and transfusion requirements have improved significantly through eras and now most involved in the field would suggest that with more minor resections blood loss is less when compared to open surgery [22,86,4]. However this is perhaps not the case for major resection and bleeding can be catastrophic and problematic when it is from a major tributary such as the RHV or venous confluence [19] and this is why some prefer the safety of a hand port when they approach the RHV during right hepatectomy.

The main advantage of LLR are the reported benefits which apply to all minimally invasive procedures. These include reduced post-operative pain relief, reduced hospital stay, less morbidity and mortality. Certainly a recent meta-analysis suggests patients have less blood loss, shorter post-operative stay and a quicker return to activities of daily living for left lateral resection or metastectomy[7] [6,86,4,10]. Without randomized studies this will be difficult to confirm as laparoscopic enthusiasts may have a tendency to send patients home earlier than usual practise and may vary between centres. Generally the disadvantage of higher costs is offset by the shorter stay [88,7,89,90].

8. Training in laparosopic liver surgery

An important consideration certainly in Europe is the recent introduction of the European Working Time Directive (EWTD) which has threatened surgical training by a reduction in working hours and doctor/patient contact. Surgical trainees are therefore not exposed to as many opportunities to learn new or advanced techniques in laparoscopic surgery. There is no doubt that laparoscopic training programs need to be developed to keep pace with the introduction of new techniques and to allow surgical trainees adequate exposure and applies to all surgical specialities.

A growth area in this field has been the introduction of various structured programs, virtual reality systems and laparoscopic simulators which have been reviewed in detail elsewhere. [91 92]. Alternative approaches to facilitate training has been the use of porcine or canine simulators [93] . Nevertheless these can be expensive to implement and can be problematic for licensing. An alternative approach which has not been widely reported is the use of a Cadaver Lab Training Facility [94].

The Newcastle Surgical Training Centre (NSTC) based at the Freeman Hospital opened in September 2007 **(Figure 9).** The laparoscopic training facility provides a specialist forum for the development of advanced laparoscopic skills and is part of the national drive to improve the delivery of near-patient technology. It is a unique, state of the art facility providing advanced cadaveric education which enables surgeons to gain cadaveric training in a unique and extremely high specification "wet lab" environment on fresh frozen cadavers. This centre is one of the very first anatomical examination units of its kind in the UK to carry a formal license from the Human Tissue Authority (HTA). The Human Tissue Act 2004 received Royal Assent in November 2004 and the act sets out standards and provides guidance to clinicians carrying out education and training in using human cadaveric materials.

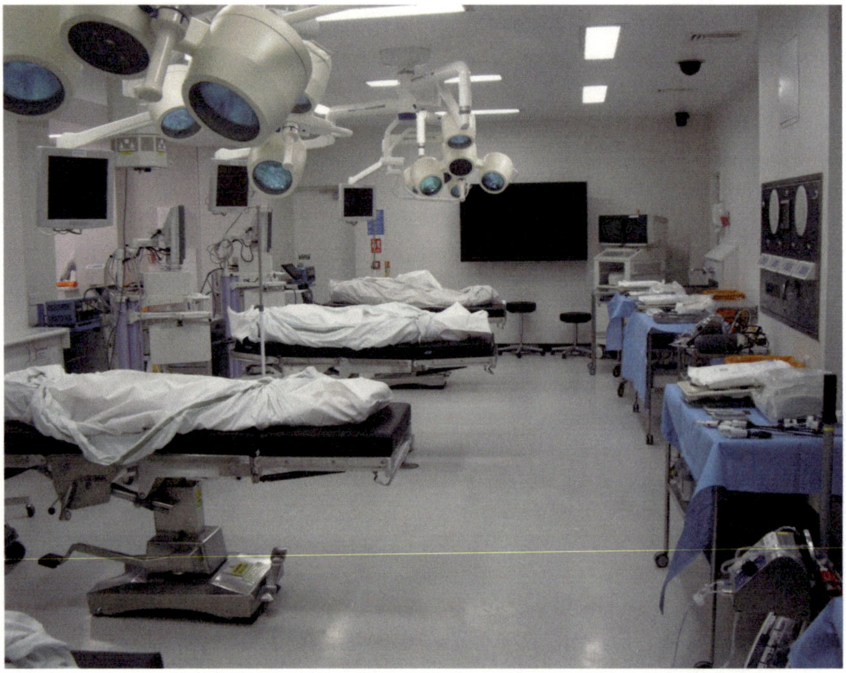

Fig. 9. Laparoscopic cadaver training lab

A course has been designed by a faculty of experienced, advanced laparoscopic surgeons providing an intensive 2 day course of lectures, debate, exchange and practical hands on with a live link to clinical laparoscopic liver resection operations. All participants are given an opportunity to perform 8 key tasks in order to develop their laparoscopic liver surgery skills. These include the following;

1. Port Positioning for left lateral liver resection
2. Tape placement around the hepatoduodenal ligament for a safe Pringle's manoeuvre
3. Dissection of hilar structures, portal vein, hepatic artery, and confluence of the hepatic ducts and common bile duct.
4. Left lateral liver mobilisation.
5. Left lateral sectionectomy with an ultrasonic aspirator and stapling of the left hepatic vein.
6. Right lobe mobilisation
7. Right hepatectomy with dissection of RHA, RPV, RHD and IVC dissection with stapling of the RHV.
8. Use of hand ports for facilitating right hepatectomy.

Although safety, efficacy and reproducibility of LLS has been established, the same cannot be said of the training and accreditation of junior surgeons. The specialist surgical societies both at National and International levels are yet to establish guidelines for training and mentoring.

With rapid progress in the field of electronics, computers and robotics, training of residents/junior surgeons through surgical simulation is slowly gaining popularity as it provides an opportunity for the trainee to develop the necessary skills for the clinical situation. Furthermore with advanced software technologies, visual fidelity , manual dexterity, hand eye co-ordination, real time response to emergency situations can now be assessed. The down side of the virtual reality simulators is their computing power and the initial set up costs. Oversimplification of complex reality isolates the trainee from the clinical situation. As far as the authors are aware there are no virtual reality simulators for LLR available for training.

Though basic psychomotor skills can be learnt on a surgical simulator or virtual reality simulator, learning to use high energy devices like diathermy or dissectors, tissue handling need a more realistic model like an animal or human cadaver. A synthetic model though attractive in terms of cost benefit falls short in recreating training outcomes. Rodents have been used extensively in both open and laparoscopic training models as they are well suited for laboratory based research activities, are expensive to buy, breed and house in a laboratory. Krahenbuhl et al. [95] have reported a safe technique of LLR in rats for liver physiology research. Canine models have also been advocated but their major drawback are anatomical constraints having multiple liver lobes but also stringent laws in the United Kingdom which prevent their routine use in the laboratory for training [96 97]. Porcine models have been used extensively in Europe because of size and more favourable anatomy. Unfortunately their overall cost and safety regulations prohibit their use in the UK. Sheep have also been used for LLR because they are anatomically similar to human [98].

The use of a cadaver in a dissection laboratory for imparting anatomical knowledge is well established [99]. Cadaver training has also been used successfully in a workshop to train residents in internal medicine to perform bedside procedures like thoracocentesis, paracentesis, lumbar puncture and bone marrow biopsy [100]. Fresh cadavers have also been used for vascular surgery training [101].

Using cadavers for learning laparoscopic procedures holds immense potential. Katz et al. [102] described a cadaver model to be superior to porcine models for urological laparoscopic training. Cadaver laparoscopic dissection has been used to enhance resident comprehension of pelvic anatomy [103]. In the UK with the introduction of the Human Tissue Act 2004, it is possible to store and use cadavers for laparoscopic training. The advantages of using cadavers are perfect for reproducing anatomical landmarks, tissue consistency and flexibility, tactile feedback and tissue handling, use of gravity and retraction to make it more realistic and almost near perfect reproduction of critical steps. Furthermore, the use of proper instruments, patient positioning and an operation room setup helps the surgeon to train in a more conducive atmosphere.

We have been conducting cadaver laparoscopic liver surgery courses for both practising and training surgeons at NSTC since 2007. We have shown that the overall rating of the course by the trainees attending has been very good.

9. References

[1] Jarnagin WR, Gonen M, Fong Y, Dematteo RP, Ben-Porat L, Little S et al. Improvement in perioperative outcome after hepatic resection: analysis of 1,803 consecutive cases over the past decade. *Ann Surg* 2002; 236(4):397-406.

[2] Rees M, Tekkis PP, Welsh FK, O'Rourke T, John TG. Evaluation of long-term survival after hepatic resection for metastatic colorectal cancer: a multifactorial model of 929 patients. *Ann Surg* 2008; 247(1):125-135.

[3] Laparoscopic partial hepatectomy for liver tumour. Surg.Endosc. 6, 99. 1-9-1992. Gagner, M., Rheault, M., and Dubuc, J. Ref Type: Generic

[4] Nguyen KT, Geller DA. Laparoscopic liver resection--current update. *Surg Clin North Am* 2010; 90(4):749-760.

[5] Nguyen KT, Gamblin TC, Geller DA. World review of laparoscopic liver resection-2,804 patients. *Ann Surg* 2009; 250(5):831-841.

[6] Simillis C, Constantinides VA, Tekkis PP, Darzi A, Lovegrove R, Jiao L et al. Laparoscopic versus open hepatic resections for benign and malignant neoplasms--a meta-analysis. *Surgery* 2007; 141(2):203-211.

[7] Rao A, Rao G, Ahmed I. Laparoscopic left lateral liver resection should be a standard operation. *Surg Endosc* 2011; 25(5):1603-1610.

[8] Croome KP, Yamashita MH. Laparoscopic vs open hepatic resection for benign and malignant tumors: An updated meta-analysis. *Arch Surg* 2010; 145(11):1109-1118.

[9] Vigano L, Tayar C, Laurent A, Cherqui D. Laparoscopic liver resection: a systematic review. *J Hepatobiliary Pancreat Surg* 2009; 16(4):410-421.

[10] Nguyen KT, Marsh JW, Tsung A, Steel JJ, Gamblin TC, Geller DA. Comparative Benefits of Laparoscopic vs Open Hepatic Resection: A Critical Appraisal. *Arch Surg* 2011; 146(3):348-356.

[11] Buell JF, Cherqui D, Geller DA, O'Rourke N, Iannitti D, Dagher I et al. The international position on laparoscopic liver surgery: The Louisville Statement, 2008. *Ann Surg* 2009; 250(5):825-830.

[12] Soubrane O, Cherqui D, Scatton O, Stenard F, Bernard D, Branchereau S et al. Laparoscopic left lateral sectionectomy in living donors: safety and reproducibility of the technique in a single center. *Ann Surg* 2006; 244(5):815-820.

[13] Suh KS, Yi NJ, Kim T, Kim J, Shin WY, Lee HW et al. Laparoscopy-assisted donor right hepatectomy using a hand port system preserving the middle hepatic vein branches. *World J Surg* 2009; 33(3):526-533.

[14] Troisi RI, Van HJ, Berrevoet F, Vandenbossche B, Sainz-Barriga M, Vinci A et al. Evolution of laparoscopic left lateral sectionectomy without the Pringle maneuver: through resection of benign and malignant tumors to living liver donation. *Surg Endosc* 2011; 25(1):79-87.

[15] Koffron AJ, Kung R, Baker T, Fryer J, Clark L, Abecassis M. Laparoscopic-assisted right lobe donor hepatectomy. *Am J Transplant* 2006; 6(10):2522-2525.

[16] Farges O, Jagot P, Kirstetter P, Marty J, Belghiti J. Prospective assessment of the safety and benefit of laparoscopic liver resections. *J Hepatobiliary Pancreat Surg* 2002; 9(2):242-248.

[17] Ardito F, Tayar C, Laurent A, Karoui M, Loriau J, Cherqui D. Laparoscopic liver resection for benign disease. *Arch Surg* 2007; 142(12):1188-1193.

[18] Morino M, Morra I, Rosso E, Miglietta C, Garrone C. Laparoscopic vs open hepatic resection: a comparative study. *Surg Endosc* 2003; 17(12):1914-1918.

[19] Troisi R, Montalti R, Smeets P, Van HJ, Van VH, Colle I et al. The value of laparoscopic liver surgery for solid benign hepatic tumors. *Surg Endosc* 2008; 22(1):38-44.

[20] Katkhouda N, Hurwitz M, Gugenheim J, Mavor E, Mason RJ, Waldrep DJ et al. Laparoscopic management of benign solid and cystic lesions of the liver. *Ann Surg* 1999; 229(4):460-466.

[21] Vibert E, Perniceni T, Levard H, Denet C, Shahri NK, Gayet B. Laparoscopic liver resection. *Br J Surg* 2006; 93(1):67-72.

[22] Koffron AJ, Auffenberg G, Kung R, Abecassis M. Evaluation of 300 minimally invasive liver resections at a single institution: less is more. *Ann Surg* 2007; 246(3):385-392.

[23] Giulianotti PC, Sbrana F, Bianco FM, Addeo P. Robot-assisted laparoscopic extended right hepatectomy with biliary reconstruction. *J Laparoendosc Adv Surg Tech A* 2010; 20(2):159-163.

[24] Elias D, Sideris L, Pocard M, Ouellet JF, Boige V, Lasser P et al. Results of R0 resection for colorectal liver metastases associated with extrahepatic disease. *Ann Surg Oncol* 2004; 11(3):274-280.

[25] Elias D, Liberale G, Vernerey D, Pocard M, Ducreux M, Boige V et al. Hepatic and extrahepatic colorectal metastases: when resectable, their localization does not matter, but their total number has a prognostic effect. *Ann Surg Oncol* 2005; 12(11):900-909.

[26] Elias D, Delperro JR, Sideris L, Benhamou E, Pocard M, Baton O et al. Treatment of peritoneal carcinomatosis from colorectal cancer: impact of complete cytoreductive surgery and difficulties in conducting randomized trials. *Ann Surg Oncol* 2004; 11(5):518-521.

[27] Gumbs AA, Gayet B. Video: the lateral laparoscopic approach to lesions in the posterior segments. *J Gastrointest Surg* 2008; 12(7):1154.

[28] Costi R, Capelluto E, Sperduto N, Bruyns J, Himpens J, Cadiere GB. Laparoscopic right posterior hepatic bisegmentectomy (Segments VII-VIII). *Surg Endosc* 2003; 17(1):162.

[29] Cho JY, Han HS, Yoon YS, Shin SH. Experiences of laparoscopic liver resection including lesions in the posterosuperior segments of the liver. *Surg Endosc* 2008; 22(11):2344-2349.

[30] Jaeck D. The significance of hepatic pedicle lymph nodes metastases in surgical management of colorectal liver metastases and of other liver malignancies. *Ann Surg Oncol* 2003; 10(9):1007-1011.

[31] Grobmyer SR, Wang L, Gonen M, Fong Y, Klimstra D, D'Angelica M et al. Perihepatic lymph node assessment in patients undergoing partial hepatectomy for malignancy. *Ann Surg* 2006; 244(2):260-264.

[32] Lochan R, White SA, Manas DM. Liver resection for colorectal liver metastasis. *Surg Oncol* 2007; 16(1):33-45.

[33] Kim SH, Lim SB, Ha YH, Han SS, Park SJ, Choi HS et al. Laparoscopic-assisted combined colon and liver resection for primary colorectal cancer with synchronous liver metastases: initial experience. *World J Surg* 2008; 32(12):2701-2706.

[34] Lee JS, Hong HT, Kim JH, Lee IK, Lee KH, Park IY et al. Simultaneous laparoscopic resection of primary colorectal cancer and metastatic liver tumor: initial experience of single institute. *J Laparoendosc Adv Surg Tech A* 2010; 20(8):683-687.

[35] Pathak S, Sarno G, Nunes QM, Poston GJ. Synchronous resection for colorectal liver metastases: the future. *Eur J Surg Oncol* 2010; 36(11):1044-1046.
[36] Reddy SK, Pawlik TM, Zorzi D, Gleisner AL, Ribero D, Assumpcao L et al. Simultaneous resections of colorectal cancer and synchronous liver metastases: a multi-institutional analysis. *Ann Surg Oncol* 2007; 14(12):3481-3491.
[37] Tanaka K, Shimada H, Matsuo K, Nagano Y, Endo I, Sekido H et al. Outcome after simultaneous colorectal and hepatic resection for colorectal cancer with synchronous metastases. *Surgery* 2004; 136(3):650-659.
[38] de SE, Fernandez D, Vaccaro C, Quintana GO, Bonadeo F, Pekolj J et al. Short-term and long-term outcomes after simultaneous resection of colorectal malignancies and synchronous liver metastases. *World J Surg* 2010; 34(9):2133-2140.
[39] Tranchart H, Diop PS, Lainas P, Pourcher G, Catherine L, Franco D et al. Laparoscopic major hepatectomy can be safely performed with colorectal surgery for synchronous colorectal liver metastasis. *HPB (Oxford)* 2011; 13(1):46-50.
[40] Casaccia M, Famiglietti F, Andorno E, Di DS, Ferrari C, Valente U. Simultaneous laparoscopic anterior resection and left hepatic lobectomy for stage IV rectal cancer. *JSLS* 2010; 14(3):414-417.
[41] Khatri VP, Petrelli NJ, Belghiti J. Extending the frontiers of surgical therapy for hepatic colorectal metastases: is there a limit? *J Clin Oncol* 2005; 23(33):8490-8499.
[42] Petrowsky H, Gonen M, Jarnagin W, Lorenz M, DeMatteo R, Heinrich S et al. Second liver resections are safe and effective treatment for recurrent hepatic metastases from colorectal cancer: a bi-institutional analysis. *Ann Surg* 2002; 235(6):863-871.
[43] Adam R, Pascal G, Azoulay D, Tanaka K, Castaing D, Bismuth H. Liver resection for colorectal metastases: the third hepatectomy. *Ann Surg* 2003; 238(6):871-883.
[44] White SA, Manas DM, Farid SG, Prasad KR. Optimal treatment for hepatocellular carcinoma in the cirrhotic liver. *Ann R Coll Surg Engl* 2009; 91(7):545-550.
[45] Mazzaferro V, Regalia E, Doci R, Andreola S, Pulvirenti A, Bozzetti F et al. Liver transplantation for the treatment of small hepatocellular carcinomas in patients with cirrhosis. *N Engl J Med* 1996; 334(11):693-699.
[46] Adam R, Azoulay D, Castaing D, Eshkenazy R, Pascal G, Hashizume K et al. Liver resection as a bridge to transplantation for hepatocellular carcinoma on cirrhosis: a reasonable strategy? *Ann Surg* 2003; 238(4):508-518.
[47] Belghiti J, Cortes A, Abdalla EK, Regimbeau JM, Prakash K, Durand F et al. Resection prior to liver transplantation for hepatocellular carcinoma. *Ann Surg* 2003; 238(6):885-892.
[48] Cherqui D, Laurent A, Tayar C, Chang S, Van Nhieu JT, Loriau J et al. Laparoscopic liver resection for peripheral hepatocellular carcinoma in patients with chronic liver disease: midterm results and perspectives. *Ann Surg* 2006; 243(4):499-506.
[49] Tranchart H, Di GG, Lainas P, Roudie J, Agostini H, Franco D et al. Laparoscopic resection for hepatocellular carcinoma: a matched-pair comparative study. *Surg Endosc* 2010; 24(5):1170-1176.
[50] Sarpel U, Hefti MM, Wisnievsky JP, Roayaie S, Schwartz ME, Labow DM. Outcome for patients treated with laparoscopic versus open resection of hepatocellular carcinoma: case-matched analysis. *Ann Surg Oncol* 2009; 16(6):1572-1577.

[51] Lai EC, Tang CN, Ha JP, Li MK. Laparoscopic liver resection for hepatocellular carcinoma: ten-year experience in a single center. *Arch Surg* 2009; 144(2):143-147.

[52] Belli G, Limongelli P, Fantini C, D'Agostino A, Cioffi L, Belli A et al. Laparoscopic and open treatment of hepatocellular carcinoma in patients with cirrhosis. *Br J Surg* 2009; 96(9):1041-1048.

[53] Zhang L, Chen YJ, Shang CZ, Zhang HW, Huang ZJ. Total laparoscopic liver resection in 78 patients. *World J Gastroenterol* 2009; 15(45):5727-5731.

[54] Belli G, Fantini C, Belli A, Limongelli P. Laparoscopic liver resection for hepatocellular carcinoma in cirrhosis: long-term outcomes. *Dig Surg* 2011; 28(2):134-140.

[55] Dagher I, Belli G, Fantini C, Laurent A, Tayar C, Lainas P et al. Laparoscopic hepatectomy for hepatocellular carcinoma: a European experience. *J Am Coll Surg* 2010; 211(1):16-23.

[56] Sahani DV, Kalva SP. Imaging the liver. *Oncologist* 2004; 9(4):385-397.

[57] Ward J, Robinson PJ, Guthrie JA, Downing S, Wilson D, Lodge JP et al. Liver metastases in candidates for hepatic resection: comparison of helical CT and gadolinium- and SPIO-enhanced MR imaging. *Radiology* 2005; 237(1):170-180.

[58] Abu HM, Pearce NW. Laparoscopic left lateral liver sectionectomy: a safe, efficient, reproducible technique. *Dig Surg* 2008; 25(4):305-308.

[59] Rao A, Rao G, Ahmed I. Laparoscopic left lateral liver resection should be a standard operation. *Surg Endosc* 2011; 25(5):1603-1610.

[60] Dagher I, O'Rourke N, Geller DA, Cherqui D, Belli G, Gamblin TC et al. Laparoscopic major hepatectomy: an evolution in standard of care. *Ann Surg* 2009; 250(5):856-860.

[61] Abu HM, Di FF, Teng MJ, Lykoudis P, Primrose JN, Pearce NW. Single-Centre Comparative Study of Laparoscopic Versus Open Right Hepatectomy. *J Gastrointest Surg* 2011.

[62] Schmidt SC, Schumacher G, Klage N, Chopra S, Neuhaus P, Neumann U. The impact of carbon dioxide pneumoperitoneum on liver regeneration after liver resection in a rat model. *Surg Endosc* 2010; 24(1):1-8.

[63] Nsadi B, Gilson N, Pire E, Cheramy JP, Pincemail J, Scagnol I et al. Consequences of pneumoperitoneum on liver ischemia during laparoscopic portal triad clamping in a swine model. *J Surg Res* 2011; 166(1):e35-e43.

[64] Fors D, Eiriksson K, Arvidsson D, Rubertsson S. Gas embolism during laparoscopic liver resection in a pig model: frequency and severity. *Br J Anaesth* 2010.

[65] Kazaryan AM, Pavlik M, I, Rosseland AR, Rosok BI, Mala T, Villanger O et al. Laparoscopic liver resection for malignant and benign lesions: ten-year Norwegian single-center experience. *Arch Surg* 2010; 145(1):34-40.

[66] Pulitano C, Catena M, Arru M, Guzzetti E, Comotti L, Ferla G et al. Laparoscopic liver resection without portal clamping: a prospective evaluation. *Surg Endosc* 2008; 22(10):2196-2200.

[67] Belli G, Fantini C, D'Agostino A, Belli A, Russolillo N, Cioffi L. [Laparoscopic liver resection without a Pringle maneuver for HCC in cirrhotic patients]. *Chir Ital* 2005; 57(1):15-25.

[68] Bryant R, Laurent A, Tayar C, Cherqui D. Laparoscopic liver resection-understanding its role in current practice: the Henri Mondor Hospital experience. *Ann Surg* 2009; 250(1):103-111.

[69] Belli G, D'Agostino A, Fantini C, Belli A, Cioffi L, Limongelli P et al. Laparoscopic hand-assisted right hemihepatectomy by ultrasound-directed intrahepatic approach. *J Hepatobiliary Pancreat Surg* 2009; 16(6):781-785.

[70] Launois B, Jamieson GG. The posterior intrahepatic approach for hepatectomy or removal of segments of the liver. *Surg Gynecol Obstet* 1992; 174(2):155-158.

[71] Belli G, D'Agostino A, Fantini C, Belli A, Cioffi L, Limongelli P et al. Laparoscopic hand-assisted right hemihepatectomy by ultrasound-directed intrahepatic approach 21. *J Hepatobiliary Pancreat Surg* 2009; 16(6):781-785.

[72] Machado MA, Makdissi FF, Herman P, Surjan RC. Intrahepatic Glissonian approach for pure laparoscopic left hemihepatectomy. *J Laparoendosc Adv Surg Tech A* 2010; 20(2):141-142.

[73] Machado MA, Makdissi FF, Galvao FH, Machado MC. Intrahepatic Glissonian approach for laparoscopic right segmental liver resections. *Am J Surg* 2008; 196(4):e38-e42.

[74] Liu CL, Fan ST, Cheung ST, Lo CM, Ng IO, Wong J. Anterior approach versus conventional approach right hepatic resection for large hepatocellular carcinoma: a prospective randomized controlled study. *Ann Surg* 2006; 244(2):194-203.

[75] Emam TA, Cuschieri A. How safe is high-power ultrasonic dissection? *Ann Surg* 2003; 237(2):186-191.

[76] Sutton PA, Awad S, Perkins AC, Lobo DN. Comparison of lateral thermal spread using monopolar and bipolar diathermy, the Harmonic Scalpel and the Ligasure. *Br J Surg* 2010; 97(3):428-433.

[77] Harold KL, Pollinger H, Matthews BD, Kercher KW, Sing RF, Heniford BT. Comparison of ultrasonic energy, bipolar thermal energy, and vascular clips for the hemostasis of small-, medium-, and large-sized arteries. *Surg Endosc* 2003; 17(8):1228-1230.

[78] Nissen NN, Grewal N, Lee J, Nawabi A, Korman J. Completely laparoscopic nonanatomic hepatic resection using saline-cooled cautery and hydrodissection. *Am Surg* 2007; 73(10):987-990.

[79] Kono M, Yahagi N, Kitahara M, Fujiwara Y, Sha M, Ohmura A. Cardiac arrest associated with use of an argon beam coagulator during laparoscopic cholecystectomy. *Br J Anaesth* 2001; 87(4):644-646.

[80] Abu HM, Underwood T, Taylor MG, Hamdan K, Elberm H, Pearce NW. Bleeding and hemostasis in laparoscopic liver surgery. *Surg Endosc* 2010; 24(3):572-577.

[81] The use of fibrin sealants in laparoscopic liver surgery. Laparoscopic . 2011. saif, r. Ref Type: Generic

[82] Buell JF, Thomas MT, Rudich S, Marvin M, Nagubandi R, Ravindra KV et al. Experience with more than 500 minimally invasive hepatic procedures. *Ann Surg* 2008; 248(3):475-486.

[83] Vigano L, Laurent A, Tayar C, Tomatis M, Ponti A, Cherqui D. The learning curve in laparoscopic liver resection: improved feasibility and reproducibility. *Ann Surg* 2009; 250(5):772-782.

[84] Lesurtel M, Cherqui D, Laurent A, Tayar C, Fagniez PL. Laparoscopic versus open left lateral hepatic lobectomy: a case-control study. *J Am Coll Surg* 2003; 196(2):236-242.

[85] Castaing D, Vibert E, Ricca L, Azoulay D, Adam R, Gayet B. Oncologic results of laparoscopic versus open hepatectomy for colorectal liver metastases in two specialized centers. *Ann Surg* 2009; 250(5):849-855.

[86] Croome KP, Yamashita MH. Laparoscopic vs open hepatic resection for benign and malignant tumors: An updated meta-analysis *Arch Surg* 2010; 145(11):1109-1118.

[87] Kazaryan AM, Marangos IP, Rosok BI, Rosseland AR, Villanger O, Fosse E et al. Laparoscopic resection of colorectal liver metastases: surgical and long-term oncologic outcome *Ann Surg* 2010; 252(6):1005-1012.

[88] Simillis C, Constantinides VA, Tekkis PP, Darzi A, Lovegrove R, Jiao L et al. Laparoscopic versus open hepatic resections for benign and malignant neoplasms--a meta-analysis. *Surgery* 2007; 141(2):203-211.

[89] Polignano FM, Quyn AJ, de Figueiredo RS, Henderson NA, Kulli C, Tait IS. Laparoscopic versus open liver segmentectomy: prospective, case-matched, intention-to-treat analysis of clinical outcomes and cost effectiveness. *Surg Endosc* 2008; 22(12):2564-2570.

[90] Vanounou T, Steel JL, Nguyen KT, Tsung A, Marsh JW, Geller DA et al. Comparing the clinical and economic impact of laparoscopic versus open liver resection. *Ann Surg Oncol* 2010; 17(4):998-1009.

[91] Fairhurst K, Strickland A, Maddern G. The LapSim virtual reality simulator: promising but not yet proven. *Surg Endosc* 2010.

[92] Vassiliou MC, Dunkin BJ, Marks JM, Fried GM. FLS and FES: comprehensive models of training and assessment. *Surg Clin North Am* 2010; 90(3):535-558.

[93] Fransson BA, Ragle CA. Assessment of laparoscopic skills before and after simulation training with a canine abdominal model. *J Am Vet Med Assoc* 2010; 236(10):1079-1084.

[94] Supe A, Dalvi A, Prabhu R, Kantharia C, Bhuiyan P. Cadaver as a model for laparoscopic training. *Indian J Gastroenterol* 2005; 24(3):111-113.

[95] Krahenbuhl L, Feodorovici M, Renzulli P, Schafer M, Abou-Shady M, Baer HU. Laparoscopic partial hepatectomy in the rat: a new resectional technique. *Dig Surg* 1998; 15(2):140-144.

[96] Frezza EE, Wachtel MS. A proposed canine model of laparoscopic nonanatomic liver resection. *J Laparoendosc Adv Surg Tech A* 2006; 16(1):15-20.

[97] Machado MA, Galvao FH, Pompeu E, Ribeiro C, Bacchella T, Machado MC. A canine model of laparoscopic segmental liver resection. *J Laparoendosc Adv Surg Tech A* 2004; 14(5):325-328.

[98] Teh SH, Hunter JG, Sheppard BC. A suitable animal model for laparoscopic hepatic resection training. *Surg Endosc* 2007; 21(10):1738-1744.

[99] Parker LM. Anatomical dissection: why are we cutting it out? Dissection in undergraduate teaching. *ANZ J Surg* 2002; 72(12):910-912.

[100] Oxentenko AS, Ebbert JO, Ward LE, Pankratz VS, Wood KE. A multidimensional workshop using human cadavers to teach bedside procedures. *Teach Learn Med* 2003; 15(2):127-130.

[101] Reed AB, Crafton C, Giglia JS, Hutto JD. Back to basics: use of fresh cadavers in vascular surgery training. *Surgery* 2009; 146(4):757-762.

[102] Katz R, Hoznek A, Antiphon P, Van VR, Delmas V, Abbou CC. Cadaveric versus porcine models in urological laparoscopic training. *Urol Int* 2003; 71(3):310-315.

[103] Cundiff GW, Weidner AC, Visco AG. Effectiveness of laparoscopic cadaveric dissection in enhancing resident comprehension of pelvic anatomy. *J Am Coll Surg* 2001; 192(4):492-497.

Part 3

Laparoscopic Appendectomy

8

Laparoscopic Appendectomy

Konstantinos M. Konstantinidis and Kornilia A. Anastasakou
Department of Surgery, Athens Medical Center
Greece

1. Introduction

Suspected acute appendicitis is the most frequent cause of emergency operations in visceral surgery worldwide. Acute appendicitis is the reason for most urgent admissions and unscheduled operations in general surgery. In the western world approximately 8% of the population are appendectomised (Addis et al., 1990). The treatment for acute appendicitis has been conventional appendectomy for more than a century. This procedure proved to be safe and effective. However, a problem that remained is the high percentage -up to 47% in women of child-bearing age- of negative appendectomies (Borgstein et. al, 1997). Laparoscopic appendectomy counts almost 30 years of presence, and its introduction has met with more hurdles than that of laparoscopic cholecystectomy. Especially during the last two decades numerous studies tried to define the role of laparoscopic appendectomy in the treatment of suspected acute appendicitis. In this chapter we aim to present our experience with the laparoscopic approach for suspected appendicitis during the last almost twenty years and discuss the diagnostic and therapeutic effects of laparoscopy in suspected appendicitis. We will present our diagnostic approach, our surgical technique, and our results, and will discuss the literature. The role of laparoscopy in fertile females will be analysed. Also the place of laparoscopy in special groups such as the elderly, the employed patients, the obese patients, the pregnant women, and the children will be discussed. Finally we will refer briefly to newer techniques including the single port laparoscopic appendectomy, the needlescopic procedure, and the incidental robotic appendectomy.

1.1 Background

1.1.1 Literature

Since the introduction of endoscopic appendectomy by Kurt Semm in 1983 (Semm, 1983) the surgical community tried to determine its advantages and disadvantages compared to the open procedure. Especially during the last twenty years there have been over 60 randomized controlled trials comparing laparoscopic and open appendectomy in adults (Vettoretto et al., 2010) as well as many meta-analyses of randomized controlled trials (Bennett et al., 2007; Chung et al, 1999; Fingerhut et al., 1999; Garbutt et al., 1999; Golub et al., 1998; Liu et al., 2010; Sauerland et al., 1998, 2002, 2004, 2010). The number of publications on laparoscopic appendectomy is still increasing, while publications on laparoscopic cholecystectomy decline. The latter shows that the laparoscopic approach in suspected acute appendicitis has not yet been fully accepted as the gold standard. There are still open issues regarding the laparoscopic approach. These have to do with the indications, the results, the costs, the standardisation of the surgical technique, the severity of leaving back a macroscopically 'innocent' appendix and the learning curve. Last but not least the debate about the place of laparoscopy in complicated appendicitis, the incidence of intraabdominal abscesses after laparoscopic appendectomy and its relationship to the severity of the disease, the surgical technique, and the surgical expertise is still vivid.

In the last years it has become apparent that the laparoscopic approach does not have the same value for all subpopulations. The investigators tried to determine the importance of the laparoscopic method in several patient groups. So, one can maintain that recent studies tend to clarify the issues regarding the worth of laparoscopy in the fertile female group, the elderly, the obese and the employed patients. The debate is still ongoing about laparoscopy in men, in complicated appendicitis, laparoscopy in pregnancy and in the paediatric population.

1.1.2 Own experience

The first laparoscopic appendectomy in our department (surgical department specialized in laparoscopy in a big private hospital in Athens) was performed in 1992. Since then we have performed over 1800 laparoscopic appendectomies. We did not analyse all these cases, but we performed a retrospective analysis in more than a thousand patients. Patients with suspected appendicitis, who were treated in the Department of General, Laparoscopic, and Robotic Surgery at the Athens Medical Center between April 1993 and March 2003 were considered for our retrospective study on laparoscopic appendectomy published in 2008 (Konstantinidis et al, 2008). The study presented the results in 1026 patients and was not comparative. Only laparoscopic patients were included as laparoscopy has been the treatment of choice since the department was founded. Patients operated on during the learning curve (100 pts.) and the few patients approached from the start by open technique (15 pts.) were not included in the study. The inclusion criteria for our study on laparoscopic appendectomy were suspected acute appendicitis (after clinical examination, laboratory tests, and imaging tests) or chronic recurrent symptoms that could be attributed to appendicitis, age 15 years or more and laparoscopy as first approach. All patients in whom we performed a laparoscopic appendectomy or an appendectomy after conversion to an open procedure were included in our analysis (908 pts). Also, diagnostic accuracy of laparoscopy was analysed separately in the subgroup of fertile women (558 pts), and was compared to diagnostic accuracy in the rest of the patients (468 pts).

After standardisation of our technique the latter did not actually change. New developments were the single incision technique and the introduction of the DaVinci robotic (TM- Intuitive Surgical Inc.) system in 2006. In this chapter we will refer to the results we had between 1993 and 2003, as we measured and published them. With this exception we will comment only on major complications and new developments.

2. Diagnostic approach, patient management and surgical technique

2.1 Diagnostic approach

We perform routine preoperative control in all patients. Women in whom differential diagnosis includes gynaecological disorders are in many cases examined by the gynaecologist and a transabdominal or transvaginal ultrasound or a CT scan is being performed whenever indicated and possible. There are also some male patients, in whom we might perform ultrasound or CT scan.

From the diagnostic point of view it has been suggested that active observation leads to a consistently lower rate of negative laparotomies and laparoscopies (Jones, 2001). Several scoring systems have also been proposed as diagnostic tools, but none of them has achieved general acceptance. In the literature very low statistical association is reported between a temperature >37° C and the presence of appendicitis (Cardal et al., 2004). An elevated WBC count > 10.000 cells/mm, while statistically associated with the presence of appendicitis, is reported to have very poor sensitivity and specificity and almost no clinical utility (Cardall et al., 2004). On the other hand the combination of either leucocyte count and CRP value (Gronroos JM & Groroos P, 1999) or leucocyte count, CRP value, and neutrophil percentage (Yang et al., 2005) is considered very important in the exclusion of appendicitis. Finally helical CT and graded compression US are reported to be useful instruments in the diagnosis of acute appendicitis as they may lower the false negative rate (Balthazar et al, 1991, 1998; Birnbaum et al., 2000; Jones et al., 2001, Pacharn et al., 2010). CT is in most studies found to be superior to US as it misses fewer cases; nonetheless, they are both reliable in suspected acute appendicitis (van Randen et al., 2011). A diagnostic pathway using routine US, limited CT, and clinical re-evaluation is proposed by Toorenvliet et al. (Toorenvliet et al., 2010). US should be the first choice especially for pregnant patients (Butala et al, 2010). Finally a multicenter study is ongoing to define the role of MRI instead of CT in the diagnostic approach of acute appendicitis (Leeuwenburgh et al., 2010).

2.2 Patient management

Our patients are being given prophylactic antibiotics (1g cefotaxime and 500mg metronidazole intravenously) and in complicated cases antibiotics are continued. Our policy is to leave back a normal looking appendix, if another pathology is found at surgery, but to remove a normal looking appendix, if there are no other findings. We normally release patients in the first postoperative day. In complicated cases the hospital stay is prolonged. Patients are examined on the tenth postoperative day as well as one month postoperatively.

2.3 Surgical team and surgical technique

The surgical team involved in diagnosis and treatment consisted of specialized surgeons trained in laparoscopy and working together over several years. The team grew with time. The operating surgeon in most cases was the director of the department (K.M.K), performing about several hundred laparoscopic procedures every year, many of them being advanced procedures. The policy of the department is to approach patients laparoscopically whenever possible. This is facilitated by the fact that almost all of the abdominal operations in this department are performed by laparoscopy, over 50% of them being advanced procedures. There are also scrub nurses and technicians with experience in laparoscopy during the day as well as after hours.

Surgical technique evolved with time, experience and appearance of new technical devices. Our technique went through several stages and has been described before (Konstantinidis et al., 2008). The technique, which was performed in the last over 1600 patients will be described here: Surgery is performed under general anesthesia with the patient lying in supine position on a multi-positional operating table. There are two monitors. The surgeon stands on the patient's left side and the assistant on the right. The abdomen is entered at the umbilicus using the open Hasson technique routinely. If there are dense adhesions another approach can be used. A 10mm reusable port is placed at the umbilicus and the 30 degree laparoscope is inserted. The abdominal cavity can now be visualized. Two further 5mm reusable trocars are inserted in the suprapubic area and the left lower quadrant under visual control. The surgeon operates with two hands and the assistant holds the laparoscope. The small bowel is retracted away from the right lower quadrant with the patient lying in the Trendelenburg position and right side up. Atraumatic forceps are used. The dissection continues, sometimes using the Plasma Kinetics™ (Gyrus Medical, Cardiff, UK) bipolar electrocautery, until the base of the cecum is visualized, and the appendix can be elevated. The mesoappendix is managed in a retrograde fashion by lifting the apex of the appendix and using the cutting bipolar electrocautery until the cecum is reached. Three ligating Endoloops PDS II™(Ethicon, Sommerville, NJ, USA) are placed, the first one at the appendicular base, the second one next to the first loop, and the third one in about 1cm distance. The appendix is then transected using scissors. Before the transaction is complete the remaining appendicular mucosa is first suctioned and then burned with caution using the bipolar electrocautery. The laparoscope is changed from the 10 to the 5mm laparoscope

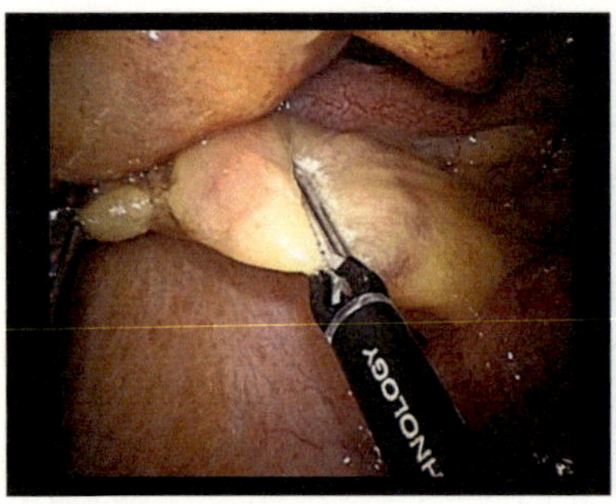

Fig. 1. Cauterisation of the mesoappendix

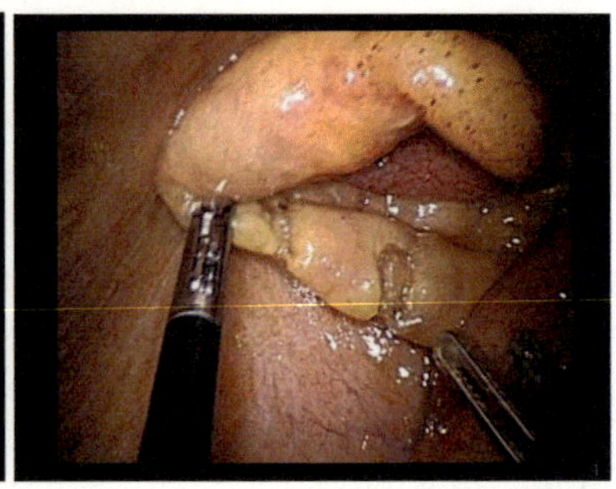

Fig. 2. Cauterisation and cutting of the mesoappendix

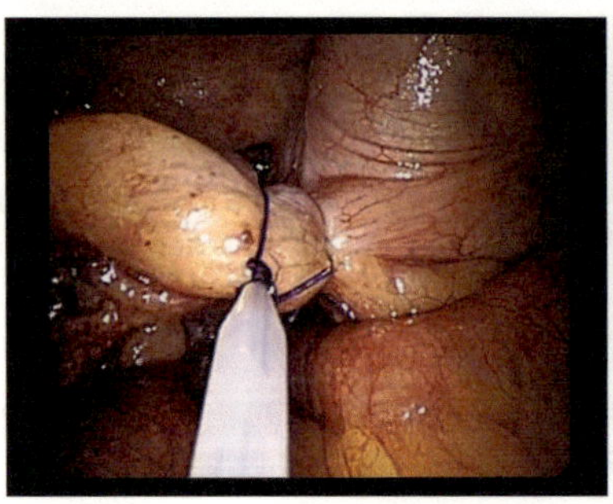

Fig. 3. Placement of the Endoloops PDS II™

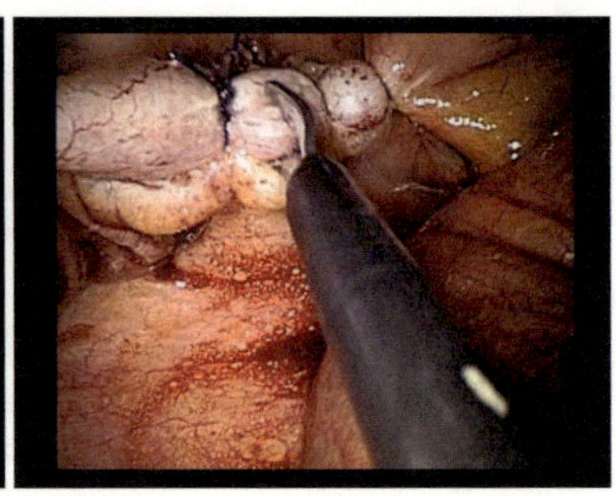

Fig. 4. Cutting of the appendix

and placed through the LLQ port. If uncomplicated, the appendix is grasped and pulled through a reducer at the umbilical port. If ruptured or gangraenous the appendix is put in a retrieval bag and the bag grasped with a traumatic grasper and pulled through the umbilical port. The site of appendectomy, right paracolic gutter, and pelvis are irrigated with about 3 to 5 liters of normal saline irrigation solution with presure. Fluid from the suprahepatic area and the pouch of Douglas is suctioned. In cases of intraabdominal abscess a drain connected to a closed suction system is placed in the abscess cavity and brought out through the subrapubic trocar. The fascial incision at the umbilicus is closed with 2.0 Vicryl™ sutures. The skin is closed with 4.0 or 5.0 absorbable subcuticular sutures, unless there is an intraabdominal contamination, in which case the skin is closed with 4.0 interrupted nylon sutures.

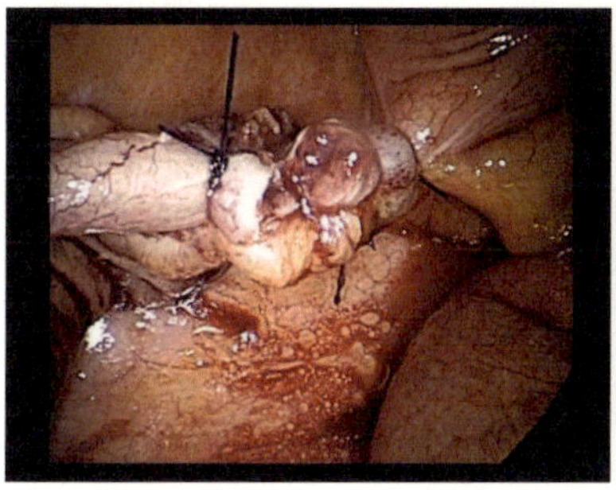

Fig. 5. Not the whole lumen of the appendix is beeing cut

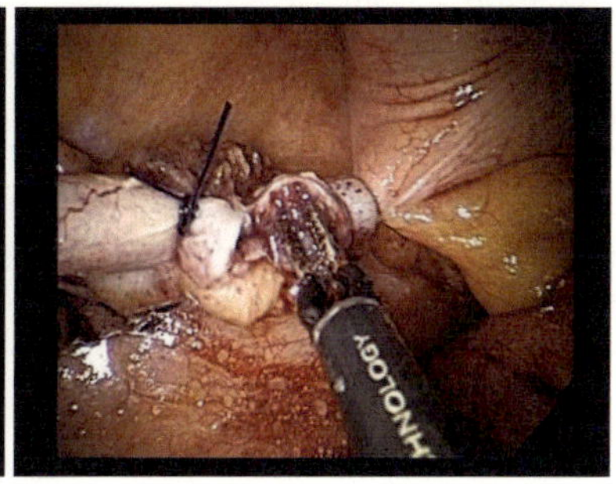

Fig. 6. Cauterisation of the appendiceal mucosa

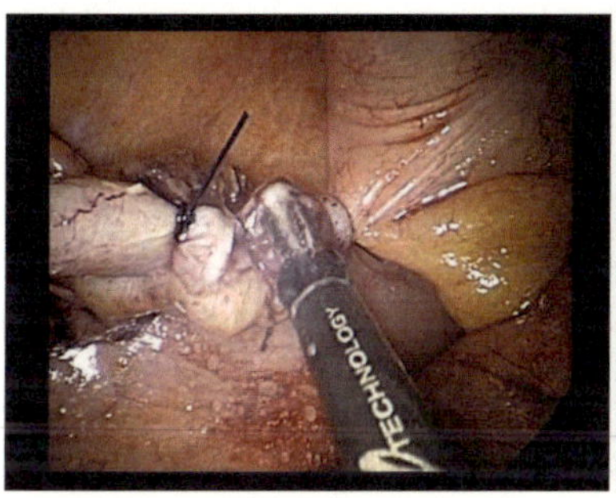

Fig. 7. Cauterisation of the appendiceal mucosa

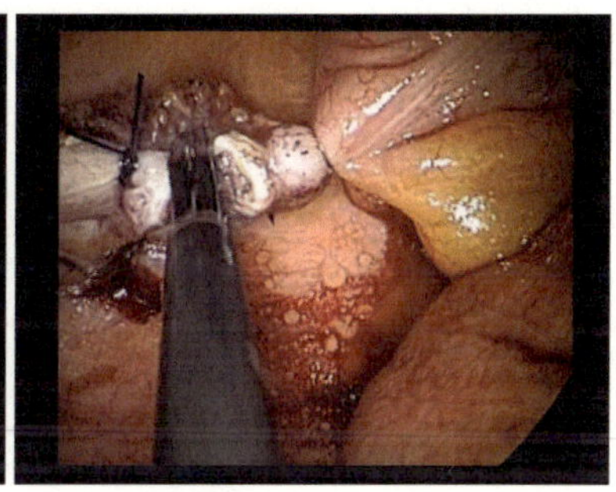

Fig. 8. Cutting of the remaining appendix with the bipolar.

Many surgeons prefer routine stapling of the appendiceal stump. The stapling is reported to be quicker, easier, and lead to less postoperative infections (Kazemier et al., 2006). On the other hand it means greater costs and the obligatory use of a 12- mm trocar. Other investigators do not report a higher complication rate with the use of endoloops as is stated in a recent review. The only difference between the two methods is considered to be operating time (Sajid et al., 2009). A protocol recruitment is now running to investigate, whether routine stapling of the stump can lead to less intraabdominal abscesses (Sauerland & Kazemier, 2007). Peritoneal lavage is contradictory, as it may lead to spillage of infection according to some investigators (Gupta, 2006) but may prevent infection if performed copiously in all quadrants according to others (Hussain, 2008). We believe that a lavage with 3-5 liters of normal saline, as we described it, using a peristaltic pump is effective and saves time. One could argue that it is more expensive, but our experience in over 1.800 patients has been that it is worth the cost. Routine use of drains is not necessary, and may in some patients lead to cecal fistulae (Petrowsky, 2004).

Finally, standardisation of surgical technique leads to reduction of operative time, conversion rate, morbidity, and to a higher surgeon satisfaction in training centers (Ng et al., 2004; Hsieh et al., 2009).

3. Results of laparoscopic appendectomy and discussion

3.1 Parameters examined in the literature

To evaluate the benefits of the laparoscopic approach in suspected appendicitis the scientific community examines several parameters. Important issues in the study of laparoscopic appendectomy are: **intraoperative findings, conversion rate to open surgery, histological findings and negative appendectomy rate, duration of operation, intra- and postoperative complications (early and late), postoperative pain, time to bowel mobilization, time until intake of solid food, duration of hospital stay, time until return to normal activities, full activities and sports, reoperations, cosmesis, and costs.** All of these parameters are dealt with in the literature and most of them were measured in our published study (Konstantinidis et al., 2008). In our patients we did not investigate the costs or the cosmetic results.

3.2 Diagnostic and therapeutic outcomes of laparoscopic appendectomy

Conversion rate ranges in meta-analyses between 0% and 23% (Lippert et al, 2002; Sauerland et al., 2004) but there are studies which report conversion rates as high as 39% (Moberg et al., 1998). In everyday praxis conversion rate typically seems to range between 10 and 20%, while in centers of excellence it is lower than 2%. It is apparent that these fluctuations are related with differences in laparoscopic experience. In most studies the operator is a surgical trainee for about 80 to 95% of open appendectomies and for about 50 to 75% of laparoscopic procedures. In our study we had a conversion rate of 0,55% in the 908 patients, in whom an appendectomy was performed. The low conversion rate in our study can be explained by the fact that we are not a teaching hospital but a private center. The operating surgeon in most of our patients has been the director of the department (K.M.K). But also the other surgeons belonging to the team are specialised and very experienced with laparoscopy. A learning curve was apparent for the first 100 appendectomies, where we had a conversion rate of 9%, but these patients were not included in the trial. Conversion rate is reported to be increased in complicated appendicitis (Wullstein et al., 2001). The most common reason for conversion is reported to be dense adhesions due to inflammation, followed by localized perforation and diffuse peritonitis (Agresta et al., 2003; Liu et al., 2002). The presence of significant fat stranding associated with fluid accumulation, inflammatory mass or localized abscess in CT scan is also reported to significantly increase the possibility of conversion (Liu et al., 2002). In our patients the reasons for conversion were dense adhesions in two patients and excessive inflammation in 3 patients.

There were also some patients, who had to be converted because of other pathologies. In our experience these were pelvic hemoperitoneum, inflammatory pelvic disease, ovarian cyst torsion, ovarian mass, ruptured diverticulitis (of the sigmoid and of the cecum) and cecal volvulus. Finally, we performed laparoscopic assisted procedures in a number of patients with Meckelitis. **The necessity to convert patients due to another pathology emphasises the role of laparoscopy as a diagnostic tool.**

There is a strong heterogeneity in **operating time** reported in the literature. Mean operating times in meta-analyses of randomised trials range between 23,5 and 102,2 min (Sauerland et al., 2004). Apart from differences in laparoscopic experience, this can be attributed to the different definitions of operating time. Nevertheless, all meta-analyses agree that the duration of surgery is longer in laparoscopic appendectomy (Benett, 2007; Chung et al., 1999; Fingerhut et al, 1999; Garbutt et al., 1999; Golub et al, 1998; Sauerland et al., 2010;

Temple et al, 1999). It is nonetheless remarkable that - as laparoscopy evolves - the results of meta-analyses performed by the same investigators show through the years a decreasing difference in operating time between the two approaches (Sauerland et al., 1998, 2002, 2004, 2010). Sauerland et al. report in their most recent meta-analysis that laparoscopic appendectomy is on the average 10 minutes longer than the open one (Sauerland et al., 2010). The median operating time in our study was 26 minutes, which compares favourably with most other studies (The time from cutting the skin at the umbilicus until putting the last skin suture was defined as operating time). We believe that the short operating time is due to the surgeon's expertise, and the training of the surgical team. We also believe that it has to do with the standardisation of the surgical technique.

It has been suggested, and seems logical, that surgical expertise has a great impact in conversion rate and operating time. The latter one as well as the lack of precision in manoeuvers by novices could affect complication rate and patients' outcome.

In our study we had an overall **complication rate** of 5,7%, consisting mostly of minor complications. At the beginning of our series we had to reoperate on a 28 year old female patient 3 days after surgery because of persisting abdominal pain. We performed a diagnostic laparoscopy. There were no findings. We attributed the pain to not properly washed instruments, with remainings of Cidex™ (Johnson& Johnson, Cincinatti, Ohio, USA) solution on them. We had no other reoperations or major complications except for one intraabdominal abscess outside our published series.

The average **wound infection rate** for laparoscopic appendectomy is reported to be 2,8% in the meta-analysis by Golub et al. (Golub, 1998) and 2,5% in a big prospective multi-center-study (Lippert et al., 2002). Wound infection rate is reduced by a half after laparoscopic appendectomy in the most recent meta-analysis (Sauerland et al., 2010) based on the study of more than 6000 cases. This is consistent with the findings of a large data base analysis of over 40.000 in the US (Guller, 2004). Wound infection rate in our study was measured separately and was 1,1%.

Intraabdominal abscesses are reported in the older meta-analyses to be equally frequent as in the open procedure (Chung et al., 1999; Garbutt et al., 1999; Temple et al.) or even increased, but without reaching statistical significance (Golub, 1998). In the most recent review **intra-abdominal abscesses** are reported to be nearly threefold after laparoscopic appendectomy(Sauerland et al., 2010), and moderate heterogeneity was detectable. There were no notable differences in the results of trials using staplers versus loop. The problem with studies reporting higher incidence of intraabdominal abscesses with laparoscopic appendectomy is that they lack standardization of the surgical technique, and also that they do not uniformly describe the different grades of disease. A recent prospective randomised study on 220 patients reports less intraabdominal abscesses with the laparoscopic approach (Wei et al., 2010). Also, a very recent review on 2.264 patients (Asarias et al., 2011) did not find a significant difference in intraabdominal abscesses between the open and the laparoscopic approach. On the other hand a multivariate analysis from the American College of Surgeons on almost 40.000 appendectomies (77% laparoscopic) found that laparoscopy was associated with an increased risk for intraabdominal abscesses in the high risk patients (12,3% vs. 8,9%) but not for the low risk patients (Fleming et al., 2010). We had no intraabdominal abscesses after laparoscopic appendectomy in our study (Konstantinidis et al., 2008). Our only experience with an intraabdominal abscess after laparoscopic appendectomy was in a 59 year old man, in whom we performed one of the first operations for a ruptured appendix in January 1993, and who was not included in our study, as mentioned before. This patient was readmitted, and reoperated laparoscopically. A large retrocecal abscess was drained without further problems in his postoperative course. We believe that surgical expertise, precise manoeuvers during the operation, technique standardisation, and irrigation with normal saline solution (5 ltrs., under presure) are very important in order to avoid intraabdominal abscesses.

Most meta-analyses agree that **postoperative pain** is reduced after laparoscopy compared to the open procedure (Chung, 1999, Chung et al., 1999; Garbutt et al., 1999; Golub et al., 1999, Sauerland et al., 2010). Our patients required a median number of 4 minor drugs and 2 narcotics until their discharge.

There is consistent evidence that laparoscopy leads to a shorter **hospital stay** than the open appendectomy (Garbutt, 1999, Liu et al., 2011, Sauerland et al., 2010), although there are great fluctuations. We assume that this has to do with different discharge policies. Also, return to normal activity, which was 7 days in our trial, seems to fluctuate very much between most investigators, but is reported to be quicker with the laparoscopic approach (Chung et al., 1999; Garbutt et al., 1999; Golub et al., 1998; Liu et al, 2010; Sauerland et al., 2010; Temple et al., 1999) as is return to full activity and sport (Sauerland et al., 2010). In our experience **recovery** as expressed through time until flatus (24 hours) and intake of solid food (48 hours), as well as time until discharge (30 hours) was very satisfactory.

There is no other pathology in surgery where as high percentages for **negative laparotomies** are tolerated as in suspected acute appendicitis. In the literature negative laparotomies in suspected acute appendicitis typically range between 20-30%, while the typical range for negative laparoscopies is 10-15% (Tate, 1996). Especially in the subgroup of fertile females authors report a negative laparotomy rate between 22-40% and a negative laparoscopy rate between 4-17% and (Sauerland et al., 2004). We assume that in experienced hands a negative laparoscopy is truly negative - at least concerning the macroscopic findings- whereas a negative laparotomy with a Mc Burney incision fails to diagnose the pathology in about half of the cases as can be confirmed by the numbers. The long-term clinical course of these patients with the missed pathology cannot always be concluded from the published literature (Vettoretto&Agresta, 2010).

The **superior visualization of the abdominal cavity** is undoubtedly the great advantage of laparoscopy and leads to a much higher diagnostic yield in comparison to the open procedure. In the most recent meta-analysis laparoscopy reduced the rate of negative appendectomies and the rate of un-established diagnoses, especially in fertile women (Sauerland et al., 2010). **Gynecological problems** are found more frequently in laparoscopy for suspected acute appendicitis than in laparotomy (Larsson, 2001). Hence, there is consensus about laparoscopy being an invaluable tool in the management algorithm of women in childbearing age (Agresta, 2003; Borgstein, 1997; Cox, 1995; Larsson, 2001; Sauerland et al., 2010; van Dalen, 2003). A recent Cochrane Review about the role of laparoscopy for the management of lower abdominal pain in women of childbearing age found in the laparoscopic group higher rates of specific diagnoses been made, lower rates of negative appendectomies and shorter hospital stays. Also, there was no evidence of an increase of adverse events with either of the two approaches (Gaitan et al., 2010). In our series laparoscopy alone could establish diagnosis in 89% of all patients, in 85,4% of fertile women and in 93,1% in all other patients except fertile women. We had to face other surgical problems than appendicitis in 11,5% of all patients. In the subgroup of fertile women we were confronted with other diagnoses in 20,4% of all patients. Most of these conditions were gynaecologic problems (19,2%), despite the fact that some of these patients were examined by the gynaecologist -which is consistent with the literature (Borgstein, 1997)- and/or had imaging studies performed. The laparoscopic approach gave us the opportunity to define these problems, as well as to deal with most of them without having to convert to an open procedure. So, even in therapeutic terms, laparoscopy offers the possibility to manage unexpected problems, while a classical Mc Burney incision has many constraints in this direction.

It has been questioned if one should remove **a normal looking appendix**, if there are no other findings at laparoscopy, especially in fertile women. Investigators who chose not to remove normal looking appendices report good results and almost no or few readmissions both in the fertile women group and in all patients (Borgstein et al., 1997; Moberg et al., 1998; Teh et al, 2000; van Dalen et al., 2003). That is why many investigators suggest not to remove a normal looking appendix (van Brock, 2001; Morino, 2006). Their argument is that removing all appendices diminishes the diagnostic value of laparoscopy, as well as beeing accompanied by morbidity, mortality, and extra hospital costs (Benjamin et al, 2002; Binjen et al, 2003; Sauerland et al., 2003). However, the assertion that mortality of incidental appendectomy exceeds that of appendectomy for appendicitis (Benjamin, 2002) did not find general acceptance (Howie, 2003). Howie reports that the estimated avoidable mortality from missed appendicitis or negative appendectomy in Scotland was virtually identical at 1,13 and 1,07 patients per 10.000 admissions. Another argument against incidental appendectomy is that it may have several adverse effects on fertility. Concerning this, a large Swedish retrospective study on 10.000 women could not confirm negative effects of appendectomy on fertility (Anderson et al, 1999). On the other hand incidental appendectomy may increase morbidity, and diminishes the diagnostic value of laparoscopy. We chose to remove all appendices if there were no other findings. This has to do with the nature of our hospital. We are a private center, and cannot always afford to reexamine patients, or, even worse, re-operate on them. It also has to do with the facilities, the laparoscopic experience of our team and the absence of major complications or mortality up to this point. In our study eighteen patients (2%) proved to have histological findings of appendicitis without having macroscopic ones. We had a negative appendectomy rate of 11,6% in fertile women and 6,4% in the rest of the patients after histological examination. In 0,8% of all excised appendices the histological examination revealed a carcinoid tumor.

Removing a macroscopically innocent appendix surely diminishes the diagnostic advantages of laparoscopy. On the other hand, the question whether or not to remove a macroscopically normal appendix cannot be easily answered. Published data show a discrepancy between the good clinical course of most patients in these series, were a macroscopically innocent appendix was not removed and the histological findings in the series were a normal appearing appendix was removed. It has been shown that a macroscopically normal appendix is not always normal (Chiarugi et al., 2001), though the literature is quite inhomogenous concerning the histological findings. It also has been shown that a histologically normal appendix is not always normal (Wang et al, 1996) . Some of these appendices in patients with acute pain in the right iliac fossa have an abnormal content of neuropeptides. This could explain the pain relief after removal of a histologically normal appendix (Di Sebastiano, 1999; Wang et al, 1996).

It seems that some patients suffer crises of **endoappendicitis**, that subsides with conservative treatment. Endoappendicitis varies from 11to 26% and the reoperation rate for the patients whose appendix was left in situ is reported to be 6%(Navez and Therasse, 2003). So it might be that the great majority of these patients will not have any problems in the future but for the individual patient the surgeon's decision to leave the appendix behind could mean a readmission, a peritonitis, a second operation, or the persistence of recurrent symptoms. So we think that the decision to remove the appendix has to be individualized and discussed with the patient prior to the operation. The experience of the laparoscopic team is very important in this context. We generally agree with the algorithm proposed by (Navez & Therasse, 2003) in the treatment of suspected acute appendicitis. The authors propose to remove a macroscopically normal appendix if one suspects an appendicitis clinically and there are no other findings. In cases of acute abdominal pain of uncertain origin and negative laparoscopy the authors propose to perform only a diagnostic laparoscopy and to avoid the terms of appendicitis or appendectomy. We also agree with the investigators that the appendix should be removed if chronic recurrent symptoms exist, and there are no other findings. We think there is enough evidence about this in the literature (Chandler et al., 2002; Mussak et al., 2002), especially in young females (Chicolm Mefire et al., 2011).

The debate on whether **complicated appendicitis** is a contraindication for the laparoscopic approach is still ongoing. Sauerland et al. reported in an earlier review (Sauerland et al., 2004) that laparoscopic approach for complicated appendicitis can probably lead to increased complications, though there is not yet enough evidence to support this. On the other hand many authors do not regard complicated appendicitis to be a contraindication for laparoscopic appendectomy. On the contrary, laparoscopic appendectomy in complicated appendicitis is reported to be safe (Ball et al., 2004; Kapischke et al., 2005; Pedersen et al., 2001; Stolzing et al., 2000; Wullstein et al., 2001) and reduce complication rate (Kapischke et al., 2005; Wullstein et al, 2001). Septic wound complications are reported to be less (Piskun et al., 2001; Stolzing et al., 2000). Intraabdominal abscesses are reported to be equally frequent (Asarias et al., 2011; Khalili et al., 1999; Wullstein et al., 2001) in the open and the laparoscopic approach. Also laparoscopic appendectomy in complicated appendicitis is supposed to lead to a shorter length of stay (Ball et al., 2004; Johnson et al., 1998; Kapischke et al., 2005; Towfigh et al., 2006) and reduced hospital costs (Johnson et al., 1998). The problem with some comparative studies is the existence of selection bias in patients undergoing laparoscopic or open appendectomy and also the fact that statistical analysis is not always done on an intention-to-treat-basis. Nevertheless Wullstein et al. in their study on 299 patients with complicated appendicitis report that laparoscopic appendectomy when compared with open appendectomy leads to a significant reduction of early postoperative complications by itself and in an intention-to-treat view (Wullstein et al., 2001). A recent systematic review with meta-analysis of 12 retrospective case-control studies found less surgical site infections in laparoscopic appendectomy for complicated appendicitis with no significant additional risk for intraabdominal abscesses (Makrides et al., 2010). More prospective, randomized trials focusing on this question are needed in the future. We did not study patients with complicated appendicitis separately in our series. Nevertheless we had to face a ruptured or gangrenous appendix in 14,1% and, in spite of that, had an overall wound infection rate of 1,1% and no intraabdominal abscesses. In our experience complicated appendicitis is not a contraindication for the laparoscopic approach.

There is evidence supporting that **cosmesis** is superior with the laparoscopic approach (Pedersen et al., 2001), and is difficult to improve (Ruiz de Angulo et al., 2011). We think that this must be especially true in obese patients and complicated appendicitis, where normally bigger incisions are needed. Also, in case of other findings that need an extension of a Mc Burney incision or a new incision, laparoscopy is surely the best choice from the cosmetic point of view.

Quality of life is also reported to be better with the laparoscopic approach, both in the early and late period (Kaplan et al, 2009).
Cost- effectiveness is difficult to measure. From the institutional perspective laparoscopic appendectomy is reported to be less cost- effective than the open procedure, even if in the future the costs of the operation and the equipment (single- use vs. reusable; Endo-GIA vs. Roeder loops) may decrease whereas from the societal perspective the laparoscopic approach seems to be more cost- effective (Heikkinen et al., 1998; Macarulla et al., 1997; Sauerland, 2010) if lost productivity is taken into consideration (Moore et al., 2004). In middle- aged patients overall costs are reported to be lower with the laparoscopic procedure (Lagares- Garcia et al., 2003). In our patients we try to reduce costs by applying reusable instruments. We also prefer to use loops for the appendicular base instead of staplers and can report excellent results and no complications.
It has been suggested that there may be fewer **adhesions** after laparoscopic appendectomy compared to the open procedure (De Wilde, 1991; Gutt, 2004). We had no patients with adhesion-related complications such as intestinal obstruction in our study. The incidence of late readmitions (>30 days) after appendectomy is of particular interest. In the literature there is increasing evidence that open appendectomy is related to late readmissions and, in some cases, reoperations for SBO but there is an inhomogeneity in the results of different studies (Anderson, 2001;Riber, 1997; Zbar, 1993). During a mean follow-up of 10 years the authors of a retrospective study on 3,230 patients report 2,94% late readmissions after open appendectomy. Almost half (45%) of readmissions were caused by nonspecific abdominal pain with no signs of small bowel obstruction. SBO was seen in 1,24% of patients and was surgically treated in 0,68%. Incisional hernias were seen in 0,4% of all appendectomies., as did patients with complicated appendicitis or negative appendectomy (Tingstend et al., 2004).
Our follow-up lasted 4 weeks. From the 63 patients operated on for chronic symptoms 5(8%) continued to have abdominal pain one month after appendectomy. There were no readmitions or reoperations for adhesion related complications or incisional hernias. We can also report that no patient of this series was readmitted in our department with a late complication such as small bowel ileus or an incisional hernia. More prospective, randomized trials comparing the incidence of late complications with the laparoscopic and open approach for suspected appendicitis in an intention-to-treat basis are needed. We also think that late complications should be included in future cost-analyses.
Laparoscopic appendectomy is reported to be a safe and suitable procedure for **surgical training** (Botha et al., 1995; Duff&Dixon, 2000; Scott-Conner et al., 1992). In our opinion it is in many cases an ideal operation for a surgical trainee starting his/her training in laparoscopy.

4. Special patient categories

4.1 Fertile females

Especially in the subgroup of fertile females authors report a negative laparotomy rate between 22-40% and a negative laparoscopy rate between 4-17% and (Sauerland et al., 2004). Females predominated among those readmitted (76%). Fertile females benefit from the laparoscopic approach at a level Ia evidence and there was no inconsistency between studies (Sauerland, 2010; Vettoretto & Agresta, 2010; Gaitan, 2011).

4.2 Obese patients

In the literature it is suggested that overweight patients seem to profit from laparoscopic appendectomy in terms of postoperative pain, postoperative recovery (Enochson et al., 2001), and septic wound complication rate (Stolzing et al., 2000, Corneille et al., 2007). In a more recent comparative study no significant differences in terms of complications were found between the two groups (Clarke et al., 2011). We did not perform a separate analysis on overweight patients.

4.3 Employed patients

Employed patients profit from laparoscopic appendectomy as it is superior to open appendectomy in terms of return to normal activities and full activity (Sauerland et al, 2010).

4.4 Elderly patients

Elderly patients have more overall complications after conventional appendectomy (especially regarding pulmonary function impairment and return to normal activities), and seem to benefit from laparoscopic appendectomy (Agresta et al., 2011; Guller et al, 2004; Kim et al., 2011; Yeh et al. 2011).

Patient Population	Level of Evidence
Women of childbearing age	LOE Ia
Employed Patients	LOE Ia
Elderly Patients	LOE IIb
Obese Patients	LOE III
Men	LOE III

Table 1. Adult patient subpopulations that profit from laparoscopic appendectomy

4.5 Pregnant patients

Acute appendicitis is the most common cause of nonobstetric acute abdomen during pregnancy. Some investigators report that the incidence is identical to that of the nonpregnant population, while others suggest that it is less, with the third trimester being particularly protective (Anderson & Lambe, 2001). Non the less, a perforation of the appendix is reported to occur twice as often in the third trimester (69%) compared with the first two (Weingold, 1983). The role of laparoscopic appendectomy during pregnancy remains controversial. Laparoscopy for suspected appendicitis is considered to have less complications and a higher diagnostic value compared to the open procedure. The ongoing debate is whether the laparoscopic procedure leads to a higher percentage of fetal loss as is reported in a systematic review from the UK (Walsh et al., 2008) or not, as is stated in a review from the United States (Jackson et al., 2008). More recent studies consider the laparoscopic approach to be safe and effective with a low rate of complications for the mother and the fetus (Corneille et al., 2010; Jeing et al., 2011; Kirshtein et al., 2009; Lemieux et al, 2009; Machado et al., 2009; Moreno-Sanz, 2007; Sadot et al.). It has to be stated that long-term consequences of the pneumoperitoneum for the fetus have not yet been studied. Also, one should stress the importance of a very good diagnostic work-up in order to avoid unnecessary procedures without missing pathologic conditions. Walsh et al. report that the negative appendectomy rate in their series was 27%, which is higher than in the nonpregnant population. Regarding the diagnostic tools it has been reported that the sensitivity of ultrasound is inversely correlated to the gestational age, while CT scan retains a high sensitivity and specificity throughout pregnancy. It seems reasonable to perform an ultrasound first, in order to exclude an obstetric pathology, and to proceed with a CT if necessary (Butala, 2010).

4.6 Pediatric patients

Pediatric patients seem to benefit from the laparoscopic approach for suspected appendicitis in the same ways adults do, and intraabdominal abscesses are not more frequent than with the open approach. However, more RCTs are needed in order to come to final conclusions. Especially in extremely obese children laparoscopy is considered to be the procedure of choice both in complicated, and not complicated cases. The operative time is reported to be shorter, there are less overall complications, and reduced analgesia requirements (Kutasy et al., 2011).

5. Novel techniques and future research implications

5.1 Novel techniques

5.1.1 Single port appendectomy

Single-port-laparoscopy for acute appendicitis is reported to be safe and effective in children (Tam et al., 2010) and adults, and may have advantages in terms of cosmetic results and patient satisfaction (Barbaros et al.; 2010; Lee YS, 2009; Raakow et al.;Tsai & Selzer, 2010). We tried this approach on two patients but could not really see the benefits. On the contrary, we believe that the single port technique is much more appropriate and ergonomic in robotic surgery. More comparative studies between the conventional technique and the single port approach are needed in order to determine its role in laparoscopic appendectomy, especially regarding long term morbidity (i.e. hernias) at the entrance site.

5.1.2 Needlescopic appendectomy

Needlescopic appendectomy can be safe and effective according to a recent review and is supposed to reduce pain compared to conventional laparoscopy (Sajid et al., 2009; Sauerland et al., 2010). Nevertheless it is associated with a longer operating time and a higher conversion rate. Multicenter, randomized controlled trials are recommended before it can be used routinely.

5.1.3 Robotic appendectomy

Incidental appendectomy is considered to eventually be necessary in women with ovarian endometrioma and chronic pelvic pain, as the majority of the appendices are found to have histopathologically confirmed pathology although being macroscopically normal (Wie et al., 2008). Incidental robotic appendectomy is reported to be safe and effective in women undergoing gynaecologic surgery, in women with chronic pelvic pain, and women with ovarian malignancy (Akl et al., 2008). In the latter group three out of seven patients were found to have appendicular metastasis. Our experience with the DaVinci (TM, Intuitive Surgical Inc.) Robotic System started in 2006, and is today the everyday routine of the department in advanced procedures. We performed incidental robotic appendectomy in three patients who underwent gynecologic surgery for endometriosis for chronic pelvic pain with good results. We believe that the robotic procedure has its place in complicated cases of appendicitis with dense peritoneal adhesions.

5.2 Implications for future research

In our opinion future research should first of all determine the role of diagnostic investigations (such as laboratory parameters, US, CT and MRI) which could lower the percentage of negative laparoscopies, especially in pregnant women and high risk patients. Also, a cost-benetit analysis of the routine appliance of US and CT in order to avoid negative laparoscopies would be reasonable. Additionally, the importance of leaving back a macroscopically innocent appendix in several patient categories (women of childbearing age, patients with chronic pain, high-risk- patients, children) if no other pathology is found should be further investigated. Another issue are intraabdominal abscesses. The role of the patients characteristics, the surgeon's expertise, the stump closure, the intraabdominal lavage and the standardization of technique in abscess formation should be further explored. The value of new techniques like the single port, the needlescopic and the robotic procedure in special cases should be investigated, as should the place of laparoscopy in obese patients and pregnant patients. Finally the late results of laparoscopic appendectomy should be explored (adhesions, SBO).

6. Conclusion

In conclusion, laparoscopy seems to be as safe as open appendectomy for acute appendicitis. Laparoscopy has many advantages, such as higher diagnostic yield, fewer postoperative wound infections, less postoperative pain, shorter hospital stay, earlier return to normal and full activity, better cosmesis, and probably decreased late complications such as adhesion formation and incisional hernias. Also one cannot overemphasize the superior visualization of the abdominal cavity and the possibility of not only diagnosing other pathologies but also dealing with them without having to use a bigger incision. Fertile women can profit the most from these advantages. But also elderly, overweight and employed patients seem to profit from laparoscopy. If the safety of leaving a macroscopically innocent appendix in situ is clarified by future studies the value of laparoscopy as a diagnostic tool will be enhanced. One expects that the further expansion of laparoscopy will lead to much more experienced surgeons, and that the progress in technology will facilitate this approach even more in the future. The reported higher incidence of intraabdominal abscesses with laparoscopy in some series could be experience- or technique-related and is likely to decrease with the evolution of laparoscopic skills among surgeons that leads to more precise operative maneuvers, and the standardisation of surgical technique. The higher operative costs in most institutions can perhaps be outweighed by a shorter hospital stay, and quicker return to normal activities with the laparoscopic approach, as well as by the possible decrease in late complications. Operative costs themselves can be reduced by the application of reusable instruments, application of loops instead of staplers, and further reduction of operating times. Finally it is important to reduce negative laparoscopies. The exact role of imaging modalities, inflammatory parameters and scoring systems in this purpose has yet to be defined.

7. Acknowledgements

The authors thank Mrs. Sofia Monastirioti for her assistance in editing the text of this chapter. We also thank Dr. Petros Hiridis for his assistance with the illustrations.

8. References

Addis, DG.; Shaffer, N.; Fowler, BS. & Tauxe, RV. (1990). The epidemiology of appendicitis and appendectomy in the United States. *Am J Epidemiol* , Vol. 8, No. 4, pp.910-925, ISSN 0963-7486

Agresta, F.; De Simone, P.; Michelet, I. & Bedin, N.(2003). Laparoscopic Appendectomy: why it should be done. *JSLS,* Vol. 16, No.1, pp. 347-352, ISSN 1679-1796

Akl, MN.; Magrina, JF.; Kho, RM.; Magtibay, PM. (2008). Robotic appendectomy in gynaecological surgery: technique and pathological findings. *Int J Med Robot,* Vol. 4, Issue 3, pp.210-213, ISSN 0029-7844

Andersson, E.; Lambe, M. & Bergstrom, R. (1999). Fertility patterns after appendicectomy: historical cohort study. *BMJ,* Vol. 318, No. 7189 pp. 963-967, ISSN 1464-3685

Andersson, RE.(2001). Small bowel obstruction after appendicectomy. *Br J Surg,* Vol.26, No. 2, pp.1387-1391, ISSN 0003-4932

Andersson, RE. & Lambe, M. (2001). Incidence of appendicitis during pregnancy. *Int J Epidemiol,* Vol., No., pp. 1281-1285, ISSN

Asarias, JR.; Schlussel, AT.; Cafasso, DE.; Carlson, TL.; Kasprenski, MC.; Washington, EN.; Lustik, MB.; Yamamura, MS.; Matayoshi, EZ. & Zagorski, SM.(2011). Incidence of postoperative intraabdominal abscesses in open versus laparoscopic appendectomies. *Surg Endosc,* Vol.136, No.4, ISSN 003-4932

Ball, CG.; Kortbeek, JB.; Kirckpatrick, AW. & Mitchell, P. (2004). Laparoscopic appendectomy for complicated appendicitis: an evaluation of postoperative factors. *Surg Endosc,* Vol.8, No.1, pp.969-973, ISSN 0003-1348

Balthazar, EJ.; Megibow, ACCJ.; Sieger, SE.; & Birnbaum, BA. (1991). Appendicits: prospective evaluation with high resolution CT. *Radiology,* Vol. 28(2), pp.21-24, ISSN 0033-8419

Balthazar, EJ.; Rofsky, NM. & Zucker, R. (1998). Appendicitis: the impact of computer tomography imaging on negative appendectomy and perforation rates. *Am J Gastroenterol,* Vol.93, No.5, pp. 768-771, ISSN 1528-8404

Barbaros, U.; Sümer, A.; Tunca, F.; Gözkün, O.; Demirel, T.; Bilge, O.; Randazzo, V.; Dinççağ, A.; Seven, R.; Mercan, S.; Budak, D. (2010). Our early experiences with single-incision laparoscopic surgery: the first 32 patients. *Surg Laparosc Endosc Percutan Tech,* Vol. 20, Issue 5, pp.306-311, ISSN 1072-7517

Benjamin, IS. & Patel, AG. (2002). Managing acute appendicitis: Laparoscopic surgery is particularly useful for women. *BMJ,* Vol.22, No.2, pp.505-506, ISSN 0749-5161

Bennett, J; Boddy, A; Rhodes, M. (2007). Choice of approach in appendicectomy: a meta-analysis of open versus laparoscopic appendicectomy. *Surg Laparosc Endosc Percutan Tech.* Vol. 14. No. 4., pp: 245-255, ISSN 1130-0108

Bijnen, CL.; Van den Broek, WT.; Bijnen, AB.; De Ruiter, P. & Gouma DJ. (2003). Implications of removing a normal appendix. *Dig Surg,* Vol.20, No.2, pp.215-219; discussion pp. 220-221, ISSN 0303-5212

Birnbaum, BA. & Wilson, SR. (2000). Appendicitis at the Millenium. *Radiology*, Vol.215, No. 2 pp.337-348, ISSN 1528-8315

Borgstein, PJ.; Gordijn, RV.; Eijsbouts, QAJ. & Cuesta, MA. (1997). Acute appendicitis – a clear-cut case in men, a guessing game in young women. *Surg Endosc,*Vol. 11 No.9, pp. 923-927, ISSN 1130-0108

Botha, AJ.; Elton, C.; Moore, EE. & Sauven P. (1995). Laparoscopic appendicectomy: a trainees perspective. *Ann R Coll Surg Eng*, Vol.3, No. 2, pp. 259-262, ISSN 1528-8242

Butala, P; Greenstein, AJ; Sur, MD; Mehta, N; Sadot, E; Divino,CM. (2010). Surgical management of acute right lower-quadrant pain in pregnancy: a prospective cohort study. *Journal of the American College of Surgeons.* Vol. 211, No.4, pp. 490-4, ISSN 1072-7515

Cardall, T.; Glasser, J. & Guss, DA. (2004). Clinical value of the total white blood cell count and temperature in the evaluation of patients with suspected appendicitis. *Acad Emerg Med,*Vol.14, No.2, pp.1021-7, ISSN 1007-9327

Chandler, B.; Beegle, M.; Elfrink, RJ. & Smith, WJ. (2002). To leave or not to leave? A retrospective review of appendectomy during diagnostic laparoscopy for chronic pelvic pain. *Mo Med*, Vol.13, No.5, pp.502-504, ISSN 1333-994

Chiarugi, M.; Buccianti, P.; Decanini, L.; Balestri, R.; Lerenzetti, L.; Franceschi, M. & Cavina, E. (2001). "What you see is not what you get". A plea to remove a "normal" appendix during diagnostic laparoscopy. *Acta Chir Belg,*Vol.19, No.5, pp.243-245, ISSN

Chichom Mefire, A; Tchounzou, R; Kuwong, PM; Atangana, JP; Lysinge, AC. & Malonga, EE. (2011). Clinical, Ultrasonographic and Pathologic Characteristics of Patients with Chronic Right-lower-quadrant Abdominal Pain that May Benefit from Appendectomy. *World Journal of Surgery.*Vol.35, No.4, pp.723-30, ISSN 1069-6563583

Chung, R.; Rowland, D.; Li ,P. & Diaz, J A. (1999). Meta-analysis of Randomized Controlled Trials of *Laparoscopic* Versus Conventional Appendectomy. *Am J Surg*, Vol.177, No.3, pp. 250-256, ISSN 1007-9327

Clarke, T.; Katkhouda, N.; Mason, RJ.; Cheng, BC.; Olasky, J.; Sohn, HJ.; Moazzez, A.; Algra, J.; Chaghouri, E. & Berne, TV. (2011). Laparoscopic versus open appendectomy for the obese patient: a subset analysis from a prospective, randomized, double-blind study. *Surg Endosc,* Vol.25, No.4, pp.1276-1280, ISSN 1432-2218

Corneille, MG.; Steigelman, MB.; Myers, JG.; Jundt, J.; Dent, DL.; Lopez, PP.; Cohn, SM. & Stewart, RM. (2007). Laparoscopic appendectomy is superior to open appendectomy in obese patients. *Am J Surg, Vol.194,* Issue 6, pp.877-880, ISSN 0803-5253

Corneille, MG.; Gallup, TM.; Bening, T.; Wolf, SE.; Brougher, C.; Myers, JG.; Dent, DL.; Medrano, G.; Xenakis, E & Stewart, RM.(2010). The use of laparoscopic surgery in pregnancy: evaluation of safety and efficacy. *Am J Surg,* Vol.20, Issue 6, pp.363-367, ISSN 1879-1883

Cox, MR.; Mc Call, JR.; Padbury, RT.; Wilson, TG. & Wattchow, DA. (1995). Tooul. Laparoscopic surgery in women with a clinical diagnosis of an appendicitis. *Med J Aust,* Vol.8, No.3, pp. 130-2, ISSN 1007-9327

De Wilde RL. (1991). Goodbye to late bowel obstruction after appendicectomy. *The Lancet, Vol.73, No.11,* ISSN 1421–9983

Di Sebastiano, P.; Fink, T. & Buchler MW. (1999). Neuroimune appendicitis. *The Lancet,* Vol. *354,* No.9172, pp. 461-66, ISSN 1021-7401

Duff, SE. & Dixon, AR. (2000). Laparoscopic appendicectomy: safe and useful in training Ann R Coll Surg Engl, Vol.172, No.1, pp. 388-391, ISSN 1469-0756

Enochson, L.; Hellberg, A.; Rudberg, C.; Fenyö; Gudbjartson, T.; Kullman, E.; Ringquist, I.; Sörensen, S. & Wenner, J. (2001). Laparoscopic vs open appendectomy in overweight patients. *Surg Endoscopy,* Vol.3, No.7, pp. 387-392, ISSN 0930-2794

Fingerhut, A.; Millat, B. & Borrie, F. (1999). Laparoscopic versus Open Appendectomy: Time to Decide. *Word J. Surg,* Vol.23, No.8, pp. 835-845, ISSN 0003-4932

Fleming, FJ.; Kim, MJ.; Messing, S.; Gunzler, D.; Salloum, R. & Monson, JR. (2010). Balancing the risk of postoperative surgical infections: a multivariate analysis of factors associated with laparoscopic appendectomy from the NSQIP database. *Ann Surg,* Vol.252, Issue 6, pp. 895-900, ISSN 0003-4932

Flum, DR.; McClure, TD.; Morris, A. & Koepsell, T. (2005). Misdiagnosis of appendicitis and the use of diagnostic imaging. *J Am Coll Surg,* Vol.201, No.6, pp. 933-9, ISSN 1468-3288

Gaitan, HG.; Ludovic Reveiz, &Cindy Farquhar (2010). Laparoscopy for the management of acute lower abdominal pain in women of childbearing age. *Cochrane Database of systematic Reviews,* Vol.1, Issue 1, ISSN 1464-780x

Gaitán HG, Reveiz L, Farquhar C.(2011). Laparoscopy for the management of acute lower abdominal pain in women of childbearing age. *Cochrane Database Syst Rev,* Vol.22, No.2, ISSN 1464-780X

Garbutt, JM.; Soper, NJ.; Shannon, WD.; Botero, A. & Littenberg, B. (1999). Meta-analysis of randomized controlled trials comparing laparoscopic and open appendectomy. *Surg Laparosc Endosc,* Vol.5, No.2, pp. 17-26, ISSN 1007-9327

Golub, R.; Siddiqui, F. & Pohl D. (1998). Laparoscopic versus open appendectomy: a metaanalysis. *J Am Coll Surg* Vol.42, No.1, pp. 545-53, ISSN 1007-9327

Gronroos, JM. & Gronross, P. (1999). Leucocyte count and C-reactive protein in the diagnosis of acute appendicitis. *Br J Surg* Vol.16, No.2, pp. 501-4, ISSN 0803-5253

Gupta, R.; Sample, C.; Bamehriz, F. & Birch, DW. (2006). Infectious complications following laparoscopic appendectomy. *Can J Surg,* Vol.49, No.6, pp. 397-400, ISSN 1435-2451

Gutt, CN.; Oniu, T.; Schemer, P.; Mehrabi, A. & Buechler, MW. (2004). Fewer adhesions induced by laparoscopic surgery? *Surg Endosc.,* Vol18., No.6, pp. 898-906, ISSN 0930-2794

Heikkinen TJ, Haukipuro H, Hulkko A. (1998). Cost-effective appendectomy. Open or laparoscopic? A prospective randomized study. *Surg Endosc,* Vol.14, No.31 ,pp.1204- 1208

Howie J BMJ (2003). 326,p49, ISSN 0253-4886

Hsieh, CS.; Chen, YL.; Lee, MH.; Chang, HC.; Chen, ST. & Kuo, SJ.(2009). A lower costly laparoscopic appendectomy: our experience of more than 2000 cases. *Int J Surg,* Vol.8, Issue 2, pp. 140-3, ISSN 1007-9327

Hussain, A.; Mahmood, H.; Nicholls, J. & El-Hasani, S. (2008). Prevention of intra-abdominal abscess following laparoscopic appendicectomy for perforated appendicitis: a prospective study. *Int J Surg,* Vol. 180, Issue 6, pp. 374-7, ISSN 1743-9159

Jackson, H.; Granger, S.; Price, R.; Rollins, M.; Earle, D.; Richardson, W. & Fanelli, R. (2008). Diagnosis and laparoscopic treatment of surgical diseases during pregnancy: an evidence-based review. *Surg Endosc*, Vol.22, No.9, pp. 1917-1927, ISSN 1432-2218

Jacob, DA.; Raakow, R. (2010). [Single-port transumbilical endoscopic cholecystectomy: a new standard?]. *Dtsch Med Wochenschr*, Vol.22, No 1, pp1363-1367, ISSN 1528-8242

Jeong, JS.; Ryu, DH.; Yun, HY.; Jeong, EH.; Choi, JW. & Jang LC. (2011). Laparoscopic appendectomy is a safe and beneficial procedure in pregnant women. *Surg Laparosc Endosc Percutan Tech*, Vol.22, Issue 1, pp. 24-27, ISSN 1534-4908

Johnson AB, Peetz ME. (1998). Laparoscopic appendectomy is an acceptable alternative for the treatment of perforated appendicitis. *Surg Endosc*, Vol.8, No.1, pp. 940-943, ISSN 0253–4886

Jones PF. (2001). Suspected acute appendicitis: trends in management over 30 years. *Br J Surg*, Vol.88, Issue 1, pp.1570-1577, ISSN 1528-8242

Kapischke M, Bley K, Tempel J, Schulz T. (2005). Open versus laparoscopic appendectomy for perforated appendicitis- a comparative study. *Zentralbl Chir*, Vol.10, No. 6, pp.137-41, ISSN 1364-5706

Kaplan, M.; Salman, B.; Yilmaz, TU. & Oguz, M. (2009). A quality of life comparison of laparoscopic and open approaches in acute appendicitis: a randomised prospective study. *Acta Chirurgica Belgica*, Vol. 106, No. 3, pp. 356-63, ISSN 0001-5458

Kazemier, G.; Hof, KH.; Saad, S.; Bonjer, HJ. & Sauerland, S.; (2006). Securing the appendiceal stump in laparoscopic appendectomy: evidence for routine stapling? *Surg Endosc*, Vol.20, No.9, pp. 1473-6, ISSN 030

Khalili, TM.; Hiatt, JR.; Savar, A.; Lau, C. & Margulies DR. (1999).Perforeted appendicitis is not a contraindication to laparoscopy. *Am Surg*, Vol.27, No.6, pp. 965- 967, ISSN 0253–4886

Kim, MJ.; Kim, MJ.; Fleming, FJ.; Gunzler, DD.; Messing, S.; Salloum, RM. & Monson, JR. (2011). Laparoscopic appendectomy is safe and efficacious for the elderly: an analysis using the National Surgical Quality Improvement Project database.*Surgical Endoscopy*, Vol.1, No. 3, (*Feb 7*). [Epub ahead of print], ISSN 1432-2323

Kirshtein B, Perry ZH, Avinoach E, Mizrahi S, Lantsberg L. (2009). Safety of laparoscopic appendectomy during pregnancy. *World J Surg*, Vol.21, Issue 1, pp.475-480, ISSN 0364

Kraemer, M.; Ohmann, C.; Leppert, R. & Yang, Q. (2000). Macroscopic assessment of the appendix at diagnostc laparoscopy is reliable. *Surg Endosc*, Vol.19, Issue 5, pp. 625-33, ISSN 0930-2794

Larsson, P-G.; Henriksson, G.; Olsson, M.; Boris, J.; Ströberg, P.; Tronstad, S-E. & Skullman, S. (2001). Laparoscopy reduces unnecessary appendicectomies and improves diagnosis in fertile women. *Surg Endosc*, Vol.15, No.2, pp. 200- 202, ISSN 1469-0756

Konstantinidis, KM.; Anastasakou, KA.; Vorias, KM.; Sambalis, GH.; Georgiou, MK.; Xiarchos, AG. (2008). *Journal of Laparoendoscopic and Advanced Surgical Techniques*, Vol. 18, No.2, pp. 248-258, ISSN 1492-6429

Kutasy, B.; Hunziker, M.; Laxamanadass, G.; Puri, P. (2011). Laparoscopic appendectomy is associated with lower morbidity in extremely obese children. *Pediatr Surg Int*, Vol. 196, Issue 2,pp.533-536, ISSN 0179-0358

Lagares-Garcia, JA.; Bandsidhar, B. & Moore, RA. (2003). Benefits of laparoscopy in middle-aged patients. *Surg Endosc*, Vol.7, No.2, pp. 68-72, ISSN 0798-0469

Lee, YS.; Kim, JH.; Moon, EJ.; Kim, JJ.; Lee, KH.; Oh, SJ.; Park, SM.; Hong, TH. (2009). Comparative study on surgical outcomes and operative costs of transumbilical single-port laparoscopic appendectomy versus conventional laparoscopic appendectomy in adult patients. *Surg Laparosc Endosc Percutan Tech,*Vol. 19, Issue 6, pp.493-496, PMID 2002-7094

Lee, SL.; Walsh, AJ. & Ho, HS. (2001). Computed tomography and ultrasonography do not improve and may delay the diagnosis and treatment of acute appendicitis. *Arch Surg,* Vol.136,No. 5, pp. 556- 562, ISSN 0014-312

Leeuwenburgh, MM.; Lameris, W.; Van Randen, A.; Bossyt, PM.; Boermeester, MA. & Stoker, J. OPTIMAP study group. (2010). Optimizing imaging in suspected appendicitis (OPTIMAP-study): a multicenter diagnostic accuracy study of MRI in patients with suspected acute appendicitis. Study Protocol. *BMC Emerg Med.* Vol.7, Issue 11, (Oct 20; 10:19), ISSN 1527-1323

Lemieux, P.; Rheaume, P.; Levesque, I.; Bujold, E. & Brochu, G.(2009). Laparoscopic appendectomy in pregnant patients: a review of 45 cases. *Surg Endosc,* Vol. 23, Issue 8, pp. 1701-1705, ISSN 1432-2218

Lippert, H.; Koch, A.; Marutsch, F.; Wolff, S. & Gastinger, I. (2002).Offene versus laparoskopische Appendektomie. *Chirurg,* Vol.101, Issue 8, pp.791-98, ISSN 723-7065

Liu, SI.; Siewert, B.; Raptopoulos, V. & Hodin, RA. (2002). Factors associated with conversion to laparotomy in patients undergoing laparoscopic appendectomy. *J Am Coll Surg,* Vol.194, Issue 3, pp. 298-305, ISSN 1527-1315

Liu, Z.; Zhang, P.; Ma, Y.; Chen, H.; Zhou,Y.; Zhang,M.; Chu, Z. & Qin, H. (2010). Laparoscopy or not: a meta- analysis of the surgical effects of lparoscopic versus open appendectomy. *Surg Laparosc Endosc Percutan Tech,* Vol.20, No.6, pp.362-70, ISSN 1471-230X

Macarulla, E.; Vallet, J.; Abad, JM.; Hussein, H.; Fernandez, E. & Nieto, B. (1997). Laparoscopic versus open appendectomy: a prospective randomized trial. *Surg Laparosc Endosc,* Vol.22, No.1, pp.335- 339, ISSN 1025 - 5583

Machado, NO.; Machado, LS. (2007). Laparoscopic cholecystectomy in the third trimester of pregnancy: report of 3 cases. *Surg Laparosc Endosc Percutan Tech,*Vol. 19, No 6, pp.439-441, ISSN 0972-2068

Markides. G.; Subar, D. & Riyad K.(2010). Laparoscopic versus open appendectomy in adults with complicated appendicitis: systematic review and meta-analysis. *World J Surg,* Vol.77, Issue 3, pp. 2026-40, ISSN 0003-1348

Moberg, AC.; Ahlberg, G.; Leijonmarck, CE.; Montgomery, A.; Reiertsen, Rosseland, AR. & Stoerksson, R. (1998). Diagnostic laparoscopy in 1043 patients with suspected acute appendicitis. *Eur J. Surg,* Vol.28, No.5, pp. 833- 840, ISSN 1102-4151

Moore, D.; Grogan, E.; Sperroff, T. & Holzman, M. (2004). Cost perspectives of laparoscopic and open appendectomy. SAGES; Poster of distinction, Vol.18, No.2, ISSN 1366-5278

Moore, CB.; Smith, RS.; Herbertson, R. &Toevs, C. (2011). Does Use of Intraoperative Irrigation with Open or Laparoscopic Appendectomy Reduce Post-Operative Intra-abdominal Abscess? *Am. Surg,* Vol.136, No.4, pp. 78-80, ISSN 1007-9327

Moreno-Sanz, C.; Pascual-Pedreño, A.; Picazo-Yeste, JS.; Seoane-Gonzalez, JB. (2009). Laparoscopic appendectomy during pregnancy: between personal experiences and scientific evidence. *J Am Coll Surg*, Vol. 205, Issue 1, pp.37-42, ISSN 1072-7515

Morino, M.; Pellegrino, L.; Castagna, E.; Farinella, E. & Mao. P.(2006). Acute nonspecific abdominal pain: A randomized, controlled trial comparing early laparoscopy versus clinical observation. *Ann Surg*, Vol.13, No.2, pp.886-888, ISSN 1528-8242

Mussack, T.; Schmidbauer, S.; Nerlich, A.; Schmidt, W. & Hallfeldt, KK. (2002). Chronic appendicitis as an independent clinical entity. *Chirurg*, Vol.33, No.3, pp.710-715, ISSN 0009-4722

Navez, B.; Therasse, A. (2003). Should every patient undergoing laparoscopy for clinical diagnosis of appendicitis have an appendicectomy? *Acta Chir Belg*, Vol.91, Issue 4, pp.87-89 ISSN 1007-9327

Neumeyer, L.; Kennedy, A. (2003). Imaging in appendicitis: a review with special emphasis on the traetment of women. *Obstet Gynecol*, Vol,102, Issue 6,pp. 1404- 1409, ISSN 0001-6002

Ng, WT.; Lee, YK.; Hui, SK.; Sze, YS.; Chan, J.; Zeng, AG.; Wong, CH. & Wong, WH. (2004). An optimal, cost-effective laparoscopic appendectomy technique for our surgical residents. *Surg Laparosc Endosc Percutan Tech*, Vol. 14, No.3, pp. 125-9, ISSN 1681-715X

Pedersen, AG.; Petersen, OB.; Wara, P.; Ronning, H.; Qvist, N. & Laurberg, S. (2001). Randomized clinical trial of laparoscopic vs open appendicectomy. *Br J Surg*, Vol.23, No. 3, pp. 200-205, ISSN 0007-1323

Piskun, G.; Kozik, D.; Rajpal, S.; Shaftan, G. & Fogler, R. (2001). Comparison of laparoscopic, open, and converted appendectomy for perforated appendicitis. *Surg Endosc*, Vol.10, No. 6, pp. 660- 662, ISSN 0972-2068

Pokala, N.; Sadhasivam, S.; Kiran, RP. & Parithivel, V.(2007). Complicated appendicitis--is the laparoscopic approach appropriate? A comparative study with the open approach: outcome in a community hospital setting. *Am Surg*, Vol.73, No.8, pp.741-2, ISSN 0303-5212

Riber, C.; Soe, K.; Jorgensen, T. & Tonnesen, H. (1997). Intestinal obstruction after appendicectomy. *Scand J Gatroenterol*, Vol.26, No.3, pp.1125- 1128, ISSN 0253–4886

Ruiz de Angulo, D.; Martínez de Haro, LF.; Ortiz, MA.; Munitiz, V.; Navas, D.; Abrisqueta, J. & Parrilla, P.(2011). Evaluation of the aesthetic results perceived by patients after 3-port laparoscopic appendectomy. *Cir Esp*, Vol.9, No.1, ISSN 1437-981

Sadot, E.; Telem, DA.; Arora, M.; Butala, P.; Nguyen, SQ. (2010). Divino CM Laparoscopy: a safe approach to appendicitis during pregnancy. *Surg Endosc*, Vol.24, No 2, pp 383-389, ISSN 0930-27

Sajid, MS.; Rimple, J.; Cheek, E. & Baig, MK. (2009). Use of endo-GIA versus endo-loop for securing the appendicular stump in laparoscopic appendicectomy: a systematic review. *Sug Laparosc Endosc Perculan Tech*, Vol.9, No.4, pp. 5-11, ISSN 1778-3852

Sauerland, S.; Lefering, R.; Holthausen, U. & Neugebauer EAM. (1998). Laparoscopic vs conventional appendectomy – a meta-analysis of randomised controlled trials. *Langenbeck's Arch Surg*, Vol.127, Issue 3, pp. 289-295, ISSN 0253–4886

Sauerland, S.; Lefering, R. & Neugebauer EAM. (2002). Laparoscopic versus open surgery for suspected appendicitis. Cochrane Review, The Cochrane Library, Vol.68, Issue 1 Cochrane Database Syst Rev. 2002;(1):CD001546, ISSN 1464-780

Sauerland, S.; Lefering, R. & Neugebauer EAM. (2004). Laparoscopic versus open appendectomy for suspected appendicitis. The Cochrane Database of Systematic Reviews,Vol.333,Issue 4.Art No.: CD001546.DOI:10.1002/14651858.CD001546.pub2, ISSN 1538-3598

Sauerland, S. et al. EAM. (2010). Laparoscopic versus open appendectomy for suspected appendicitis. *The Cochrane Database of Systematic Reviews*, Vol.19, No.6, CD001546, ISSN 1538-3598

Sauerland S, Kazemier G. Appendix stump closure during laparoscopic appendectomy (Protocol). *Cochrane Database of Systematic Reviews* 2007, Issue 2. Art. No.: CD006437. DOI: 10.1002/14651858.CD006437, ISSN 1469-493

Semm K (1983). Endoscopic appendectomy. *Endoscopy*, Vol.21, Issue 1, pp.59-64, ISSN 1528-8242

Scott-Conner, CE.; Hall, TJ.; Anglin, BL. & Muakassa FF. (1992). Laparoscopic appendectomy. Initial experience in a teaching program. *Ann Surg*, Vol.20, No.1, pp.660- 667, ISSN 1681-715

Stoltzing, H. & Thon, K. (2000). Perforated appendicitis: is laparoscopic operation advisable? *Dig Surg*, Vol.17, No.6, pp.610-616, ISSN 1364-5706

Tate, J. J. T. (1996). Laparoscopic appendicectomy. Leading articles. *Br J Surg*, Vol.83, Issue 9, pp. 1169-70 ISSN 2036-3605

Teh, SH.; O'Ceallaigh, Mckeon, JG.; O'Ceallaigh, S.; Mckeon. JG.; O'Donohoe, MK.; Tanner, WA. & Keane, FB. (2000). Should an appendix that looks "normal" be removed at diagnostic laparoscopy for acute right iliac fossa pain? *Eur J Surg*, Vol.166, Issue 5 pp.388- 389, ISSN 1102–4151

Temple, LK.; Litwin, DE. & Mc Leod, RS. (1999). A meta-analysis of laparoscopic versus open appendectomy in patients suspected of having acute appendicitis. *Can J Surg*, Vol.22, No.2, pp.377- 383, ISSN 1528-8242

Terasawa, T.; Blackmore, C.; Bent, S. & Kohlwes, J. (2004). Systematic Review: Computed Tomography and Ultrasonography To Detect Acute Appendicitis in Adults and Adolescents. *Ann Intern Med*, Vol.141, No.7, pp.537-546, ISSN 1748-880

Tingstedt, B.; Johansson, J.; Nehez, L.& Andersson, R. (2004). Late abdominal complaints after appendectomy-readmissions during long-term follo-up. *Dig Surg*, Vol.21, No.1, pp. 23-27, ISSN 1007-9327

Toorenvloiet, BR.; Wiersma, F.; Bakker, RF.; Merkus, JW.; Breslau, PJ. & Hamming, JF. (2010). Routine ultrasound and limited computed tomography for the diagnosis of acute appendicitis. *World Journal of Surgery*. Vol.34, No. 10, pp: 2278-85, ISSN 1432-2323

Towfiigh, S.; Chen, F.; Mason, R.; Kathkouda, N.; Chan, L. & Berne, T. (2006). Laparoscopic apppendectomy significantly reduces length of stay for perforated appendicitis. *Surg Endosc*, Vol. 18, No. 2, pp. 495-499, ISSN 1007-9327

Tsai, AY.; Selzer, DJ. (2010). Single-port laparoscopic surgery. *Adv Surg*, Vol.23, Issue 1, pp.1-27, ISSN 1528-8242

Van Randen, A.; Lameris, W.; Van Es, HW.; Van Heesewijk, HP.; Van Ramhorst, B.; Ten Hove, W.; Bouma, WH.; Van Leeuwen, MS.; Van Keulen, EM.; Bossyt, PM.; Stoker, J. & Boeremeester, MA; on behalf of the OPTIMA study group. (2011). *Eur Radiol. Vol.8, No.25,* Mar 2 [Epub ahead of print]. ISSN 0033-8419

Van Dalen, R.; Bagshaw, PF.; Dobbs, BR.; Robertson, GM.; Lynch, AC. & Frizelle, FA. (2003). The utility of laparoscopy in the diagnosis of acute appendicitis in women of reproductive age. *Surg Endosc*, Vol.2, No.2, pp. 1311- 1313, ISSN 0930-2794

Van den Broeck, WT.; Bijnen, AB.; Van Eerten, PV.; De Ruiter P. & Gouma DJ. (2000). Selective use of dignostic laparoscopy in patients with suspected appendicitis. *Surg Endosc*, Vol.14, No.10, pp. 938- 941, ISSN 0930-2794

Vettoretto, N. & Agresta F. (2011). A brief review of laparoscopic appendectomy: the issues and the evidence. *Tech Coloproctol*, Vol.15, No.1, pp.1-6, ISSN 1428-045X

Walsh, CA.; Tang, T. & Walsh SR. (2008). Laparoscopic versus open appendicectomy in pregnancy: a systematic review. *Int J Surg*, Vol., No., pp. 339-344, ISSN

Wang, Y.; Reen, DJ. & Puri P. (1996). Is a histologically normal appendix following emergency appendicectomy always normal? *The Lancet*, Vol.347, Issue 9008, pp. 1076-79, ISSN 1543-2165

Weston, AR.; Jackson, TJ. & Blamey, S.(2005). Diagnosis of appendicitis in adults by ultrasonography or computed tomography: Asystemic review and meta-analysis. *International Journal of Technology Assessment in Health Care*, Vol.21, No.3, pp. 368-379, ISSN: 1948-5204

Wei, HB.; Huang, JL.; Zheng, ZH.; Wei, B.; Zheng, F.; Qiu, WS.; Guo, WP.; Chen, TF. & Wang, TB.(2010). Laparoscopic versus open appendectomy: a prospective randomized comparison. *Surg Endosc*, Vol.59, No.1, pp. 266-9, ISSN 0930-2794

Wie, HJ.; Lee, JH.; Kyung, MS.; Jung, US.; Choi, JS. (2008). Is incidental appendectomy necessary in women with ovarian endometrioma? *Aust N Z J Obstet Gynaecol*, Vol.48, No 1, pp.107-111, ISSN 0004-8666

Wullstein, C. Barkhausen, S. & Gross, E. (2001). Results of laparoscopic vs. conventional appendectomy in complicated appendicitis. *Dis Col Rectum*, Vol.44, No.11, pp. 1700-1705, ISSN 0100-6991

Yang, HR.; Wang, YC.; Chung, PK.; Chan, WK.; Jeng, LB. & Chen, RJ. (2005). Role of leucocyte count, neutrophil percentage, and C-reactive protein in the diagnosis of acute appendicitis in the elderly. *Am Surg*,Vol.2, No.1, pp. 344-7, ISSN 1681-715

Yeh, CC.; Wu, SC.; Liao, CC.; Su, LT.; Hsieh, CH. & Li, TC. (2011). *Surgical Endoscopy*, Mar 18, [epub ahead of print], Vol.17, No. 13, ISSN 1007-9327

Zbar, RI.; Crede, WB.; McKhann, CF. & Jekel, JF. (1993). The postoperative incidence of small bowel obstruction following standard, open appendectomy and cholecystectomy: a six year retrospective cohort study at Yale- New Haven Hospital. *Conn Med*, 57, Vol.9, No.12, pp. 123- 127, ISSN 1715-5258

9

Appendicitis and Appendicectomy

Sami M. Shimi
Department of Surgery, Ninewells Hospital and Medical School, University of Dundee Scotland, United Kingdom

1. Introduction

The term appendicitis was first used by an epic publication by FITZ (Harvard Medical School) in 1886. FITZ outlined the clinical diagnosis and suggested early removal of the appendix. This new concept was not readily accepted. The first recorded appendicectomy was reported from Australia and was done on a kitchen table in Toowoonba in 1893. Appendicectomy in the UK did not gain early acceptance until 1902, when Sir Frederick Treves operated on King Edward VII twelve days before his coronation.

2. Epidemiology

The epidemiology of appendicitis has caused a lot of intrigue. Although appendicitis was unknown before the 18th Century, there was a striking increase in its prevalence from the end of the 19th Century. There were suggestions that it was a side effect of modern western life. Although evidence for this was lacking, the rapid emergence of appendicitis in developed countries in the 20th Century and its rarity in rural areas and in undeveloped countries was sited as evidence. By the mid 1920s appendicitis became sufficiently common.
Several theories have been advanced to account for the prevalence of the disease. One theory suggested that diet was responsible for the geographical distribution of appendicitis. It was however clear that diet could not fully explain the epidemiology of appendicitis. An alternative hypothesis proposed that improved hygiene in developed countries reduced the exposure of infants to enteric organisms would, modify the immune response to virus infections which might then cause appendicitis. Although this theory was accepted for many years, the hygiene hypothesis does not adequately explain the recent decline in the frequency of appendicitis in the latter half of the 20th Century. It remains uncertain whether there has been a real change in the incidence of appendicitis or whether the presentation and course of the disease has indeed changed.
The current incidence of appendicitis is about 100 per 100,000 person-years in Europe/America. Whereas the appendectomy rate is still decreasing, the incidence of appendicitis is now nearly stable. During the last 30 years the incidence of perforated appendicitis has not changed (approximately 20 per 100,000 person-years). Established risk factors for acute appendicitis are age (peak: 10-19 years), sex, and ethnic group/race. Classical theories (diet, hygiene) present illuminating models to explain the rise and fall of incidence in the last century; however, from a contemporary perspective the evidence is insufficient. The study of the epidemiology of appendicitis is complicated by the influence

of referral, infrastructure, and surgical treatment strategy on the incidence of acute appendicitis. Therefore, there is a strong need for good prospective studies with high-quality data.

3. Pathology

Several factors are claimed to predispose to acute inflammation of the appendix, including faecolith, food residues, lymphoid hyperplasia (in children) and the presence of a carcinoid tumour. Specific viral and bacterial inflammation can also affect the appendix. In addition the appendix can be involved by ulcerative colitis and Crohn's disease. In early acute appendicitis there is acute inflammation of the mucosa which undergoes ulceration. Pus may be present in the lumen. At this stage the patient experiences an ill defined central abdominal pain. Microscopically, the appendix is usually swollen and the overlying vessels are dilated and prominent. As the acute inflammation develops, it spreads through the full thickness of the appendix wall to reach the serosal surface. This causes a localised acute peritonitis, which is perceived as a sharp pain localised to the right iliac fossa. At this stage the appendix microscopically shows dilated serosal vessels and a rough, yellow, fibrinous exudate on the surface. By this stage the inflammation and the infection has spread to involve all layers of the appendix wall. The build up of fluid exudate within the wall increases tissue pressure and this, together with the toxic damage to blood vessels and subsequent thrombosis can lead to superimposed ischemia. In addition the muscle layer is replaced by an acute inflammatory infiltrate with degranulation of neutrophils contributing to toxic damage. Both the ischemia, toxic products and infection contribute to weakness of the wall of the appendix and the distal part of the appendix can become gangrenous and perforate. This liberates bowel contents in to the peritoneal cavity and causes generalised peritonitis which leads to severe deterioration in the clinical condition. If the general condition of the patient is satisfactory, the omentum might cover the site of perforation and local abscess formation follows. Infiltration into blood vessels and lymphatics leads to the consequences of blood spread which is suppurative pylephlebitis (inflammation and thrombosis of the portal vein), liver abscess and septicaemia. The inflammation can also become chronic, or obstruction to the neck of the appendix may lead to mucus retention in its lumen causing a mucocoele of the appendix. This does not often give rise to clinical problems but on rare occasions may rupture and disseminate mucus secreting epithelial cells in to the peritoneal cavity - pseudomyxoma peritonei.

The presence of gangrene or perforation seems to be associated with the presence of faecoliths. These are intraluminal laminated appendiceal calculi. They result from dehydration and compaction of faecal pellets. Approximately 50% of cases of gangrenous or perforated appendicitis are associated with a faecolith in contrast with uncomplicated appendicitis in which a faecolith is rarely present. It is thought that a faecolith increases the likelihood of obstruction of the appendix and thereby allows the accumulation of pus. Overall about 20% of all patients with acute appendicitis have perforation at the time of operation. At the extremes of age (below 5 and above 60 years) the rate of perforation is in the region of 60%.

Perforation rates of 20% to 30% have been reported consistently over the past 70 years despite the technologic advances over this interval. Recent evidence suggesting that perforation precedes surgical evaluation in the majority of cases indicates that reduction of perforation rates will have to be addressed through encouraging earlier evaluation and greater access to care. However, modern surgical therapy has been responsible for reducing the mortality of appendicitis from 26% overall to less than 1% over the same period. The mortality rate of 0.08% reported is testament to the benefits of advancing technology in managing a persistent rate of perforation and its attendant complications. Perforation continues to disproportionately affect those individuals at the extremes of age. This is most likely due to delays in presentation and diagnosis related to an inability to communicate in the younger population. In the older population, a combination of delayed presentation, confounding medical conditions and a decreased index of suspicion may contribute to this observation.

Emergency appendectomy was originally advocated because of the very high mortality of perforated appendicitis and the assumption that acute appendicitis evolved to perforated disease, a pathophysiologic hypothesis that has never been proven. This notion was first proposed by Reginald Fitz, the originator of the term appendicitis, in 1886. Fitz was the first to identify inflammation of the appendix as a cause for right lower quadrant infections, previously known as thyphilitis. In making the argument that the appendix causes this entity, however, Fitz incidentally noted that one-third of patients undergoing autopsy in the pre-appendectomy era had evidence of prior appendiceal inflammation, suggesting that appendicitis often resolved spontaneously without surgery. Later evidence from submariners who developed appendicitis while at sea and received delayed surgical therapy has shown that in most cases the acute disease can resolve with non-operative antibiotic and supportive therapy.

Perforated and non-perforated appendicitis have followed radically different epidemiologic trends over the past 2 decades. While perforated appendicitis slowly but steadily increased in incidence, non-perforated appendicitis stabilised or declined. If perforated appendicitis was simply the result of appendicitis that was not surgically treated early enough, the trends should have been more nearly parallel throughout all the time periods studied. Time series analysis showed that on a year-to-year basis, there was a significant positive correlation between perforated and non-perforated appendicitis for men but not for women. These unassociated epidemiologic trends suggest that the pathophysiology of these diseases is different. If true, it might follow that many patients presenting with non-perforated appendicitis might experience spontaneous resolution without perforation. There is historical, clinical, and immunologic evidence to support this hypothesis.

An alternative hypothesis suggests that several factors (ie, prehospital time, availability of operating room for emergency surgery, time of presentation) have been shown to be significantly associated with perforated appendicitis. Compared with uncomplicated appendicitis, perforated appendicitis is associated with a two- to tenfold increase in mortality

4. Diagnosis

The diagnosis of appendicitis is predominantly a clinical one. The history and examination are pivotal to determining the correct diagnosis. The pain can be a generalised colicky abdominal pain that became more localised to the right iliac fossa over the course of three days. Owing to the embryological origin of the appendix as a midline structure, the majority of patients with acute appendicitis first notice a pain which starts in the region of the umbilicus. This is usually a dull ache or it may be colicky pain when the appendix lumen is obstructed. The pain may change from an intermittent pain to a constant localised sharp pain. After a period of time the pain shifts to the right lower quadrant of the abdomen owing to the inflamed appendix irritating the parietal peritoneum. Approximately 30% of patients do not experience this shift of pain and their symptoms commence in the right iliac fossa. Nausea and vomiting are common and anorexia is inevitable. About 20% of patients will also have diarrhoea especially when the appendix lies in the pelvis.

There can be other features in the history suggestive of appendicitis. This includes episodes of vomiting, fever and anorexia. Points to exclude in the history are changes to bowel habits and urinary symptoms. In some cases the inflamed appendix can irritate the bladder due to the close proximity. This however can be supported by a negative urinalysis. The possibility of mesenteric adenitis should be considered in children. This is triggered by viral pathogens and manifests initially as a respiratory tract infection or generalised malaise and fever prior to the onset of abdominal symptoms. Although mesenteric adenitis is more common in children, it still should be considered in young adults as such a diagnosis would not require surgical intervention. It presents very similarly to acute appendicitis however subtle differences do exist. Often the pain of mesenteric adenits can move location when the patient moves whereas in appendicitis it is fixed to the right iliac fossa. Inflammatory bowel disease such as Crohn's often presents with ileocaecal disease and can present similarly to appendicitis. In such cases a mass could be palpated in the right iliac fossa, without any extraintestinal signs. The clinical history alone is not enough to diagnose the condition therefore examination and investigation are essential.

Most patients with appendicitis have a low grade fever and some tachycardia. A very high temperature (above 39 ^{o}C) indicates probable abscess formation or other cause of infection. The site of maximum tenderness is usually at McBurney's point. In patients with inflammation of a retro-caecal appendix the pain may be considerably higher and more lateral. Alternatively in pelvic appendicitis, the pain may be lower and almost midline. The abdomen may show signs of guarding in 90% of patients with acute appendicitis. In patients with perforation of the appendix they will have generalised peritonitis and the area of guarding may extend beyond the right iliac fossa. Rebound tenderness is a useful sign. In some patients an appendix mass could be felt on abdominal examination.

On general examination fever is an important sign indicative of an inflammatory condition. A foetor is also detected in 50 % of patients. In children, general observation of discomfort associated with movement or posture is also indicative. Abdominal examination should reveal tenderness over the right iliac fossa with or without rebound tenderness or guarding which indicates signs of peritonism. Specific signs of Appendicitis include McBurneys and Rovsing's signs. The appendix lies in the right iliac fossa and is attached to the posteromedial wall of the caecum where the teniae coli unite. The surface marking for the root of the appendix is relatively constant and is situated approximately one third of the distance from the anterior superior iliac spine to the umbilicus. This is referred to as McBurneys point as shown in the diagram (Figure 1).

In general, the clinical features of appendicitis can vary depending on the position of the appendix. The commonest position of the appendix is retrocaecal. In this position, psoas muscle irritation (exacerbation of pain on hip extension) can be evident. In the subcaecal and pelvic position, supra pubic pain and urinary frequency may be the predominant symptoms with right sided tenderness on rectal or vaginal examination. In the pre and post ileal position, diarrhoea or vomiting may be the presenting features due to irritation of the ileum. On examination for appendicitis it is important to determine if the pain is worst at McBurneys point. Furthermore the patient may describe pain over this area on coughing. Specific localisation of tenderness over this anatomical landmark is indicative that the inflammation is no longer limited to the lumen of the appendix which poorly localises pain.

It is suggestive that there is irritation at the peritoneum where it comes into contact with the appendix. Rovsing's sign can be demonstrated by palpating the left iliac area which results in stretching of the underlying peritoneum. This induces pain in the right iliac fossa due to irritation of the inflamed peritoneum. Digital rectal examination can elicit tenderness on the ipsilateral side to the appendix.

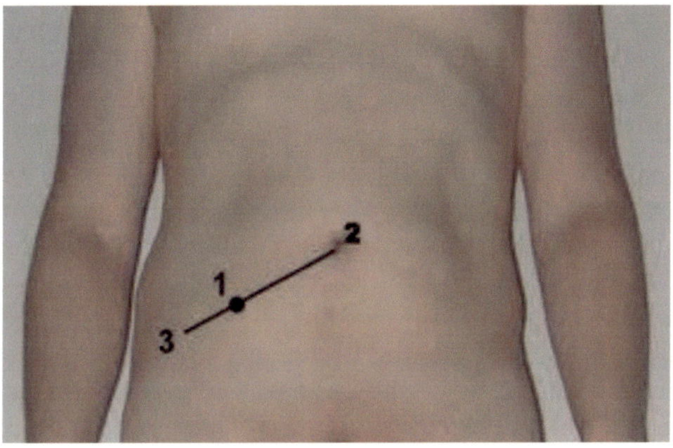

Fig. 1. Diagramatic illustration of McBurneys point (1) with regards to the umbilicus (2) and the anterior superior iliac spine (3).

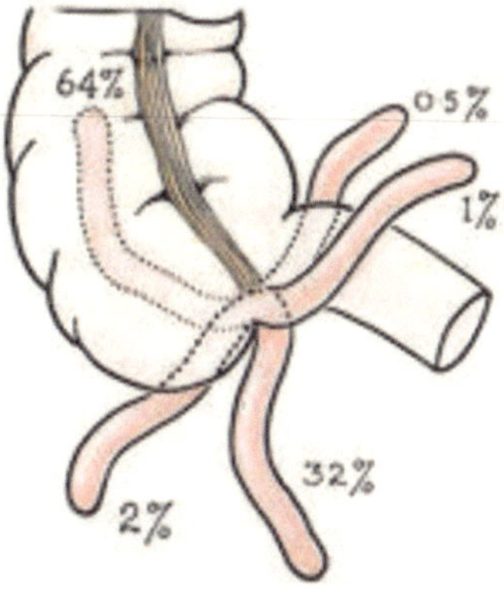

Fig. 2. Various positions of the vermiform appendix.

In females of child bearing age it is important to consider the possibility of pregnancy particularly if the patient was sexually active. An ectopic pregnancy should be considered in the potential differential diagnosis which can often present with pain in the lower quadrants. The pain associated with ectopic pregnancies often radiates to the shoulder. A history of the patient's menstrual cycle and sexual activity and contraception can help in elimination of this differential. It is important to assess beta HCG levels on admission as this would determine further management. Ultasonography and CT scanning are the best non-invasive means of investigating appendicitis. The scan may show an abnormal appendix or an appendicolith with a diameter of over 6mm. The blood results will often have a rise in the inflammatory markers including white cell count and C-Reactive protein (CRP).

It is important to ensure that the patient has received adequate analgesia and has had blood tests to ensure clotting is normal before surgery. The patient would also require a 'group and save' due to a small risk of bleeding during or after surgery. Antibiotics are often prescribed as prophylaxis to help reduce the risk of wound infections. The patient may require an NG tube if vomiting to prevent the risk of aspiration.

In order to make the diagnosis of appendicitis and at the same time avoid unnecessary appendicectomies a variety of diagnostic modalities were advanced. A review of the literature suggested that the clinical diagnosis of acute appendicitis based on symptoms, physical findings, and serological tests is relatively inaccurate. Despite having high sensitivity (up to 100%), clinical evaluation has relatively low specificity (73%). This means that surgeons are likely to overestimate the presence of appendicitis in patients who present acutely. Several reports have found the use and diagnostic accuracy (specificity and sensitivity) of ultrasound and computed tomography (CT) to be limited in the preoperative evaluation of patients with suspected appendicitis especially in the emergency setting.

The most common US technique used to examine patients with acute abdominal pain is the graded-compression procedure. With this technique, interposing fat and bowel can be displaced or compressed by means of gradual compression to show underlying structures. Furthermore, if the bowel cannot be compressed, the noncompressibility itself is an indication of inflammation. Curved (3.5–5.0-MHz) and linear (5.0–12.0-MHz) transducers are used most commonly, with frequencies depending on the application and the patient's stature. The reported sensitivity of ultrasonic detection of appendicitis lies between 55 and 98% and the specificity between 78 and 100%.

Computed Tomography (CT) has a higher sensitivity and specificity for the diagnosis of appendicitis. The CT technique used to examine patients with acute abdominal pain generally involves scanning of the entire abdomen after intravenous administration of an iodinated contrast medium. Although abdominal CT can be performed without contrast medium, the intravenous administration of contrast material facilitates good accuracy with a positive predictive value of 95% reported for the diagnosis of appendicitis and a high level of diagnostic confidence, especially in rendering diagnoses in thin patients, in whom fat interfaces may be almost absent. Although rectal or oral contrast material may be helpful in differentiating fluid-filled bowel loops from abscesses in some cases, the use of oral contrast material can markedly increase the time to complete the test in the emergency setting and may be contraindicated for patients who potentially may require anesthesia and surgery. The lack of enteral contrast medium does not seem to hamper the accurate reading of CT images obtained in patients with acute abdominal pain as it does in postoperative patients. Exposure to ionizing radiation is a disadvantage of CT. This risk however should be weighed against the direct diagnostic benefit. CT has been shown to reduce the negative-finding appendectomy rate from 24% to 3%. However, only routine CT in comparison to selective use of CT would achieve such results. CT seems to be more sensitive (96% vs. 76%) and accurate (94% vs. 91%) than US in diagnosing acute appendicitis, whereas they are almost equal when it comes to specificity (89% vs. 91%). CT imaging tailored to evaluate acute appendicitis has proven to be particularly successful with a sensitivity of 100%, specificity of 95%, positive predictive value of 97%, negative predictive value of 100%, and accuracy of 98%.

Based on the clinical diagnosis, surgical exploration for suspected appendicitis is advocated early to prevent progression or perforation with its associated morbidity and mortality.

Active observation is advocated for patients with equivocal symptoms, signs and laboratory results. Surgical exploration has been accompanied by an incidental appendicectomy in a considerable number of cases. Authors of large prospective studies report a 15%-32% removal rate of normal appendices at surgery. The reported negative appendicectomy rate for men varies from 7 % to 15 %, whereas that for women of child bearing age lies between 22 % and 47 % . This high rate of unnecessary appendicectomies has considerable morbidity and high cost to the health care system. A large population based study found that patients undergoing negative appendicectomy have prolonged hospitalisation, increased infectious complications and higher rates of case fatality when compared with patients with appendicitis. The national cost of hospitalisation was also higher. This may be due to concomitant disease which necessitated the presentation of right iliac fossa pain which otherwise remains undiagnosed after appendicectomy.

A number of studies have emphasised the value of laparoscopy as a diagnostic and operative tool particularly in young women. Diagnostic laparoscopy has been found reliable in the assessment of the appendix and has reduced the number of unnecessary appendicectomies. In addition, it has been useful in the diagnosis of alternative pathology when it exists.

In order to reduce total costs, some studies have suggested a selective approach in the use of diagnostic laparoscopy. There is evidence however that unless diagnostic laparoscopy is used routinely, the number of negative appendicectomies remains high.

5. Management

Historically we have seen progression in the management of right iliac fossa pain from purgation to early appendicectomy. Early surgical dictum necessitated appendicectomy for patients with right iliac fossa pain admitted to hospital with convincing signs and symptoms. Appendicectomy was clearly overdone in the past as the delay in diagnosis of appendicitis contributed to an increase in morbidity and mortality. Indeed delayed diagnosis of appendicitis was the most common cause of litigation against emergency surgeons. In regard to laparoscopic appendicectomy, early reports suggested a high rate of complications particularly intra-abdominal abcess formation which was associated with laparoscopic appendicectomy. A more recent Cochrane review however, has found an equal rate of complications in open and laparoscopic appendicectomy. However, patients operated on by laparoscopy, realised the benefits of laparoscopy in terms of less pain, early discharge from hospital and return to normal activities.

Natural orifice translumenal endoscopic surgery (NOTES) has become an exciting area of surgical development. Significant limitations to this surgical concept include lack of surgical expertise and appropriate flexible instrumentation although both aspects are being addressed. An alternative and competing technology to NOTES is single-incision laparoscopic surgery (SILS). A number of reports have produced encouraging results for single incision appendicectomy but this technique remains in its infancy. A number of skeptics have expressed reservations about the applicability of these two techniques for appendicectomy and it will be a matter for the surgical community uptake and adoption of these two techniques over the next few years.

In terms of the cost of the utility of laparoscopic appendicectomy, the overall costs might be justified since the use of laparoscopy can increase diagnostic power, provide less postoperative pain and fewer wound infections, decrease hospital stay and return to normal activities, and decrease the number of postoperative adhesions. At least six randomized studies have addressed the cost issue. Some found that overall costs for laparoscopic appendectomy were less (but not significantly so), most of the other studies have shown consistently that laparoscopy is more expensive. There was however a wide range of costs. One study found a mean difference of £148 in operating room charges, which does not compensate the costs for the mean difference in analgesics requirement between laparoscopic and open appendicectomy. On the other hand, there is no doubt in the superiority of diagnostic laparoscopy and laparoscopic appendicectomy in terms of quality but only if the incidence of post-operative complications could be reduced. The key to this dilemma lies in separating simple appendicitis from complicated appendicitis. The former will almost invariably have a low incidence of post-operative complications while those with complicated appendicitis (perforation or abcess) seem to have a higher rate of complications after laparoscopic appendicectomy.

5.1 Management of appendix abcess

Patients presenting with an appendix mass should be treated non-surgically in the first instance. Once the abscess has been confirmed radiologically, percutaneous drainage is the best treatment of choice. Occasionally this drainage can be followed by the development of a faecal fistula but this is usually a low output fistula which normally heals spontaneously. If percutaneous drainage is inadequate, it may be necessary to carry out operative drainage. In patients who have had an appendix mass treated conservatively, about 15% will develop recurrent appendicitis. An interval appendicectomy should be considered.

If appendix mass was found at laparoscopy or laparotomy an attempt should be made to drain the abscess and leave the appendix in situ. Old surgical dogma which continues to apply is that it is 'fool hardy to remove the appendix in the presence of an appendix abcess'. The main reasons for this is the generalised inflammation of the adjacent caecum and small bowel. Attempts at appendicectomy in this scenario, invariably result with intra and post operative complications. Such attempts usually result in a more extensive resection of the adjacent small bowel and caecum. Given the emergency presentation of these patients, the potential for complications is large.

5.2 Negative, incidental and elective appendicectomy

If a normal appendix was found at laparoscopy, most surgeons would leave the appendix in-situ as an appendicectomy may carry some procedures specific complications. However some skilled surgeons have excellent results with removing a normal appendix laparoscopically. Based on the results of negative appendicectomies published, the complication rate tends to be low. However, if a right iliac fossa incision has been made over the appendix for open appendicectomy, it would seem reasonable to carry out an appendicectomy. This is mainly due to a future assumption that appendicectomy has been carried out when a patient presents at a later stage. It is also claimed that 20% of normal looking appendices may have evidence of mucosal appendicitis. Further, although rare, carcinoma of the appendix occurs in rare cases when the appendix looks microscopically normal.

There is little evidence to support the concept of chronic appendicitis. A number of patients mainly young females will have repeated acute presentations with right iliac fossa pain in the absence of raised inflammatory markers. Labels such as chronic appendicitis and 'grumbling appendix' have been applied to these patients. However, there is no evidence to support this diagnosis. In some of these patients a faecolith was found in the lumen of the appendix which could in theory account for some of the symptoms without necessarily causing full fledged appendicitis. However, elective appendicectomy does not necessarily obviate the long term symptoms of many of these patients any more than a placebo effect. Consequently, the concept of elective appendicectomy for chronic right iliac fossa pain seems unjustified.

5.3 Non-operative management

Acute appendicitis is considered a surgical emergency. The incidence decreases with increasing adult age, and the overall incidence in the general population has probably been decreasing during the last 50 years. Classically, appendectomy is performed to avoid perforation, which typically occurs within 48 hours. With the development of the preoperative use of antibiotics, early investigators reported that the peritonitis associated with appendicitis usually resolved before appendectomy. A number of publications have reported cases of appendicitis treated conservatively with a small number of deaths, a further number requiring abscess drainage, and a large number of failures requiring appendectomy. Several more recent studies have shown that perforated appendicitis can be treated nonoperatively with IV antibiotics with the performance of percutaneous drainage if an abscess is present. Success rates have been reported as between 88% and 100%, with the incidence of recurrent appendicitis 5% to 38%. The use of conservative (non-surgical) management of appendicitis is currently reserved to situations where access to surgical management is limited such as on board of ships, fishing vessels, submarines, space missions, polar and Antarctic expeditions . Medical evacuation is performed when possible, and is expedited if improvement does not occur. For some programs, prophylactic appendectomy has been considered. The benefits and long term risks of performing a prophylactic appendectomy in an otherwise healthy individual must however be carefully considered.

There are no studies that have looked at the complications associated with prophylactic appendectomy.

5.4 Management of acute appendicitis

Based on current evidence, all patients presenting with convincing symptoms and signs of appendicitis with raised serological markers of inflammation, should have a diagnostic laparoscopy to confirm the diagnosis where possible. Patients found to have evidence of appendicitis by virtue of serosal inflammation and / or the presence of fibrinous exudates should be considered for appendicectomy. The consideration for open or laparoscopic appendicectomy hinges on the experience of the surgeon, the availability of suitable assistance and appropriate instruments and the express wishes of the patient if these have been made in advance. In equivocal cases, all surgeons would search for an alternative source to account for the patient's symptoms and signs and in the absence of an alternative source, appendicectomy should be considered.

In patients found to have perforated appendicitis surgeons should attempt to evaluate the risks and benefits of laparoscopic surgery for the individual patient based on the amount of contamination of the peritoneal cavity, the spread and intensity of inflammation against the general condition of the patient together with surgical technical factors including the experience of the surgeon and the availability of appropriate instruments.

In all patients undergoing appendicectomy, prophylactic antibiotics should be used. In patients who have had a perforated appendix, appendicectomy should be followed by peritoneal lavage. When perforation has occurred it is common practice to continue intravenous antibiotics for a period postoperatively depending on the degree of infection and contamination. Recent evidence suggests that metronidazole would be sufficient for simple appendicitis. Additional broad-spectrum antibiotics may be necessary for complicated appendicitis. If an adequate peritoneal lavage has been carried out, abdominal drains do not confer any benefit.

5.4.1 Technique of open appendicectomy

An open procedure involves a muscle splitting gridiron incision at McBurneys point. The muscle layers are separated along the line of the fibres allowing for the identification and opening of the peritoneum. Upon entry into the peritoneum the caecum is identified and appendix is located. This can be achieved through using the merging of the teniae coli as a reference point. The vessels in the meso-appendix are ligated until the appendix is free. The base of the appendix can then be ligated with two loops of absorbable sutures and the appendix divided between the two loops. The appendix can then be removed. Some surgeons invaginate the appendix stump either using a purstring absorbable suture or a Z stitch. The majority of surgeons do not invaginate the appendix stump but use electro-coagulation on the visible edge of the mucosa. After ensuring haemostasis, a thorough wash is carried out. The wound is then closed in layers.

5.4.2 Laparoscopic appendicectomy

In 1983, Semm performed the first laparoscopic appendectomy. Ever since then, the efficiency and superiority of laparoscopic approach compared to the open technique has been the subject of much debate. The idea of minimal surgical trauma, resulting in significantly shorter hospital stay, less postoperative pain, faster return to daily activities, and better cosmetic outcome has made laparoscopic surgery for acute appendicitis very attractive. However, several retrospective studies, several randomized trials and meta-analyses comparing laparoscopic with open appendectomy have provided conflicting results. Some of these studies have demonstrated better clinical outcomes with the laparoscopic approach, while other studies have shown marginal or no clinical benefit and higher surgical costs. The European Association of Endoscopic Surgeons have published their guidelines on laparoscopic appendicectomy. In summary, the EAES have found that laparoscopic appendicectomy is feasible and safe with a slightly longer operating time than open appendicectomy. However, they expressly state that the safety of laparoscopic appendicectomy during pregnancy is not established. Laparoscopic appendicectomy has advantages over open appendicectomy but there is potential for serious injuries. EAES recommends that at least 20 cases of laparoscopic appendicectomy should be done before surgeon's accreditation for this procedure.

5.4.3 Technique of laparoscopic appendicectomy

The patient is placed in a Trendelenburg position, with a slight rotation to the left. The surgeon should stand on the patients left side and the primary monitor should be placed on the right side of the patient (opposite the surgeon). The patients arms should be tucked at the sides to allow sufficient room for the surgeon and camera operator to move cepahalad as required. Pneumoperitoneum is produced by continuous pressure of 10-12 mmHg of carbon dioxide *via* a Verres canula, positioned in the sub-umbilical area. Following gas insufflation, a 12 mm canula for the 30 degree angled laparoscope should be placed in the periumbilical area (preferably on the left). Alternatively, a 12 mm canula can be introduced by the Hasson's technique (introduction of first trocar into the peritoneum through a sub-umbilical small incision) for initial insufflations of gas. Two additional canulae are required. A 12 mm canula should be placed in the suprapubic area at the midline point to accommodate the grasping or stapling device and/or to facilitate specimen extraction, and a third 5 mm canula in the right (or left) lower abdominal quadrant is introduced under direct vision. When the third cannula is placed on the right, it must be sufficiently far from the appendix to allow a safe and comfortable working distance. The abdominal cavity is thoroughly inspected in order to exclude other intra-abdominal or pelvic pathology. If the appendix is normal, it is important to seek other sources to account for the patient's presentation. If no other cause is identified, it will be up to the discretion of the surgeon at the operating table to decide on removing an apparently normal looking appendix. This has to be guided by prior knowledge of the patient's history, acute presentation, examination findings and serological markers of inflammation.

The appendix should be identified at the base of the caecum. Atraumatic bowel graspers should be used to lift the caecum. Part of the appendix should start coming to view. A second pair of atraumatic graspers (or blunt suction probe) should be used to separate the appendix from adherent tissue by blunt dissection. The mesoappendix should be identified and divided with bipolar forceps (or mono-polar diathermy and scissors). Alternatively, the meso-appendix could be divided using clips, *Ligature,* ultrasonic dissector or endoscopic stapler. The base of the appendix should then be identified and secured with one or two ligating loops of absorbable sutures placed at the base of the appendix close to the caecum. This is followed by blunt dissection distal to the second loop using a curved dissector. The appendix should then be divided between the 2 loops. The visible part of the mucosa is usually electro-coagulated. There is no need to bury the appendix stump. Alternatively, the base of the appendix could be stapled using one of the commercially available staplers. This achieves both closure and division of the appendix. In all cases, the specimen should be removed through the trocar without contact with the wound. Alternatively, if the appendix is too bulky, it should be placed in an endobag (a variety are available on the market) which can be extracted through one of the larger canulae sites. All removed tissue should be sent for histopathology. A thorough wash is then carried out. Although this should centre on the operative site, it should cover all sites of contamination encountered at the initial evaluation. Any faecoliths or necrotic material which have escaped from a perforated appendix should be removed if encountered. On occasion it may be necessary to look for inter-bowel fluid or pus collections and wash these out as well. The procedure should terminate by abdominal desufflation and removal of all cannulae. Patients should have two additional doses of antibiotics post operatively unless widespread contamination and peritonitis was evident. In these cases, antibiotics coverage should be continued for several days post operatively until the patient is no longer septic.

If bleeding is encountered during the procedure, an additional trocar may be required to place a suction device while looking for the source of bleeding. Once this is identified, control of bleeding may be achieved using clips or ligatures.

The use of staplers and more complex energy devices in appendicectomy saves time but adds to the cost of the operation. In general, they are not recommended unless time is a significant issue or these are used due to complexity or difficulty encountered during the procedure.

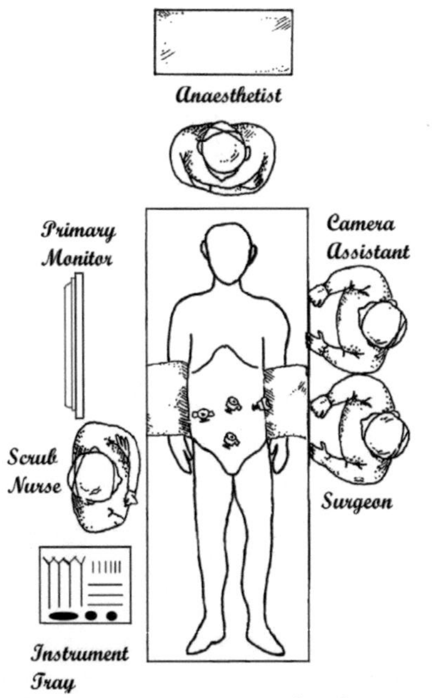

Fig. 3. Operating room set-up for diagnostic laparoscopy and appendicectomy.

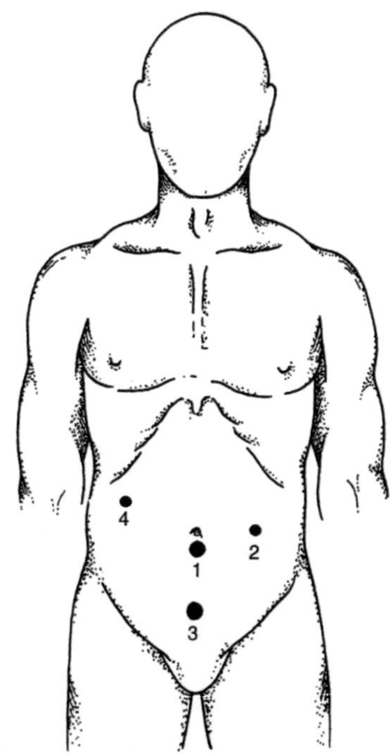

Fig. 4. Trocar positions for appendicectomy. Trocar 1 is used for the laparoscope. Trocars 2 and 3 are the main dissection sites. Trocar 4 can be added if necessary.

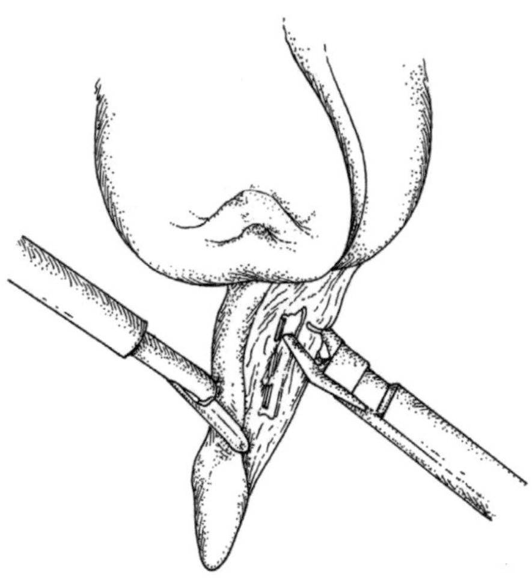

Fig. 5. Vesseles in the meso-appendix are dissected and clipped.

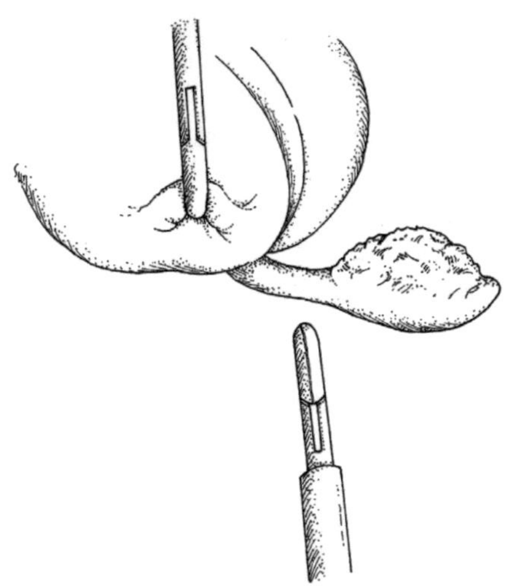

Fig. 6. The appendix is freed by blunt dissection to its base on the caecum.

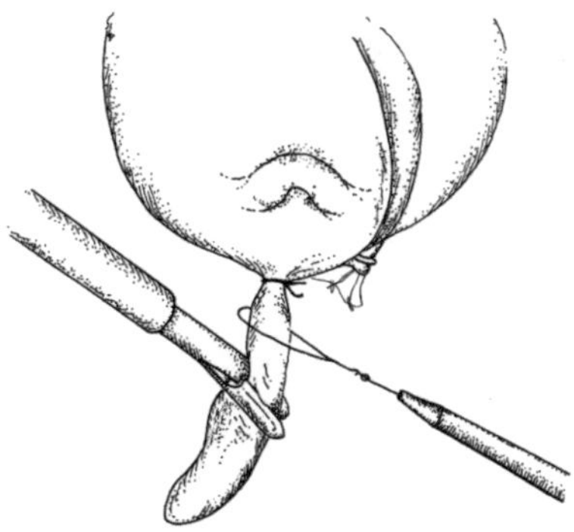

Fig. 7. Two pre-tied loops of absorbable sutures are applied to the base of the appendix.

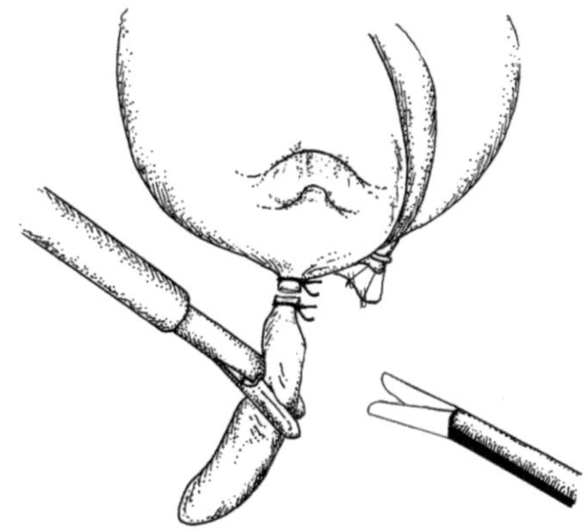

Fig. 8. The appendix is divided between loops and then delivered.

5.5 Laparoscopic versus open appendicectomy

Despite numerous prospective randomised trials, systematic reviews and meta-analysis the superiority of laparoscopic over open appendicectomy remains unclear particularly for complicated appendicitis. Previous studies have produced conflicting conclusions regarding the incidence of postoperative adverse events after laparoscopic and open appendicectomy. Retrospective cohort studies, randomised controlled trials and meta-analysis have demonstrated similar rates of overall morbidity. However, significant differences have been demonstrated in a few studies. With regards to operating time, there is a clear trend of extended operating time with laparoscopic appendicectomy in earlier studies with a further trend towards parity between the two procedures. This is a reflection of the experience of surgeons with the technique. With regards to hospital stay, the length of hospital stay after surgery was shortened in laparoscopic appendicectomy by a fraction of a day. This difference although numerically significant is of little practical significance.

Early return to full activity is accepted as an obvious advantage of laparoscopic appendicectomy which is supported by a large scale meta-analysis conducted by the Cochrane Colorectal Cancer Group. Clearly the smaller incisions of laparoscopic appendicectomy contribute to reduce trauma to the abdominal wall and less pain allowing faster recovery. Fast resumption of a normal diet following laparoscopic appendicectomy was another appealing advantage, resulting from minimal manipulation of bowel. The difference between laparoscopic and open appendicectomy in terms of resumption of normal diet intake represents a fraction of a day. Although this is significant numerically it is of doubtful practical significance. Reduced postoperative pain is another quality attribute of laparoscopic surgery. Although difficult to assess, a number of meta-analysis found that laparoscopic appendicectomy offered significant advantages in relieving postoperative pain mainly due to its minimal abdominal wall trauma. Reduction of wound infection is a significant advantage of laparoscopic appendicectomy. The chance of wound infection is greater in open appendicectomy partly because the inflamed appendix is removed from the abdominal cavity directly through the wound whereas in laparoscopic appendicectomy it is extracted via a bag or trocar. In addition the port-site wounds in laparoscopic appendicectomy are considerably smaller with less potential space and less interruption of blood supply around wound.

Several explanations have been advanced for the reduction of ileus following laparoscopic appendicectomy. Firstly, decreased handling of the bowel during the procedure leads to less postoperative adhesion and such adhesions may be responsible for ileus. Secondly patients after laparoscopic appendicectomy had less opiate analgesics which inhibited bowel movements in the postoperative period. Thirdly earlier mobilisation after laparoscopic appendicectomy may also contribute to the reduction of ileus. Several meta-analysis have found that the incidence of intra-abdominal infections, intra-operative bleeding and urinary tract infections after laparoscopic appendicectomy was higher compared with open appendicectomy. It is not clear why intra-operative bleeding and urinary tract infections are higher after laparoscopic appendicectomy. With regards to intra-abdominal infections and abscess formation, there was suggestions that aggressive manipulation of the infected appendix and increased use of irrigation fluid might have increased the incidence of intra-abdominal infections after laparoscopic appendicectomy. The majority of studies however have not separated the results for simple uncomplicated appendicitis. It does however appear that patients with complicated appendicitis managed by laparoscopic appendicectomy have a higher tendency for intra-abdominal abscess formation.

The conversion rate from laparoscopic to open appendicectomy is around 10%. This is not surprising when considering the proportion of complicated appendicitis and the emergency setting of the procedure.

Appendicectomy carries a fairly low risk of mortality. Consequently many studies do not report mortality rates or multi-variate analysis on these rates. Amongst studies that do report mortalities, the event rate ranges between 0.16 and 0.24.

During pregnancy, laparoscopic appendectomy was found to be safe and effective and at least equivalent to open appendicectomy. Despite the raised intra-abdominal pressure associated with pneumoperitoneum, laparoscopic appendicectomy is associated with good maternal and fetal outcome. Further confirmatory studies are awaited before the safety of laparoscopic appendicectomy can be accepted.

5.6 Long-term complications and implications

Both the acute inflammatory condition of appendicitis and the surgical operation carried out to remove the appendix can potentially promote adhesion formation particularly around the fallopian tubes which may lead to tubal dysfunction in females of child bearing age. There is controversy surrounding the association between previous appendicectomy with subsequent infertility in females. Some reports found perforated appendicitis in childhood is not an appreciable cause of subsequent tubal infertility, while other reports found a high incidence of tubal infertility in women previously treated for appendicitis complicated by perforation, pelvic peritonitis or abscess. Three studies considered non-perforated appendicitis as well as perforated appendicitis on subsequent infertility and their result suggest that neither acute appendicitis nor perforation of the appendix was associated with a significant risk of infertility. Other studies, considered the question of the association between appendectomy and infertility. Some studies showed no association between a history of appendicectomy and subsequent infertility while others found a higher incidence of infertility in patients who have had a previous appendicectomy. One of these studies analysed fertility after removal of a normal appendix. This study found that women whose appendix was found to be normal at appendectomy in childhood seem to belong to a subgroup with a higher fertility than the general population. The majority of these studies suffer from small numbers, selected populations, design or analysis flaws. A recent systematic review and appraisal of the evidence for evaluating if perforation of the appendix was a risk factor for tubal infertility and ectopic pregnancy found 4 studies with an appropriate epidemiological design with reasonable quality. It found that the risk of the association for perforation of the appendix ranged from a high of 4.8 % for tubal infertility to an insignificant association for ectopic pregnancy. The reviewed studies were consistent in demonstrating a modest increase in risk, with all results in the same direction of increased risk. Based on diagnostic tests for causation, the authors of the review did not accept a causal relationship between perforation of the appendix and tubal infertility or ectopic pregnancy although they have accepted the association and the risk of the exposure. A subsequently published case control study did not provide substantial evidence that perforation of the appendix was an important risk factor for female tubal infertility. A further study examined fertility after appendectomy during pregnancy. This study found that appendectomy during pregnancy of a normal, inflamed or perforated appendix did not affect subsequent fertility. A recent epidemiological study concluded that appendicitis appears to be low risk factor in subsequent infertility. However, Appendicectomy is associated with increased fertility. On the basis of this data, a policy of liberal and prompt laparoscopy used routinely on young women presenting with signs and symptoms of appendicitis is encouraged. If the appendix is found to be inflamed or equivocal, then appendicectomy is justified.

This epic study is likely to be cited for encouraging the practice of laparoscopic appendicectomy for all cases presenting with right iliac fossa pain. This is based on the fact that early mucosal appendicitis is thought to be a real entity and this is not apparent at the time of laparoscopy. However, caution must be exercised due to apparent complications of laparoscopic appendicectomy.

5.7 Post operative monitoring and management of complications

All patients require adequate post-operative monitoring. Those patients who had percutaneous drainage of appendix abcess also require monitoring. In addition to vital parameters, these patients require daily evaluation of the wound and abdomen by clinical examination. Serial measurement of inflammatory parameters is also useful in showing trends of improvement or otherwise. This should be continued until patients are discharged from hospital.

Superficial wound infection can start to manifest 48 hours after surgery. Patients who show signs of wound infection by virtue of inflammation of wound edges, should continue on antibiotics treatment until the wound inflammation settles. As a marker of progress of the inflammation, the area of cellulitis surrounding the wound should be marked on the skin and monitored for progression or regression. In addition, palpation of the wound itself may suggest accumulation of infected material under the wound, in the superficial tissues. In such cases, the wound should be opened either fully or partially to allow drainage of the infected material. In some cases, operative drainage under anaesthesia should be considered.

Patients who do not show signs of improvement after appendicectomy or those who show further deterioration, either clinically or serologically, should be considered for three dimensional imaging. In these patients, the attending surgeon is looking for evidence of intra-abdominal collection to account for the apparent lack of improvement. However, in rare cases, there may be evidence of iatrogenic injury particularly during laparoscopic appendicectomy or other missed diagnosis. In such patients, there should be a low threshold for repeat laparoscopy or laparotomy. Any evidence of intra-abdominal collection should be managed by drainage and peritoneal lavage. Iatrogenic injuries will require expert surgical correction and appropriate post-operative management. A missed diagnosis will require appropriate management.

Patients who had either percutaneous or laparoscopic drainage of an appendix abcess require careful monitoring for resolution of the inflammation and regression of the abcess. This is done clinically in the first instance but repeat three-dimensional imaging using contrast enhanced CT is usually more accurate than clinical evaluation. Failure of resolution of the inflammatory abcess or phelgmon associated with the abcess indicates either insufficient drainage together with incomplete or inappropriate antibiotics treatment. In such cases, the three dimensional imaging as well as bacteriological sensitivity testing of retrieved purulent material will guide further management. In some patients, revision of antibiotics requirement is necessary and in others revision of drainage is essential. In some patients, operative intervention is necessary due to intra-abdominal spread or rupture of the abcess. In these patients, the objective of operative intervention whether by laparotomy or laparoscopy is adequate drainage of any collection together with peritoneal lavage. When the abcess has been adequately drained, there is usually an accompanying improvement in the general condition of the patient. The drain should be withdrawn when no further purulent material is obtained. The patients can usually return to normal activity and can be safely discharged from hospital. However, due to the relatively high incidence of recurrent appendicitis, patients should be given a date for appendicectomy. This delayed appendicectomy should be done when all signs of inflammation have disappeared and should be attempted laparoscopically by an experienced surgeon.

6. Conclusion

Despite the recent decline in the incidence of appendicitis, it remains the commonest surgical emergency. It is estimated that 10% of the population will have appendicitis during their life time. Approximately 20 % of those will have complicated appendicitis. The diagnosis of appendicitis remains clinical. However, reliance on clinical examination alone will result in an unnecessary number of patients having exploratory surgery. Clinical history and examination supplemented with routine inflammatory marker analysis improves the diagnostic accuracy. Although ultrasound and computed tomography are relatively accurate in the diagnosis of appendicitis, it is important to emphasise that CT is more accurate than ultrasound but carries a radiation burden. The use of both radiological investigations is limited in the emergency setting. The diagnosis of appendicitis is most difficult at the extremes of age and it is in these patients that additional investigations may be justified. In all other cases, if the history and examination is compatible with appendicitis with raised inflammatory markers, patients (both males and females) should have a diagnostic laparoscopy which can proceed to laparoscopic appendicectomy if the appendix was found to be inflamed. If an appendix abcess was found, the abcess should be drained. If the appendix was found to be perforated, conversion to open appendicectomy should be considered. In all cases, adequate peritoneal lavage should be carried out. Post-operatively, all patients should have antibiotics for different periods depending on the degree of inflammation and contamination found at operation. Post-operatively, all patients should be monitored for the emergence of adverse events. Patients who develop signs of peritoneal infection or who fail to improve should have a CT in the first instance. Wound infections should be managed by open drainage and antibiotics. Intra-abdominal infection should be managed by laparoscopy/ laparotomy, drainage of collection and peritoneal lavage together with systemic antibiotics.

Laparoscopic appendicectomy is safe for the majority of cases of simple appendicitis. If at laparoscopy, the appendix is found to have perforated, the surgeon should make a careful evaluation of whether to continue with laparoscopic surgery or convert to open surgery. In either situation, the surgical objective is appendicectomy together with adequate peritoneal lavage of all areas of the peritoneal cavity.

7. References

Ball CG, Kortbeek JB, Kirkpatrick AW, and Mitchell P. Laparoscopic appendectomy for complicated appendicitis: an evaluation of postoperative factors. Surgical Endoscopy. 2004; 18: 969-973.

Garbarino S, Shimi SM. Routine diagnostic laparoscopy reduces the rate of unnecessary appendicectomies in young women. Surg Endosc. 2009 Mar;23(3):527-33. Epub 2008 Mar 26.

Hale DA, Molloy M, Pearl RH, Schutt DC, Jaques DP. Appendectomy: a contemporary appraisal. Annals of Surgery 1997 Vol. 225, No. 3, 252-261

Ingraham AM, Cohen ME, Bilimoria KY, Pritts TA, Ko CY, and Esposito TJ. Comparison of outcomes after laparoscopic versus open appendectomy for acute appendicitis at 222 ACS SQIP hospitals. Surgery 2010; 148: 625-37.

Livingston EH, Woodward WA, Sarosi GA, and Haley RW. Disconnect Between Incidence of Nonperforated and Perforated Appendicitis: Implications for Pathophysiology and Management. Ann Surg. 2007 June; 245(6): 886–892.

Stoker J, van Randen A, Lameris W, and Boermeester MA. Imaging patients with acute abdominal pain. Radiology 2009; 253: 31-46.

Kirshtein B, Perry ZH, Avinoach E, Mizrahi S, Lantsberg L. Safety of laparoscopic appendectomy during pregnancy. World J Surg. 2009 Mar;33(3):475-80.

Li X, Zhang J, Sang L, Zhang W, Chu Z, Li X, and Liu Y. Laparoscopic versus convential appendectomy – a meta-analysis of randomised controlled trials. BMC Gastroenterology 2010; 10: 129.

Markides G, Subar D, Riyad K. Laparoscopic versus open appendectomy in adults with complicated appendicitis: systematic review and meta-analysis. World J Surg. 2010 Sep;34(9):2026-40. Review.

Needham PJ, Laughlan KA, Botterill ID, Ambrose NS. Laparoscopic appendicectomy: calculating the cost. Ann R Coll Surg Engl. 2009 Oct;91(7):606-8.

Park HC, Yang DH, Lee BH. The laparoscopic approach for perforated appendicitis, including cases complicated by abscess formation. J Laparoendosc Adv Surg Tech A. 2009 Dec;19(6):727-30.

Sauerland S, Jaschinski T, Neugebauer EA. Laparoscopic versus open surgery for suspected appendicitis. Cochrane Database Syst Rev. 2010 Oct 6;(10):CD001546. Review.

Part 4

Laparoscopic Hernia Repair Surgery

10

Laparoscopic Hernia Repair

Eva Deerenberg, Irene Mulder and Johan Lange
Erasmus University Medical Centre
The Netherlands

1. Introduction

A hernia is a protrusion of abdominal content (preperitoneal fat, omentum or abdominal organs) through an abdominal wall defect. Anatomically the most important features of a hernia are the hernial orifice and the hernia (peritoneal) sac, if present. The hernial orifice is represented by the primary defect in the aponeurotic layer of the abdomen, and the hernial sac by the bulging peritoneum. The neck of the hernial sac is located at the hernial orifice. As the French anatomist Henri Fruchaud (1894-1960) already stated, hernias of the abdominal wall occur in areas where aponeurosis and fascia are lacking the protective support of muscles (Fruchaud, 1953). Most of these weak areas are anatomically present in the abdominal wall congenitally, others may be acquired during life, for example by surgery. The uncovered weak aponeurotic areas are subject to elevated intra-abdominal pressures and give way if they deteriorate or represent anatomic varieties. The common sites of herniation of the abdominal wall are the groin, the umbilicus, the linea alba, the semilunar line of Spigel, the diaphragm and surgical incisions. In addition, more exceptionally obturator hernias and hernias of the triangle of Petit are also encountered. Hernias can broadly be classified into congenital and acquired types. Congenital hernias typically occur at the groin, although they may be observed at other locations such as the umbilicus or diaphragm.

Abdominal wall hernias represent a common issue in general surgical practice. The definitive treatment of all hernias, regardless of their origin or type, is surgical repair. It is suggested that a strategy of watchful waiting rather than surgery can be considered in patients with asymptomatic or minimally symptomatic inguinal and incisional hernia. The risks of delayed surgery are primarily related to the risks of incarceration and strangulation, which necessities emergency surgery. Elective surgical repair should be considered if the hernia is symptomatic, in case of an increased risk for incarceration or if the size of the hernia complicates dressing or activities of daily living. Hernias that are less likely to incarcerate include upper abdominal hernias, hernias with an abdominal wall defect larger than 7-8cm and hernias less than 1 cm in diameter. The likelihood of incarceration decreases as the hernia defect increases in size since it is less likely that intestinal or visceral contents will become caught by a narrow neck of the hernia sac. In large incisional ('giant') hernias more skin problems (ischemia, necrosis and ulcerations) are observed and represent an indication for operation.

The surgical treatment of hernias is already performed since Hellenistic times when Celsus performed hernial sac extirpations. The founder of modern hernia surgery is Bassini from Padova (Italy), who performed the first anatomic hernia groin repair in 1887 (Bassini, 1887).

The results of anatomical hernia repair were a large step forward, however recurrences kept frustrating surgeons since. Over de last decades it has become clear that prosthetic reinforcement by a non-resorbable synthetic polymer mesh is required for most hernia repairs. Abdominal wall hernias can be repaired with mesh reinforcement by open or laparoscopic approach. The first report of the use of a laparoscope in the repair of an abdominal wall hernia was made by Ger in 1982 (Ger, 1982). Bogojavalensky in 1989 was the first to report on the use of a prosthetic mesh during laparoscopic hernia repair (Bogojavalensky, 1989).

The objective of successful hernia repair is achieving a cost-effective repair with a low recurrence rate, minimal operative and acute and chronic postoperative pain with a rapid return to normal activities. Laparoscopic repair has the potential benefits of smaller wounds, with less wound infections and better cosmetic results, and the possibility to perform the procedure in the outpatient clinic. Patients are thought to experience less postoperative discomfort and a faster recovery time. Additional benefit, especially in incisional hernia surgery, is the possibility to diagnose and treat multiple hernias in one procedure. During laparoscopic repair a mesh is placed intraperitoneally which makes contact between the mesh and viscera inevitable. The contact with the viscera can lead to adhesion formation and associated complications like small bowel obstruction, enterocutaneous fistula, infertility and chronic pain. Other possible complications of the laparoscopic approach in general are bowel and bladder injuries, artery laceration, neuralgia and trocar site herniation. During laparoscopic hernia repair it is hardly ever possible to restore functional anatomy of the abdominal wall and manage skin redundancy or the hernia sac.

The risk of recurrence is determined by surgical-technical factors (i.e. mesh use, choice and placement), the experience of the surgeon, the occurrence of a wound infection and patient related factors. Literature shows that recurrence rates are low in experienced hands. Several co-morbidities have been identified that increase the risk of recurrence and wound infection following hernia repair: smoking, diabetes, coronary artery disease, chronic obstructive pulmonary disease (COPD), nutritional status, immunosuppression, chronic corticosteroid use, low serum albumin, obesity and advanced age. A prolonged operative time and the use of an absorbable synthetic mesh are also significant independent predictors of wound infection and associated recurrences.

1.1 Mesh characteristics

The first prosthetic mesh for hernia repair, introduced in 1900, was a hand-made silver wire filigrees. In the second half of the 20th century nylon, (expanding) PTFE, polypropylene and polyester meshes were introduced. The current large diversity of synthetic polymer and biologic materials available for the reinforcement of hernia repair, without high level evidence for clinical use, complicates the selection of an appropriate prosthesis. The material must be reactive enough to stimulate fibroblast ingrowth, yet inert enough to minimize foreign body reaction, adhesion formation, allergic reaction and to avoid infection. The mesh must have enough strength to prevent early recurrence but enough flexibility to accommodate activity. The mesh should also have optimal laparoscopic handling characteristics. Until now the ideal mesh does not exist and the location of implantation (intra- or extraperitoneally) should be taken into account when choosing a mesh. When choosing a synthetic mesh for laparoscopic hernia repair it is important to consider all characteristics that generate the host response, like absorbability, pore size and weave.

- **Absorbability.** Absorbable materials are less likely to become infected than non-absorbable materials, and are less harmful to viscera. However the main disadvantage of absorbable meshes is that the resultant scar tissue weakens after the mesh is absorbed and the necessary long-term repair strength is not provided, in contrast with permanent non-absorbable meshes. Partial absorbable meshes are thought to decrease the amount of foreign material while maintaining mechanical strength, but data about the clinical (long-term) performances are not available yet. Total non-absorbable meshes can be more stiff and heavy, possibly causing discomfort for the patient.
- **Pore size.** Porosity of a mesh is the main determinant of tissue reaction. The space between fibrils influences cellular infiltration, risk of infection, and mesh density and flexibility. Meshes with large pores allow increased tissue ingrowth and are more flexible than meshes with small pores. In a microporous mesh the granulomas around individual fibrils can become confluent which leads to encapsulation of the mesh and makes the mesh inflexible. Microporous meshes are more at risk of becoming infected, as large immune cells cannot infiltrate to phagocytose bacteria. Due to the strong chronic host response, macroporous meshes show good incorporation, but are more likely to give rise to adhesions and erosions than microporous meshes when use intra-abdominally. With increasing size of the pores, the chance of bulging of a macroporous mesh used for bridging increases.
- **Weave.** Multifilament meshes are soft, flexible and resistant to wrinkling. They result in strong integration in the host, but are more susceptible to infection. Monofilament meshes are less susceptible to infection, but have the disadvantage of causing significant adhesions when used intra-abdominally.
- **Anti-bacterial of anti-adhesive treatment.** Synthetic meshes with additional coatings (i.e. silver or antiseptics) to reduce the risk of infection or adhesions (i.e. cellulose or collagen layer) have been developed. The anti-adhesive layer functions as a barrier between the viscera and the mesh and reduces the risk of adhesion formation.

Biological meshes made of donor collagen (porcine, bovine or human) are suggested to be used especially in a contaminated or infected environment when closure is required. These new developed collagen meshes are thought to be replaced by the patients own collagen in time (remodelling), with an associated low adhesion formation and low infection risk.
They are less suitable for bridging; because due to gradual absorption, the risk of recurrence is high. Unfortunately collagen meshes cannot be introduced through a laparoscopy port yet and more research on outcome and recurrence rates should be done. Finally until now surgeons and hospitals are also reluctant as costs of biological meshes are very high compared to synthetic meshes.

1.2 Mesh fixation

During laparoscopic hernia repair the mesh can be placed intra- or extraperitoneally. For extraperitoneally placed meshes, commonly used during groin hernia repair, minimal to no fixation is required. This because when intraperitoneal pressure is evenly distributed over the large peritoneal surface from the inside the mesh is kept in place without need for fixation. However, some surgeons fixate the mesh in case of a direct inguinal hernia larger than 2 cm. Fixation is then performed with tackers to the muscles and the periostal fascia of the pubic bone. Care must be taken to avoid the lateral space as all three inguinal nerves are located within.

An intraperitoneally implanted mesh, commonly used in ventral hernia repair, can be fixated using different techniques. Proper fixation of the mesh is important to prevent recurrence, but no consensus about the ideal fixation method exists. The ideal fixation method would guarantee sufficient strength to withstand the pressures generated in the abdomen during coughing and straining. The first used fixation method was represented by stapling, using titanium staples with a penetration depth of 2 to 4.8 mm. These staples could cause chronic pain by compression and twisting of tissue containing nerves. Currently, the most frequently used techniques involve fixation with transabdominal sutures and tackers; titanium helical coils with a maximal tissue penetration depth of 3.8 mm. Fixation with tackers is fast and strong, but complications of adhesions to the tackers and nerve injury and intestinal lesions have been observed. Transabdominal sutures penetrate all layers of the abdominal wall, providing a significant stronger fixation than fixation with tackers only. The disadvantages of transabdominal sutures are the time consuming procedure and the increased risk of chronic postoperative pain by incorporating large bites of tissue.

When fixating a mesh it is important to use an appropriate amount of fixation points, avoiding loosening and incarceration of omentum or bowel loops. Transabdominal sutures should be placed no more than 5 cm apart. An overlap of 3 cm of the fascial defect is sufficient when transabdominal sutures are used. If no sutures are used the minimal overlap of the fascial defect should be 4 to 5 cm. The tackers or staples should be placed every 2 cm. Newly developed are absorbable tackers that absorb within one year. These absorbable tackers may lower the complication rate, but a tack is initially an invasive anchor that can result in nerve damage and postoperative pain. Completely non-invasive mesh fixation, such as with glue sealing, is gaining popularity in inguinal hernia repair, but use of glue in laparoscopic ventral hernia repair is not a common procedure yet. This fixation technique may be promising, but mesh dislocations, when positioned intraperitoneally, are reported.

2. Hernias of the groin region

The groin is the area of junction of the lower abdomen and the thigh at the myopectineal orifice of Fruchaud. The myopectineal orifice is bounded by the oblique and transversus abdominis muscles cranially, the iliopsoas muscles laterally, the rectus abdominis muscles medially and the pubic pecten caudally. This orifice is the weak spot through which neurovascular, muscular and testicular structures pass the abdominal wall during embryologic development. Protruding through the abdominal wall occurs at this point of the abdominal floor because no muscular covering reinforced by transversalis fascia is present.

The most common symptoms of a groin hernia are heaviness or a dull sense of discomfort in the groin that is most pronounced when the intra-abdominal pressure is raised, for example by straining or lifting. The pain is caused by the contents of the hernia pressing to the tight ring at the neck of the hernia sac. As the intra-abdominal pressure increases, the contents of the hernia are forced into the ring constricting them causing ischemia. Another cause of pain may be from stretching of the ilioinguinal or iliohypogastric nerves hard enter. In case of clinical suspicion of a groin hernia without palpable swelling herniography or MRI have the highest sensitivity and specificity. In daily practice ultrasonography with Valsalva manoeuvre is most often used.

The inguinal area is formed during embryologic development when the gubernaculum develops. This ligament exists between the ovary or testis and labioscrotal swelling and passes through the abdominal wall at the future inguinal canal. After twelve weeks of gestation the ventral peritoneal processus vaginalis follows the gubernaculum, equally piercing the abdominal wall. The processus vaginalis gives rise to the deep and superficial inguinal rings and pushes up the scrotal skin, the subcutaneous layers and the different investing layers of the spermatic cord. The spermatic cord consists of the internal spermatic fascia, cremasteric fascia and external spermatic fascia as continuations of transversalis fascia, internal and external oblique muscles, respectively. Thus, the cranial end of the inguinal canal is the internal or deep inguinal ring, which is a normal defect of the transversalis fascia. Its superior margin is represented by the transversus abdominis arch and the inferior margins are formed by aponeurotic fibers from the iliopubic tract, the inferior epigastric vessels, and the interfoveolar ligament of Hesselbach. The external or superficial inguinal ring is a triangular opening in the aponeurosis of the external oblique muscle. The superior and inferior crura, which form the margins of the ring, are held together and reinforced by intercrural fibers.

2.1 Anatomy of the groin

In the male within the 'triangle of doom' between the testicular vessels and vas deferens, the external iliac vessels are encountered. They are enveloped by lymphatic and fatty tissue. The deep circumflex iliac artery and vein originate from the external iliac vessels and run parallel to the iliopubic tract (ligament of Thomson), which is the thickened caudal margin of the transversalis fascia. This structure, which extends from the anterior superior iliac spine to the pubic tubercle, dorsally parallels the inguinal ligament. The latter is not visible from the posterior view.

The inferior epigastric artery and (two) veins are, especially in the laparoscopic extraperitoneal approach, the hallmark of safe exposure and entering of the 'proper preperitoneal space'. As the external iliac vessels are located within the endo-abdominal fascia, the inferior epigastric vessels pass to the dorsal aspect of the rectus abdominis muscles after perforation of the transversalis fascia, at the lateral boundaries of the rectus abdominis muscles. The frequently occurring accessory obturator artery and vein (corona mortis: 'circle of death'), connecting the obturator and inferior epigastric vessels, cross the superior pubic bone. They are at risk during dissection of the medial part of the pectineal ligament of Cooper, especially in femoral hernia surgery.

The genital branch of the genitofemoral nerve innervates the ventral genital skin and the cremaster muscle. After having accompanied the external iliac artery on the psoas muscle, it enters the inguinal canal through the deep inguinal ring, running dorsally to the round ligament of the uterus or the testicular vessels. Laterally to the deep inguinal ring, the lateral femoral cutaneous nerve crosses dorsally to the iliopubic tract, innervating the skin at the lateral side of the thigh. The femoral branch of the genitofemoral nerve and the lateral femoral cutaneous nerve are observed within the 'triangle of pain', also known as Kathouda's 'quadrant of doom'. The triangle is located between the gonadal vessels and iliopubic tract, at Bogros' space. Bogros' space is located between the transversalis fascia of ventral abdominal wall and the iliopsoas muscles, laterally to the inferior epigastric and external iliac vessels. In this area the application of staples for mesh prosthesis fixation is hazardous. The other nerves from the lumbar plexus (iliophypogastric, ilio-inguinal, obturator and femoral nerves) are only encountered if, inadvertently, dissection is performed between the transversus abdominis and iliopsoas muscles and the transversalis fascia. The nerves encountered in the triangle of pain from medial to lateral are the femoral branch of the genitofemoral nerve, the femoral nerve, the cutaneous branch of the femoral nerve and the lateral femoral cutaneous nerve. The anatomic landmarks and structures of importance are illustrated in the RISE (Rotterdam Institute of Surgical Endoscopy)-circle, figure 1 (Lange & Kleinrensink, Surgical Anatomy of the Abdomen, Elsevier gezondheidszorg, 2002).

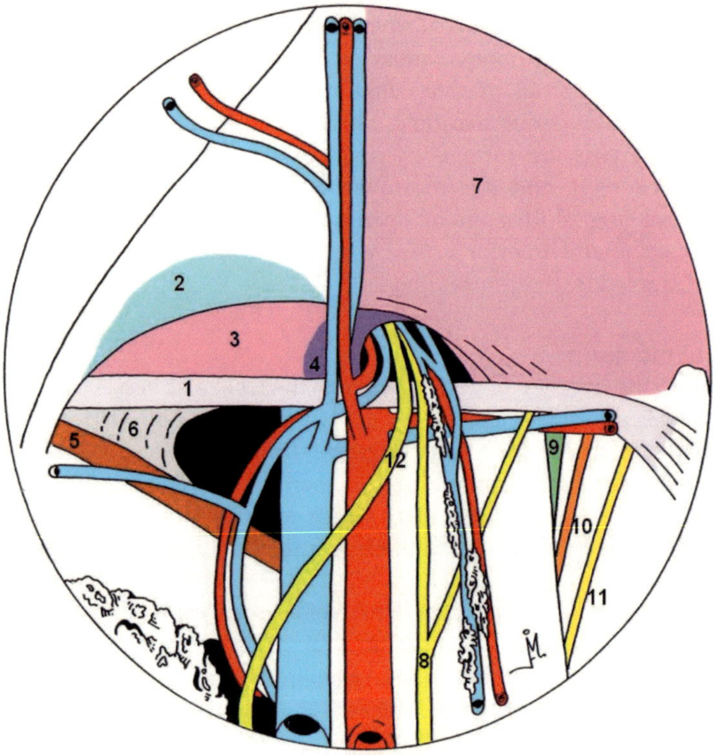

Ventromedial quadrant (direct hernia):
Base; iliopubic tract (of Thomson)(1)
Conjoint tendon(2)
Transeversalis fascia (caudal part of Hesselbach's triangle)(3)
Interfoveolar ligament (of Hesselbach)(4)
Branches of inferior epigastric vessels

Ventrolateral quadrant (indirect hernia):
Deep inguinal ring
Interfoveolar ligament (of Hesselbach)
Transversus abdominis muscle(7)

Dorsomedial quadrant (femoral hernia at femoral canal/lacuna vasorum):
Pectineal ligament (of Cooper)(5)
Lacunar ligament (of Gimbernat)(6)
Bladder
Corona mortis
External iliac vein
Prevesical space (of Retzius)

Dorsolateral quadrant (Kathouda's quadrant of doom):
Nerves of triangle of pain:
Femoral branch of genitofemoral nerve(8)
Femoral nerve(9)
Cutaneous branch of femoral nerve(10)
Lateral femoral cutaneous nerve (11)
Testicular vessels
Iliopectineal arch (ligament)
Vas deferens(12) or round ligament of uterus

Fig. 1. RISE (Rotterdam Institute of Surgical Endoscopy)-circle. Anatomic landmarks and structures of importance in inguinal hernia repair (Lange & Kleinrensink, Surgical Anatomy of the Abdomen, Elsevier gezondheidszorg, 2002).

The contents of the inguinal canal differ between male and female. In the male the spermatic cord is surrounded by the cremasteric fascia and cremaster muscle. Within the cord, the spermatic vessels and vas deferens are surrounded by the internal spermatic fascia. The spermatic vessels are the internal spermatic (testicular) artery, the deferential artery and the external spermatic (cremasteric) artery and vein, accompanied by the venous pampniform plexus. Between the internal spermatic and cremasteric fascia, the genital branch of the genitofemoral nerve and the cremasteric vessels are observed. The external spermatic fascia envelops the cord caudally to the superficial inguinal ring. The contents of the inguinal canal in the female include the round ligament of the uterus, the artery of the round ligament of the uterus (Samson's artery), the genital branch of the genitofemoral nerve, the ilio-inguinal nerve and lymphatics.

2.2 Different types of groin hernia

Groin hernias are divided in inguinal and femoral hernias depending on their position in relation to the inguinal ligament. This structure is formed by the external abdominal oblique aponeurosis and the fascia lata of the thigh. It is located in between the anterior superior iliac spine and the pubic tubercle of the pubic bone.

- **Inguinal hernias** are located cranially to the inguinal ligament. The occurrence of inguinal hernias can be explained by the persistence of a processus vaginalis (indirect or lateral hernia), by a deficient fascia transversalis (direct or medial hernia) or by a combination of both.
- **Femoral hernias** occur through the opening located caudally to the ligament inguinal and medially to the femoral vein.
- **Scrotal hernias** are sometimes classified separately but are in fact large indirect inguinal hernias with a hernia sac reaching into the scrotum.

To distinguish an inguinal hernia from a femoral hernia clinically, or an indirect hernia from a direct hernia, is often impossible and is of little importance since the operation is nowadays the same.

2.3 Inguinal hernia

The inguinal hernia is one of the most frequently occurring hernias with an estimated 20 million hernias repair operations around the world. Estimated incidence rate in the UK is 13 per 10,000 population per year (Primatesta & Goldacre, 1996). Indications for laparoscopic hernia repair are debatable. In case of a primary unilateral hernia an open mesh procedure is currently recommended by the European Hernia Society because of lower recurrence rate, costs and the possibility of local anaesthesia when compared with laparoscopic repair (Simons et al., 2009; Neumayer et al., 2004). From a socio-economic perspective, an endoscopic procedure is probably most cost-effective in patients participating in labour, especially in bilateral hernia. Furthermore chronic postoperative inguinal pain seems to be less generated by laparoscopic repair compared to conventional technique. All patients fit for general surgery without significant contraindications, including extreme age or significant cardiac, pulmonary or systemic illness, should be offered the option of a laparoscopic hernia repair (Simons et al., 2009).

2.3.1 Classification

To date, there is a lack of consensus among general surgeons and hernia specialists on classification systems for inguinal hernias. The traditional system classifies them into direct and indirect inguinal hernias. The persistence of a processus vaginalis is often described as a lateral or indirect hernia and a deficient transversalis fascia as a medial or direct hernia. In general clinical distinguishing is often difficult and irrelevant because treatment does not differ.

- **Indirect inguinal hernias** are the most common groin hernias in men and women. The hernia develops at the internal ring laterally to the inferior epigastric artery, in contrast to direct hernias which arise medially to the inferior epigastric vessels. Most indirect inguinal hernias are congenital, even though they may not become symptomatic until later in life (van Wessem et al., 2003). Indirect hernias develop more frequently on the right, because the right testicle descends later to the scrotum than the left.
- **Direct inguinal hernias** occur through the transversalis fascia at (the caudal part of) Hesselbach's triangle, formed by the inguinal ligament inferiorly, the inferior epigastric vessels laterally, and the rectus abdominis muscle medially. They occur as a result of a weakness of this part of the transversalis fascia, representing the floor of the inguinal canal. This weakness appears to be most often a congenitally diminished strength of collagen.

To be able to compare results most researchers choose to classify hernias by the classification of Nyhus (Nyhus, 1993):

- Type 1: Lateral/ indirect hernia with normal internal inguinal ring
- Type 2: Lateral/ indirect hernia with wide internal inguinal ring and normal transversalis fascia
- Type 3a: Medial/ direct hernia
- Type 3b: Pantaloon- or combined hernia
- Type 4: Recurrent hernia

2.3.2 Laparoscopic repair

The two laparoscopic techniques that are currently most frequently performed are the transabdominal preperitoneal repair (TAPP) and the total extraperitoneal repair (TEP). Both TAPP and TEP use a mesh in the preperitoneal space as described by Stoppa to replace the visceral sac. These laparoscopic techniques were originally developed for repair of difficult and recurrent inguinal hernias, which were known to have high recurrence rates (Stoppa et al., 1984). Performance of a laparoscopic repair may be technically challenging if the patient has had prior prostatic surgery or lower abdominal radiotherapy. Currently no indications exist in which TAPP is preferred over TEP.

One of the major challenges in learning laparoscopic hernia repair is the relative unfamiliarity of most surgeons to the anterior abdominal wall anatomy from a posterior view. This unfamiliarity is mainly responsible for the steep learning curve, which is associated with an increased incidence of complications. Although peroperative complications are rare in laparoscopic repair, they occur more often early during the learning curve and are more critical. Reported complications include trocar injury to bowel and bladder, vascular injury to the inferior epigastric and femoral vessels, nerve entrapment, transection of vas deferens, and trocar site haemorrhage (Davis & Arregui, 2003). After 250 laparoscopic repairs the recurrence rate is half of the rate of surgeons who have performed fewer repairs (Neumayer et al., 2004). If in future training would not be only incidental but more structurally organised with emphasis on anatomy including a defined proctorship it might be expected that learning curves will be much shorter.

2.3.3 TAPP

The TAPP approach was first described by Arregui and colleagues in 1992 (Arregui et al., 1992). Performing a TAPP, firstly laparoscopic access into the peritoneal cavity is obtained. After identification of the inguinal hernia the peritoneum is incised several centimetres above the peritoneal defect. The peritoneum is incised from the edge of the median umbilical ligament toward the anterior superior iliac spine. Repair of bilateral hernias can be performed through two separate peritoneal incisions or one long transverse incision between the superior iliac spines. Subsequently the preperitoneal avascular space between the posterior and anterior fascia transversalis is dissected to provide visualization of the myopectineal orifice of Fruchaud and size of the abdominal wall defect. In case of an indirect hernia, the cord structures are isolated and dissected free from the surrounding tissues. Simultaneously, the indirect hernia sac is identified on the anterolateral side and adherent to the cord. The cord must be skeletonized with care to minimize trauma to the vas deferens and the spermatic vessels. If the sac is sufficiently small, it can be reduced into the peritoneal cavity. If the hernia sac is large it should be completely dissected and divided beyond the internal ring, and the subsequent peritoneal defect closed with an endoloop suture. The distal end of the transsected sac should be left open to avoid formation of a hydrocèle. When reducing a direct hernia sac, a "pseudosac" may be present, which consists of fascia transversalis that overlies and adheres to the peritoneum and invaginates into the preperitoneal space during the dissection. This layer must be separated from the true hernia sac in order for the peritoneum to be released back fully into the peritoneal cavity. Once the pseudosac is freed, it will typically retract anteriorly into the direct hernia defect.

A large piece of mesh, of at least 15 x 10 cm, is used to cover the myopectineal orifice, including the direct, indirect and femoral hernia spaces. It is important to dissect the preperitoneal space to prevent folding of the edge of the mesh within this space. In addition the mesh should be placed with a slight overlap of the midline to ensure adequate coverage of the entire posterior floor of the groin. The intraperitoneal pressure that is evenly distributed over the large surface of the mesh keeps it in place making fixation of the mesh controversial provided that elimination of fixation does not lead to an increased rate of recurrence. The use of tackers or sutures is associated with increased chronic inguinal pain, use of postoperative narcotic analgesia, hospital length of stay and the development of postoperative urinary retention (Koch et al., 2006; Taylor et al., 2008). Suitable structures for fixation are the contralateral pubic tubercle and the symphysis pubis, Cooper's ligament or the tissue just above it and the posterior rectus sheath and transversalis fascia at least 2 cm above the hernia defect. Fixation is never performed below the iliopubic tract laterally to the internal spermatic vessels, to minimize the chance of damage to the lateral cutaneous nerve of the thigh or the femoral branch of the genitofemoral nerve. Finally the mesh is covered by securing the peritoneal flap back to its original position. The peritoneum should be closed to eliminate the risk of formation of adhesions between the mesh and the intestine. The configuration of the mesh is also important. A slit in the mesh, although attractive in concept, can lead to constriction of the cord structures or allow herniation through the slit.

When using the TAPP technique, in addition to femoral hernias, especially sacless sliding fatty inguinal hernias may be overlooked because of intact peritoneum. Therefore, in cases of clinically diagnosed inguinal hernias, the preperitoneal space should be inspected intraoperatively to avoid unsatisfactory results (Hollinsky & Sandberg, 2010). The main drawback of the TAPP procedure is that it requires entering of the peritoneal cavity with increased risk of injury to intra-abdominal organs. Further it requires subsequent incising the peritoneum with eventually peritoneal closure. The TEP was developed to avoid opening the peritoneal cavity with the associated risks.

2.3.4 TEP

The first to describe total extraperitoneal endoscopic repair of a inguinal hernias was Ferzli in 1992 (Ferzli et al., 1992). The procedure is initiated with a subumbilical incision followed by blunt dissection of the subcutaneous layer up to the anterior rectus sheath. The anterior rectus sheath is horizontally incised and with retractors the rectus abdominis muscle is searched and gently moved aside to bring the posterior rectus sheath in sight. The dissection of the preperitoneal space up to the symphysis is continued with a balloon. When using a balloon ('space maker') the thin fibrous layer of the posterior lamina of the fascia transversalis will rupture automatically to expose the 'proper preperitoneal space'. Subsequently a blunt tipped trocar is inserted into the preperitoneal space and a pneumoperitoneum is established. Additional trocars are inserted under direct vision. Further identification and repair of the inguinal hernia is identical to TAPP repair.

2.3.5 Acute repair

Acute repair of inguinal hernia is necessary in case of incarceration or strangulation. The cumulative probability of hernia getting strangulated after three months is 2.8% (Gallegos et al., 1991). The risks of postoperative complications following emergency surgery are high, and in elderly patients, mortality can be as high as 5% (Nilsson et al., 2007; Primatesta & Goldacre, 1996). Mostly open surgery is performed is case of incarceration to reduce the strangulated content, dissect the hernia sac and repair the abdominal wall defect. In 1993 Watson was the first to report acute laparoscopic reduction of the hernia with resection of the bowel (Watson et al., 1993). This reluctance may be attributable to the technical difficulties encountered in reducing the hernia sac and contents and the increased risk for iatrogenic injuries. The overall rate of complication, recurrence and hospital stay are very close to the rates documented in open repair for incarcerated hernias.

In case of a direct hernia, a releasing incision is made in the anteromedial aspect of the defect to avoid the inferior epigastric vessels. In indirect henias, the vessels are controlled, clipped and transected to facilitate the way for the releasing incision performed anteriorly in the deep (internal) ring at the 12 o'clock position toward the superficial (external) ring facilitating reduction of the incarcerated sac and its contents.

2.4 Laparoscopic repair of inguinal hernia in children

Laparoscopic repair of indirect hernia is nowadays one of the most frequently executed paediatric surgical procedures. Laparoscopic repair has the same advantages in children as in adults; less pain, faster recovery and better cosmesis. The overall incidence of inguinal hernias in childhood ranges from 0.8% to 4.4% (Bronsther et al., 1972), with predominantly indirect inguinal hernias. Incidence is higher in boys than in girls and in premature infants weighing less than 1000 grams with an incidence between 5 and 30% (Harper et al., 1975; Rajput et al., 1992). Inguinal hernias in children are mostly the result of a patent processus vaginalis because of an arrest of embryologic development. The processus vaginalis closes between the 36th and 40th week of gestation, which explains the increased incidence of hernia in premature infants. Because the descend of the left testis takes place before the right testicle the closure of the processus vaginalis is equally asymmetric, which results in 60% of patent processus vaginalis occurrence on the right side. However only in 25-50% of patients with a patent processus vaginalis a clinically significant hernia will become apparent (Lau et al., 2007; van Veen et al., 2007). Diagnosis of inguinal hernia in children is often based on anamnestic information from the parents or physical examination showing a bulge in the groin with crying or coughing. For timing of elective surgery no evidence is available, but surgical repair is usually performed as soon as possible after diagnosis even if the hernia is asymptomatic. This because of fear of incarceration, although its exact risk has not been studied in paediatric watchful waiting studies. Additionally between 24 and 30 % of patients present with incarcerated inguinal hernia (Moss & Hatch, 1991; Puri et al., 1984). Manual reduction is successful in a majority of patients (Moss & Hatch, 1991; Puri et al., 1984; Stringer et al., 1991). Many paediatric surgeons hospitalize children after successful manual reduction of incarcerated inguinal hernia and repair the hernia within 24-48 hours. The short delay allows the involved tissues to return to their normal texture before surgery. However some surgeons prefer immediate laparoscopy to inspect for vascular compromise of bowel, testicular or ovarian tissue with repair of the hernia.

The laparoscopic technique of inguinal hernia repair in children involves a high ligation of the indirect hernia sac without application of a mesh. First the spermatic cord is identified followed by dividing and tracing the sac in the inguinal channel without mobilization of the spermatic cord, with finally ligation of the hernia sac. In girls the surgeons must confirm before ligation that the hernia sac does not contain ovary, fallopian tube, or uterus. In addition to ligation and excision, plication of the floor of the inguinal canal may be necessary when the inguinal ring has been enlarged by repetitive herniation. In paediatric patients surgeons choose for primary repair because of the unknown effect of prosthesis material and because paediatric tissues have greater elasticity making primary repair more straightforward than in the adult population. A debate exists on exploration of the contralateral processus vaginalis during surgery to diagnose and treat asymptomatic contralateral hernia. The incidence of bilateral patent processus vaginalis has been described in literature between 5 and 12% (Manoharan et al., 2005; Miltenburg et al., 1997; Tackett et al., 1999). In open surgery routine contralateral exploration is not recommended, because exploration increases the risk of testicular atrophy and infertility after cord injury. However in laparoscopic hernia repair, evaluation and treatment of the contralateral processus vaginalis is feasible without significant risk of injury to the vas and vessels. Additionally it decreases the need for later contralateral surgery. Femoral hernias in children are rare, occurring in less than 1% of children with groin hernia. They often present as recurrent hernias after inguinal hernia repair, most likely because the surgeon was misled by the findings of a processus vaginalis at the initial surgery and missed the femoral hernia defect.

2.5 Sportsmen hernia

The term sportsmen hernia describes a condition characterized by chronic groin pain, without a demonstrable defect in the inguinal canal or abdominal wall, mostly observed in athletes. The pain flares with activity and results from chronic, repetitive trauma or stress to the musculotendinous portions of the groin. The exact pathophysiology is unclear and various theories have emerged in literature considering the presences of an occult hernia, a tear or microtears in the transversalis fascia or muscle strain. The theory that posterior weakness in the inguinal wall is the prime cause of groin pain in athletes is supported by the

fact that reinforcement of the posterior wall often resolves the groin pain (Malycha & Lovell, 1992; Paajanen et al., 2004; van Veen et al., 2007; Ziprin et al., 2008).
Sportmen hernia are found almost exclusively in men and only sporadically in women (Hackney, 1993; Moeller, 2007). For patients presenting with groin pain there are numerous other potential causes for groin pain, including hip articulation problems, taking in consideration the complex anatomy and biomechanics of the symphisis region. This makes the sportsmen hernia largely a clinical diagnosis of exclusion by physical examination and usage of radiological imaging. Sportsmen hernia can often be treated conservatively with rest, anti-inflammatiory medication and physiotherapy. However when pain persist after conservative treatment, laparoscopic mesh placement has shown to be a good option.

2.6 Femoral hernia

Femoral hernias account for 2 to 4% of groin hernias. Femoral hernia present more often in women and account for 23% of groin hernia operations in women, as compared with 1% in men (Dahlstrand et al., 2009). The reason for the higher incidence in women may relate to comparatively less bulky musculature at baseline and weakness of the pelvic floor muscles from previous childbirth. Additionally, the angle of the superior ramus of the pubic bone with the inguinal ligament is less acute in women, explaining for a wider femoral canal.
Femoral hernias frequently present acutely with signs of incarceration and require emergency surgery, with 40% emergency surgery in women and 28% in men. Subsequently bowel resection is required more often than in elective repair, 23% in emergency repair versus 0.6% in elective repair. Additionally, the risk for mortality is 5.4 times increased when compared to elective operations. This highlights the importance of repairing femoral hernias soon after presentation in an elective setting and suggests that there is no indication for watchful waiting in patients with femoral hernias. Strangulated Richter's type femoral hernias occur relatively frequent and carry a significant morbidity and mortality. The diagnosis of such strangulated femoral hernias is invariably delayed because they develop without intestinal obstruction and with minimal local manifestation until the entrapped knuckle of small bowel is gangrenous. A bruit over the femoral vein is an indication that the adjacent femoral hernia is incarcerated or strangulated because the hernia compresses the vein. Both open and laparoscopic approaches have been described for repair of femoral hernia. If a large volume of intra-abdominal contents has protruded into the hernia sac, or if there is bowel in the defect, laparoscopy is the operation of choice. Intra-abdominal contents are best removed by preperitoneal approach. Additionally during laparoscopy the viability of the bowel can be inspected.

3. Hernias of the ventral abdominal wall

Ventral hernias result from defects in the ventral abdominal wall and are typically classified by etiology and location. They can develop as a result of prior surgery (incisional and trocar site hernia) or at anatomical congenital weak locations (umbilical, epigastric and Spigelian hernia). The abdominal wall exists of five muscles (external oblique, internal oblique, transversus abdominis, rectus abdominis and pyramidal muscles) that protect the viscera. Herniation of the abdominal wall during activity is prevented by the transverse abdominal muscles. In adults the external oblique muscle is aponeurotic up to the level of the umbilicus. The caudal boundary of the posterior layer of the rectus sheath is the linea semicircularis, usually located 5 cm caudally to the umbilicus. Cranially to it, the medial aponeuroses of the three lateral muscles give rise to the anterior and posterior layers of the rectus sheath, enveloping the lateral border of the rectus sheath. Cranially to the umbilicus, the muscular part of the transversus abdominis muscle extends more medially than the muscular parts of the oblique muscles. Cranially to the umbilicus the abdominal cavity has an integral muscular cover, except for the linea alba in the midline. Caudally to the umbilicus, the medial borders of the external oblique and transversus abdominis muscles decline laterally, and the medial border of the internal oblique muscle medially. The transversus abdominis muscle is connected to the rectus sheath by its aponeurosis, the fascia of Spigel, which is cutaneously represented by the linea semilunaris (Lange & Kleinrensink, Surgical Anatomy of the Abdomen, Elsevier gezondheidszorg, 2002).

3.1 Technique of laparoscopic ventral hernia repair

After establishing a pneumoperitoneum and introducing trocars, laparoscopic ventral hernia repair is started with lysis of intra-abdominal adhesions with caution to prevent bowel injury. After reduction of the hernial content, the hernia sac is commonly left in situ. In doing so seroma formation can occur. The fascial defect is measured and a piece of mesh able to cover the defect with an overlap of at least 3 to 5 cm is cut in shape. The intra-abdominal pressure should be lowered to make the abdominal wall more natural shaped and to allow a flat placement of the mesh. The mesh is tension-free implanted and fixated with tackers (every 2 cm) and possibly additional transabdominal sutures (at least every 5 cm). Tackers can be placed in one row or a double row (double-crown technique). Drains are not typically used after laparoscopic hernia repair. Complications than can occur are related to laparoscopy (i.e. bowel injury and subsequent enterotomy), nerve injury by tackers or transabdominal sutures, adhesion formation to the mesh and fixation material, mesh infection and mesh dislocation.

3.2 Incisional hernia

An incisional hernia develops when the fascial tissue fails to heal at the incision site of a prior laparotomy. Incisional hernia is a common complication and represents about 80% of all ventral hernias. The highest incidence of incisional hernias is observed after midline laparotomy, the most common incision for abdominal surgery. In decreasing order of incidence, incisional hernias are diagnosed after upper midline incisions, lower midline incisions, transverse incisions and subcostal incisions. Incisional hernias are also described after paramedian, McBurney, Pfannenstiel and flank incisions.

Conditions that impair wound healing make patients susceptible to the development of an incisional hernia, such as wound infection, diabetes mellitus, obesity, immunosuppressive drugs, aneurysm of the abdominal aorta, connective tissue disorders and smoking. Approximately 15-20% of all patients will develop an incisional hernia after midline laparotomy (Hoer et al., 2002; Millbourn et al., 2009; Mudge & Hughes, 1985). The incidence rises up to 35% in patients with an aneurysm of the abdominal aorta (Adye & Luna, 1998; Bevis et al., 2010). Besides patient co-morbidities, technical failure contributes to the development of incisional hernia. After midline laparotomy the fascia should be closed with a non absorbable or slowly-absorbable continuous suture in a suture length to wound length ratio of 4:1 or more to lower the rate of incisional hernia (Hodgson et al., 2000; van 't Riet et al., 2002).

Around 40% of incisional hernias are symptomatic and approximately 1 out of every 3 incisional hernias is repaired in an elective or emergency setting. In the United States, approximately 4 to 5 million laparotomies are performed annually, leading to 400,000 to 500,000 incisional hernias, of which approximately 200,000 repairs are performed (Burger et al., 2004).

3.2.1 Classification

Different classification systems for incisional hernias are available. The European Hernia Society developed a classification for incisional hernias which takes in account the location, size and possible recurrence of the incisional hernia (Muysoms et al., 2009). This classification allows comparison of publications and future studies on treatment and outcome of incisional hernia repair. Incisional hernias are classified by:

- Location:
  - Midline: M1 (subxiphoidal), M2 (epigastric), M3 (umbilical), M4 (infraumbilical) and M5 (suprapubic)
  - Lateral: L1 (subcostal), L2 (flank), L3 (iliac) and L4 (lumbar)
- Width: W1 (smaller than 4 cm), W2 (4 to 10 cm), W3 (10 cm or more)
- Recurrence: yes or no

The Ventral Hernia Working Group (USA) developed a hernia grading system based on the characteristics of the patient and the wound (Ventral Hernia Working et al., 2010). Using this system a surgeon can assess the risk for surgical-site occurrences (infection, seroma, wound dehiscence, and the formation of enterocutaneous fistulae) for individual patients and thereby select the appropriate surgical technique, repair material, and overall clinical approach for the patient. The grading system with assessment of risk for surgical site occurrences:

- Grade 1, Low risk: patients without a history of wound infection and a low risk of complications
- Grade 2, Co-morbid: patients with one or more co-morbidities of smoking, obesity, diabetes mellitus, COPD, immunosuppression.
- Grade 3, Potentially contaminated: patients with a previous wound infection, stoma present or operation with violation of the gastrointestinal tract.
- Grade 4, Infected: patients with an infected mesh or septic dehiscence.

3.2.2 Recurrence after laparoscopic repair

Luijendijk (2000) and Burger (2004) stressed the importance of mesh reinforcement for incisional hernia repair, with long-term recurrence rates of 60% in the suture repair group and 32% in the mesh group. Recurrence rates following laparoscopic and open ventral hernia repair with prosthetic reinforcement are comparable (Bingener et al., 2007; Goodney et al., 2002; Sajid et al., 2009). Wound infection is one of the main contributors to the recurrence rate after laparoscopic ventral hernia repair, but surgical-technical failure is underestimated. Technical failure (i.e. inadequate mesh fixation, mesh overlap and lateral detachment) accounts for approximately 50% of the recurrences and infection for an additional 25% (Awad et al., 2005). This explains the major decrease of recurrences in experienced hands, compared to non-experts. By laparoscopic ventral hernia repair the intraperitoneally placed mesh is pushed outward and held in place by the natural intra-abdominal pressure. Another benefit of the laparoscopic approach is identifying small fascial defects, known as "Swiss cheese" defects, which may be missed during open repair. These small fascial defects are thought to be the major source of incisional hernia recurrence and therefore identification is important for a successful hernia repair.

3.3 Trocar site heria

Trocar site hernias (TSH) have an overall low incidence of less than 1% in adults. The incidence of TSH increases with the size of the used trocar. Almost all TSH develop from trocars of 10 mm or above. Most TSH are located at the umbilical port site, where the largest trocars are used and the fascia is expanded to remove surgical specimen. To prevent TSH the fascia of trocar sites of 10 mm or above should be sutured with a non-absorbable or slowly-absorbable suture, especially in the umbilical area. Co-morbidities as diabetes, smoking and obesity might be risk factors for TSH (Helgstrand et al., 2010). The use of a Veress Needle (instead of an open introduction technique) and a sharp trocar (compared to a conical shaped trocar) are associated with a higher incidence of TSH. In young children the reported incidence of TSH is higher than in adults (5% vs 1%). Herniation of the small sized bowels through trocar ports of 3-5 mm is described, which shows the importance of closing all trocar port fascias in paediatric patients.

3.4 Umbilical hernia

A congenital umbilical hernia develops when the umbilical scar fails to heal at birth. The incidence of congenital umbilical hernia is 10-30%, with a higher incidence in African American children than in Caucasian children. During the first 1.5 year of life most umbilical hernias close and at the age of 5 almost all children have complete closure of the umbilical ring. Repair should not be considered before an age of 3 years and only in children with large hernias that do not decrease in size or are symptomatic. In the rare case of incarceration, repair is necessary to avoid strangulation (Katz, 2001). Umbilical hernias in adults are an acquired defect in over 90% and are three times more frequently seen in women than in men. The development of an umbilical hernia is associated with obesity, abdominal distension, ascites and pregnancy. In females umbilical hernias are more frequent among multipara and are often easily reducible. Men often present with an incarcerated umbilical hernia, most often containing herniated omentum or preperitoneal fat. Laparoscopic umbilical hernia repair with an onlay patch is a safe and efficacious technique, and compared to open repair has the advantages of a lower rate of wound complications, reduced postoperative pain, shorter hospital stay and a diminished morbidity rate (Lau & Patil, 2003; Toy et al., 1998). Hernia repair in the presence of ascites due to cirrhosis should be considered elective, since emergency repair has an associated morbidity of 70% and mortality of 5% (Telem et al., 2010). Even in patients with mild to moderate cirrhosis correction can be safely performed (Heniford et al., 2000).

3.5 Epigastric hernia

An epigastric hernia is a defect in the linea alba located between the xyphoid process and umbilicus. Epigastric hernias are comparable to umbilical hernias, but smaller in size, often less than 1 cm (Lang et al., 2002). Epigastric hernias are acquired defects with an incidence of 3-5%, three times more frequent in men than in women and mostly diagnosed between 40-60 years. Associated factors for the development of epigastric hernias are increased intra-abdominal pressure and muscle or linea alba weakness. During laparoscopy an epigastric hernia can be difficult to visualize due to lack of peritoneal involvement through the hernia defect. Frequently epigastric hernias present incarcerated and in general only contain omentum or preperitoneal fat. Because of the small defect the hernia defect mostly need to be enlarged to reduce the hernial sac and its content.

3.6 Spigelian hernia

A Spigelian hernia is relatively rare, but more often diagnosed since the introduction of CT-scan and laparoscopy. The Spigelian hernia occurs along the semilunar line at the level of the absence of the posterior rectus sheath (semicircular line, below the umbilicus). Almost all Spigelian hernias are interparietal due to the intact external oblique aponeurosis covering the hernia. A large Spigelian hernia is most often found laterally and inferior to its defect in the space directly posterior to the external oblique muscle.

The Spigelian hernia has different factors of etiology (Lange & Kleinrensink, Surgical Anatomy of the Abdomen, Elsevier gezondheidszorg, 2002):

- Muscular gap between linea semilunaris and medial boundaries of oblique and transversus abdominis muscles, caudally to umbilicus,
- Maximal width of aponeurosis of transversus abdominis muscle at crossing of semicircular and semilunar lines.
- Parallelism of fibers of internal oblique and transversus abdominis muscles between arcuate line and Hesselbach's triangle.
- Blending of aponeuroses of internal oblique and transversus abdominis muscle into one separate structure, caudally to arcuate line.

Clinical diagnosis of a Spigelian hernia is challenging, but imaging with ultrasonography or CT-scan will confirm the presence of the hernia. Up to 20% of Spigelian hernias present incarcerated and therefore elective repair is indicated when diagnosed. The technique of laparoscopic repair is similar to other ventral hernia repairs. Compared to open repair, laparoscopic repair of Spigelian hernias is associated with a decreased morbidity, shorter hospital stay and low recurrence rate (Moreno-Egea et al., 2002).

4. Diaphragmatic or hiatal hernia

The diaphragm consists of striated muscle and has a collagenous central tendon, which is cranially blended with the pericardium. The esophageal hiatus is a 2-3 cm long muscular tunnel with a diameter of 3.5 cm, located 2-3 cm to the left at the peripheral muscular part of the diaphragm. The right crus and dorsal median arcuate ligament encircle the esophagus. Through the esophageal hiatus, besides the esophagus, pass the vagus trunks, sensory phrenico-abdominal branch of left phrenic nerve to the pancreas and peritoneum, esophageal vessels and retro-esophageal fat.

The natural anti-reflux mechanism is complex with several synergistic elements. A crucial element in preventing reflux is the circular muscular lower esophageal sphincter (LES) of 3.5 cm, extending from the distal esophagus down to the angle of His. The LES is autonomically controlled by vagal stimulation through intramural plexuses and enterohormones. Normally at least 1 cm of the LES is held intra-abdominally by the circular bilaminar phrenico-esophageal ligament. The ventral descending leaf connects the adventitia and muscular coat of the distal esophagus to the hiatus and is continuous with the lesser omentum at the right side of the esophagus. The supradiaphragmatic ascending leaf is

elastic and permits movement during swallowing and breathing. The extrinsic component of the anti-reflux mechanism is the pinching action of the right crus of the diaphragm. The right crus narrows the hiatus and increases the angle between the ventrally bended distal esophagus and the cardia. The LES and crus normally supplement each other in preventing acid reflux during swallowing or acute increased intra-abdominal pressure (Lange & Kleinrensink, Surgical Anatomy of the Abdomen, Elsevier gezondheidszorg, 2002).
A diaphragmatic or hiatal hernia occurs after enlargement of the hiatus and is a common disorder of the digestive tract. Cranial movement of the esophagus with protrusion of abdominal content (stomach in general) into the thoracic cavity can occur through the widened hiatus. This natural antireflux function is often disrupted by the presence of a hiatal hernia and is strongly associated with gastro-esophageal reflux disease (GERD). Hiatal hernias larger than 3 cm are a risk factor for erosive GERD and Barrett's esophagus.

4.1 Classification

Anatomically four different types of hiatal hernias can be recognised:

- Type 1: Sliding hernia. The gastroesophageal junction migrates into the thoracic cavity.
- Type 2: Paraesophageal hernia. Herniation of the gastric fundus anterior to a normally positioned gastroesophageal junction.
- Type 3: Mixed sliding and paraesophageal hernia.
- Type 4: Herniation of additional organs. The whole stomach and sometimes additional visceral organs (i.e. colon, omentum or spleen) migrate into the thoracic cavity. This can result in a stomach in upside-down position.

Up to 95% of all hiatal hernias can be classified as a type 1, sliding hernia. Type 3 and type 4 hiatal hernias tend to be large or giant hernias. Large or giant hernias are defined as at least 30%-50% of the stomach herniating into the thoracic cavity. Patients with hiatal hernia can experience symptoms of GERD, as epigastric pain, dysphagia, heartburn, but in more severe cases gastric hemorrhaging, vomiting and cardiopulmonary problems with dyspnea. Paraesophageal hernias account for less than 5% of all hiatal hernias but can have potentially life-threatening complications, such as obstruction, dilatation, necrosis with perforation or bleeding of the stomach.

4.2 Laparoscopic repair

Patients with sliding hernias and GERD should be considered for elective surgical repair. The objectives of hiatal hernia surgery for GERD are repair of the intrinsic component of the anti-reflux mechanism by bringing back LES into the hiatal tunnel and repair of the extrinsic component of the anti-reflux mechanism by narrowing the hiatus. Paraesophageal hernias (type 2, 3 and 4) should be repaired when symptomatic, due to the associated possible life-threatening complications. The laparoscopic approach to hiatal hernia repair has the benefit of easy exposure of the hiatus area and a good vision into the mediastinum. To restore the intrinsic component of anti-reflux mechanism a laparoscopic fundoplication is performed. The laparoscopic Nissen fundoplication (360° wrap) is the most frequently applied procedure. Other possible fundoplications are the posterior Toupet (270° wrap) and anterior Dor (180° wrap). The laparoscopic Nissen fundoplication is equally effective in patients with GERD or with paraesophageal hernia and is the preferred fundoplication procedure. The failure rate of a Nissen fundoplication for GERD is between 2-30%, depending whether failure is defined as resumption of conservative treatment or failure requiring reoperation.

The failure rate of a Nissen fundoplication for paraesophageal hernia is 7-33%, depending whether failure is defined anatomically or symptomatically. Patient satisfaction after laparoscopic Nissen fundoplication with 5-year follow-up is 86-96% (Lafullarde et al., 2001; Smith et al., 2005). Complications associated with laparoscopic hiatal hernia surgery include stenosis, pulmonary complications (pneumonia, pneumothorax, pulmonary edema) and gastrointestinal complications (bleeding, perforation, dysphagia).

4.2.1 Laparoscopic fundoplication technique

The patient should be positioned supine on a split leg table with arms out and in a steep reverse Trendelenburg position to help expose the hiatus. After establishing a pneumoperitoneum five trocars are inserted. A liver retractor is used to retract the left liver lobe and expose the anterior surface of the proximal stomach near the gastroesophageal junction. The hepatogastric omentum should be opened over the caudate lobe of the liver, just above the hepatic branch of the vagal nerve, exposing the right crus of the diaphragm. Caution should be taken for an aberrant left hepatic artery in this area, present in approximately 20% of patients. Over left, anteriorly the phrenoesophageal ligament can be divided to its apex on the right. The right and left crus are dissected from its base to the crural arch and the retroesophageal window is gently opened, protecting the posterior vagal nerve. A penrose drain can be used to retract the esophagus during further dissecting, until at least 2-3 cm of distal esophagus can be pulled below the diaphragm without tension. During this dissection caution should be taken not to injure the anterior and posterior vagal nerves, left or right pleura and aorta. The gastric fundus should be mobilized from 10-15 cm inferior to the angle of His, isolating and dividing the short gastric vessels, working back to the gastroesophageal junction. It is important to avoid excessive traction when dividing all posterior gastric arteries and other attachments, to prevent tearing of the short gastric arteries or splenic capsule. In some patients the proximal fundus and upper pole of the spleen are closely attached, making this part of the dissection quite difficult. The mobilized gastric fundus is brought through the retroesophageal window and around the distal esophagus anteriorly to ensure adequate mobilization. If the gastric fundus is released and exits the retroesophageal window, further mobilization is necessary. The fundoplication can be completed around a 50-60 French dilator. The internal diameter of the wrap should exceed the external diameter of the esophagus. Two or three non-absorbable sutures are placed with bites taking full thickness gastric fundus and partial thickness anterior esophageal wall, avoiding the anterior vagal nerve. When completed the wrap should be no greater than 2 cm in length and optimally a bit of distal esophagus should be visible distally to the wrap. Additional sutures from the wrap to the diaphragm can be placed. The crus can be closed using non-absorbable stitches.

4.2.2 Paraesophageal hernia repair

Laparoscopic repair of a paraesophageal hernia consists of reduction of the stomach and gastroesophageal junction into the abdominal cavity, complete excision of the peritoneal hernia sac from the mediastinum, and repair of the esophageal hiatus. Following a Nissen fundoplication, the crus should be closed using non-absorbable sutures. In case of a large hiatus, additional anterior or lateral crural stitches can be added. An additional anterior gastropexy can be performed in case of a very large or shortened esophagus. The anterior stomach wall and the antrum should be sutured to the abdominal wall.

Laparoscopic repair of paraesophageal hernias is superior to open repair, with an associated decreased length of hospital stay, complication rate and recurrence rate (Draaisma et al., 2005). Long-term good functional results are observed in 75% and (symptomatic) recurrences in 15% after large paraesophageal hernia repair (Poncet et al., 2010). Postoperative complications associated with laparoscopic large paraesophageal hernia repair are intrathoracal wrap migration, relative stenosis of the cardia, gastric volvulus or strangulation, pneumothorax, pneumonia and dysphagia. A synthetic mesh can be used to reinforce the hiatal repair, but is still controversial. A mesh might be associated with a decreased recurrence rate, but may give rise to serious complications like prosthetic migration, esophageal perforation, dysphagia and mesh infection. Since the majority of paraesophageal hernias are mixed sliding and paraesophageal hernias, an insufficient LES with GERD-symptoms may remain after surgery and antireflux medication is still required.

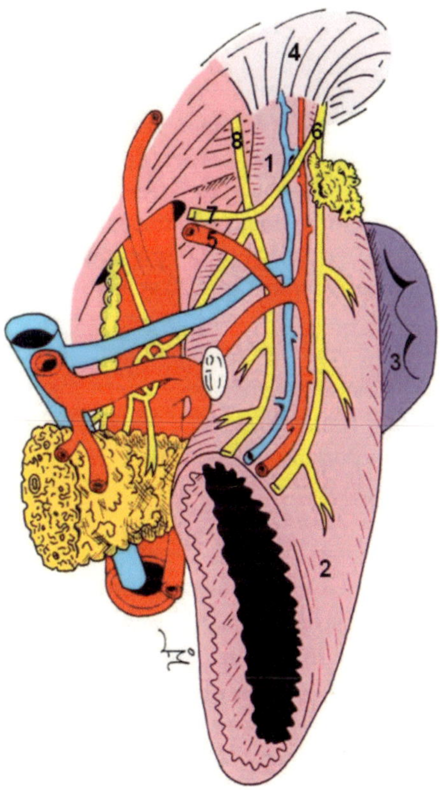

Esophagus (1)
Gastric fundus (2)
Splenic capsule (3)
Phrenico-esophageal ligament (4)
Abberant left hepatic artery (5)
Anterior vagus nerve (6)
Hepatic branch (7)
Posterior vagus nerve (8)

Fig. 2. Anatomic landmarks and structures of importance in hiatal hernia repair (Lange & Kleinrensink, Surgical Anatomy of the Abdomen, Elsevier gezondheidszorg, 2002)

4.3 Treatment of recurrence

The reported failure following laparoscopic Nissen fundoplication for GERD and paraesophageal hernia is between 2-33%. Although failure of fundoplication is unusual when performed by an experienced surgeon, wrap herniation ('slipped Nissen') is the most common mechanism of failure. Other causes of failure are represented by disrupted fundoplication, slipped fundoplication, crural stenosis, too tight wrap, misplaced fundoplication or twisted fundoplication. In carefully selected patients who have recurrent or persistent symptoms (heartburn, dysphagia, chest pain, regurgitation, asthma, hoarsness or laryngitis) after laparoscopic or open fundoplication a laparoscopic redo fundoplication can be safely performed by an experienced surgeon. The overall conversion rate of redo laparoscopic fundoplication is 10%. Complications occur in approximately 15%, slightly increasing with multiple redos. After redo laparoscopic fundoplication 70% of patients is GERD-related symptom free (Smith et al., 2005).

5. Parastomal hernia

Occurrence of parastomal herniation is a common complication after stoma formation. The reported incidence of parastomal hernias varies from 28% in ileostomies to 56% in colostomies (Carne et al., 2003; LeBlanc et al., 2005; Rieger et al., 2004). A parastomal hernia is more likely to occur when the stoma emerges through the semilunar line rather than the rectus sheath. Although most hernias become present within two years after stoma construction, the risk of herniation extends up to 20 years.

5.1 Classification

Parastomal hernias can be classified in four types:

- Subcutaneous type: subcutaneous hernia sac
- Interstitial type: hernia sac within the aponeurotic layers of the abdomen
- Perstomal type: bowel prolapsing through a circumferential hernia sac enclosing the stoma
- Intrastomal: hernia sac between the intestinal wall and the everted intestinal layer

Symptoms patients may experience are pain, poor fitting of stoma-material resulting in leakage of stomal contents, obstruction, incarceration and cosmetic disfigurement. Fortunately, most parastomal hernias can be treated conservatively and surgical intervention is only indicated in 15% of patients with parastomal hernias (Hansson et al., 2003). Recurrence rates after surgical repair are reported up to 76%, and can be explained by the underlying defect in wound healing and collagen metabolism in most patients.

5.2 Laparoscopic repair

Parastomal hernia repair with prosthetic mesh is recommended, since recurrence rates are unsatisfactory high after suture repair or relocation of the stoma. Complications that can arise with mesh placement for parastomal hernia are mesh-infection, fistula formation and adhesion formation. Laparoscopic repair is effective in correction of these hernias and has the advantages of improved vision and definition of the fascial edges of the hernia.

Laparoscopic techniques for repair of parastomal hernia with prosthetic mesh can be divided in 'keyhole techniques' and modified 'Sugarbaker techniques'. All involve introduction of trocars, extensive adhesiolysis, and identifying and measuring the fascial

defect. A mesh should provide at least 5 cm of overlap of the fascial edges and should be secured with tacks or constructed with transfascial sutures.
Several different 'keyhole techniques' have been described, which have in common that a mesh is placed with a central hole or slit in the mesh to allow the bowel to pass through the mesh to the stoma site. One of the main drawbacks is shrinkage of the mesh that can result in obstruction or recurrent herniation by enlargement of the hole. In the modified Sugarbaker technique no hole is made in the mesh but the bowel to the stoma is lateralized and covered by the mesh (Berger & Bientzle, 2007; Mancini et al., 2007; Sugarbaker, 1985). The mesh is secured to the abdominal wall at the margin of the mesh at 5 cm intervals. A second row of tackers is placed at the margin of the hernia defect with additional tackers at each side of the colon. Both techniques are promising, however long term results are not yet available. Perhaps prevention of development of parastomal hernia by placement of a lightweight sublay mesh is the key (Janes et al., 2004).

6. References

Adye, B., & Luna, G. (1998). Incidence of abdominal wall hernia in aortic surgery. *Am J Surg, 175*(5), 400-402.

Arregui, M. E., Davis, C. J., Yucel, O., & Nagan, R. F. (1992). Laparoscopic mesh repair of inguinal hernia using a preperitoneal approach: a preliminary report. *Surg Laparosc Endosc, 2*(1), 53-58.

Awad, Z. T., Puri, V., LeBlanc, K., Stoppa, R., Fitzgibbons, R. J., Jr., Iqbal, A., et al. (2005). Mechanisms of ventral hernia recurrence after mesh repair and a new proposed classification. *J Am Coll Surg, 201*(1), 132-140.

Bassini, E. (1887). Sulla cura radicale dell'ernia inguinale. *Arch Soc Ital Chir, 4*, 380.

Berger, D., & Bientzle, M. (2007). Laparoscopic repair of parastomal hernias: a single surgeon's experience in 66 patients. *Dis Colon Rectum, 50*(10), 1668-1673.

Bevis, P. M., Windhaber, R. A., Lear, P. A., Poskitt, K. R., Earnshaw, J. J., & Mitchell, D. C. (2010). Randomized clinical trial of mesh versus sutured wound closure after open abdominal aortic aneurysm surgery. *Br J Surg, 97*(10), 1497-1502.

Bingener, J., Buck, L., Richards, M., Michalek, J., Schwesinger, W., & Sirinek, K. (2007). Long-term outcomes in laparoscopic vs open ventral hernia repair. *Arch Surg, 142*(6), 562-567.

Bogojavalensky, S. (1989). laparoscopic treatment of inguinal and femoral hernia (video presentation). In: Proceedings of the 18th Annual Meeting of the American Association of Gynecological Laparoscopists. *Washington DC, USA.*

Bronsther, B., Abrams, M. W., & Elboim, C. (1972). Inguinal hernias in children--a study of 1,000 cases and a review of the literature. *J Am Med Womens Assoc, 27*(10), 522-525 passim.

Burger, J. W., Luijendijk, R. W., Hop, W. C., Halm, J. A., Verdaasdonk, E. G., & Jeekel, J. (2004). Long-term follow-up of a randomized controlled trial of suture versus mesh repair of incisional hernia. *Ann Surg, 240*(4), 578-583; discussion 583-575.

Carne, P. W., Robertson, G. M., & Frizelle, F. A. (2003). Parastomal hernia. *Br J Surg, 90*(7), 784-793.

Dahlstrand, U., Wollert, S., Nordin, P., Sandblom, G., & Gunnarsson, U. (2009). Emergency femoral hernia repair: a study based on a national register. *Ann Surg, 249*(4), 672-676.

Davis, C. J., & Arregui, M. E. (2003). Laparoscopic repair for groin hernias. *Surg Clin North Am, 83*(5), 1141-1161.

Draaisma, W. A., Gooszen, H. G., Tournoij, E., & Broeders, I. A. (2005). Controversies in paraesophageal hernia repair: a review of literature. *Surg Endosc, 19*(10), 1300-1308.

Ferzli, G. S., Massad, A., & Albert, P. (1992). Extraperitoneal endoscopic inguinal hernia repair. *J Laparoendosc Surg, 2*(6), 281-286.

Fruchaud, H. (1953). [The effect of the upright position proper to man upon the anatomy of the inguinal region: surgical consequences; anatomic bases of surgical treatment of inguinal hernia]

Du retentissement de la position debout propre a l'homme sur l'anatomie de la region de l'aine: consequences chirurgicales; les bases anatomiques du traitement chirurgical des hernies de l'aine. *Mem Acad Chir (Paris), 79*(25-6), 652-661.

Gallegos, N. C., Dawson, J., Jarvis, M., & Hobsley, M. (1991). Risk of strangulation in groin hernias. *Br J Surg, 78*(10), 1171-1173.

Ger, R. (1982). The management of certain abdominal herniae by intra-abdominal closure of the neck of the sac. Preliminary communication. *Ann R Coll Surg Engl, 64*(5), 342-344.

Goodney, P. P., Birkmeyer, C. M., & Birkmeyer, J. D. (2002). Short-term outcomes of laparoscopic and open ventral hernia repair: a meta-analysis. *Arch Surg, 137*(10), 1161-1165.

Hackney, R. G. (1993). The sports hernia: a cause of chronic groin pain. *Br J Sports Med, 27*(1), 58-62.

Hansson, B. M., van Nieuwenhoven, E. J., & Bleichrodt, R. P. (2003). Promising new technique in the repair of parastomal hernia. *Surg Endosc, 17*(11), 1789-1791.

Harper, R. G., Garcia, A., & Sia, C. (1975). Inguinal hernia: a common problem of premature infants weighing 1,000 grams or less at birth. *Pediatrics, 56*(1), 112-115.

Helgstrand, F., Rosenberg, J., & Bisgaard, T. (2010). Trocar site hernia after laparoscopic surgery: a qualitative systematic review. *Hernia.*

Heniford, B. T., Park, A., Ramshaw, B. J., & Voeller, G. (2000). Laparoscopic ventral and incisional hernia repair in 407 patients. *J Am Coll Surg, 190*(6), 645-650.

Hodgson, N. C., Malthaner, R. A., & Ostbye, T. (2000). The search for an ideal method of abdominal fascial closure: a meta-analysis. *Ann Surg, 231*(3), 436-442.

Hoer, J., Lawong, G., Klinge, U., & Schumpelick, V. (2002). [Factors influencing the development of incisional hernia. A retrospective study of 2,983 laparotomy patients over a period of 10 years]

Einflussfaktoren der Narbenhernienentstehung. Retrospektive Untersuchung an 2.983 laparotomierten Patienten uber einen Zeitraum von 10 Jahren. *Chirurg, 73*(5), 474-480.

Hollinsky, C., & Sandberg, S. (2010). Clinically diagnosed groin hernias without a peritoneal sac at laparoscopy--what to do? *Am J Surg, 199*(6), 730-735.

Janes, A., Cengiz, Y., & Israelsson, L. A. (2004). Randomized clinical trial of the use of a prosthetic mesh to prevent parastomal hernia. *Br J Surg, 91*(3), 280-282.

Katz, D. A. (2001). Evaluation and management of inguinal and umbilical hernias. *Pediatr Ann, 30*(12), 729-735.

Koch, C. A., Greenlee, S. M., Larson, D. R., Harrington, J. R., & Farley, D. R. (2006). Randomized prospective study of totally extraperitoneal inguinal hernia repair: fixation versus no fixation of mesh. *JSLS, 10*(4), 457-460.

Lafullarde, T., Watson, D. I., Jamieson, G. G., Myers, J. C., Game, P. A., & Devitt, P. G. (2001). Laparoscopic Nissen fundoplication: five-year results and beyond. *Arch Surg, 136*(2), 180-184.

Lang, B., Lau, H., & Lee, F. (2002). Epigastric hernia and its etiology. *Hernia, 6*(3), 148-150.

Lange & Kleinrensink, *Surgical Anatomy of the Abdomen*, Elsevier gezondheidszorg, 2002.

Lau, H., & Patil, N. G. (2003). Umbilical hernia in adults. *Surg Endosc, 17*(12), 2016-2020.

Lau, S. T., Lee, Y. H., & Caty, M. G. (2007). Current management of hernias and hydroceles. *Semin Pediatr Surg, 16*(1), 50-57.

LeBlanc, K. A., Bellanger, D. E., Whitaker, J. M., & Hausmann, M. G. (2005). Laparoscopic parastomal hernia repair. *Hernia, 9*(2), 140-144.

Luijendijk, R. W., Hop, W. C., van den Tol, M. P., de Lange, D. C., Braaksma, M. M., JN, I. J., et al. (2000). A comparison of suture repair with mesh repair for incisional hernia. *N Engl J Med, 343*(6), 392-398.

Malycha, P., & Lovell, G. (1992). Inguinal surgery in athletes with chronic groin pain: the 'sportsman's' hernia. *Aust N Z J Surg, 62*(2), 123-125.

Mancini, G. J., McClusky, D. A., 3rd, Khaitan, L., Goldenberg, E. A., Heniford, B. T., Novitsky, Y. W., et al. (2007). Laparoscopic parastomal hernia repair using a nonslit mesh technique. *Surg Endosc, 21*(9), 1487-1491.

Manoharan, S., Samarakkody, U., Kulkarni, M., Blakelock, R., & Brown, S. (2005). Evidence-based change of practice in the management of unilateral inguinal hernia. *J Pediatr Surg, 40*(7), 1163-1166.

Millbourn, D., Cengiz, Y., & Israelsson, L. A. (2009). Effect of stitch length on wound complications after closure of midline incisions: a randomized controlled trial. *Arch Surg, 144*(11), 1056-1059.

Miltenburg, D. M., Nuchtern, J. G., Jaksic, T., Kozinetz, C. A., & Brandt, M. L. (1997). Meta-analysis of the risk of metachronous hernia in infants and children. *Am J Surg, 174*(6), 741-744.

Moeller, J. L. (2007). Sportsman's hernia. *Curr Sports Med Rep, 6*(2), 111-114.

Moreno-Egea, A., Carrasco, L., Girela, E., Martin, J. G., Aguayo, J. L., & Canteras, M. (2002). Open vs laparoscopic repair of spigelian hernia: a prospective randomized trial. *Arch Surg, 137*(11), 1266-1268.

Moss, R. L., & Hatch, E. I., Jr. (1991). Inguinal hernia repair in early infancy. *Am J Surg, 161*(5), 596-599.

Mudge, M., & Hughes, L. E. (1985). Incisional hernia: a 10 year prospective study of incidence and attitudes. *Br J Surg, 72*(1), 70-71.

Muysoms, F. E., Miserez, M., Berrevoet, F., Campanelli, G., Champault, G. G., Chelala, E., et al. (2009). Classification of primary and incisional abdominal wall hernias. *Hernia, 13*(4), 407-414.

Neumayer, L., Giobbie-Hurder, A., Jonasson, O., Fitzgibbons, R., Jr., Dunlop, D., Gibbs, J., et al. (2004). Open mesh versus laparoscopic mesh repair of inguinal hernia. *N Engl J Med, 350*(18), 1819-1827.

Nilsson, H., Stylianidis, G., Haapamaki, M., Nilsson, E., & Nordin, P. (2007). Mortality after groin hernia surgery. *Ann Surg, 245*(4), 656-660.

Nyhus, L. M. (1993). Individualization of hernia repair: a new era. *Surgery, 114*(1), 1-2.

Paajanen, H., Syvahuoko, I., & Airo, I. (2004). Totally extraperitoneal endoscopic (TEP) treatment of sportsman's hernia. *Surg Laparosc Endosc Percutan Tech, 14*(4), 215-218.

Poncet, G., Robert, M., Roman, S., & Boulez, J. C. (2010). Laparoscopic repair of large hiatal hernia without prosthetic reinforcement: late results and relevance of anterior gastropexy. *J Gastrointest Surg, 14*(12), 1910-1916.

Primatesta, P., & Goldacre, M. J. (1996). Inguinal hernia repair: incidence of elective and emergency surgery, readmission and mortality. *Int J Epidemiol, 25*(4), 835-839.

Puri, P., Guiney, E. J., & O'Donnell, B. (1984). Inguinal hernia in infants: the fate of the testis following incarceration. *J Pediatr Surg, 19*(1), 44-46.

Rajput, A., Gauderer, M. W., & Hack, M. (1992). Inguinal hernias in very low birth weight infants: incidence and timing of repair. *J Pediatr Surg, 27*(10), 1322-1324.

Rieger, N., Moore, J., Hewett, P., Lee, S., & Stephens, J. (2004). Parastomal hernia repair. *Colorectal Dis, 6*(3), 203-205.

Sajid, M. S., Bokhari, S. A., Mallick, A. S., Cheek, E., & Baig, M. K. (2009). Laparoscopic versus open repair of incisional/ventral hernia: a meta-analysis. *Am J Surg, 197*(1), 64-72.

Simons, M. P., Aufenacker, T., Bay-Nielsen, M., Bouillot, J. L., Campanelli, G., Conze, J., et al. (2009). European Hernia Society guidelines on the treatment of inguinal hernia in adult patients. *Hernia, 13*(4), 343-403.

Smith, C. D., McClusky, D. A., Rajad, M. A., Lederman, A. B., & Hunter, J. G. (2005). When fundoplication fails: redo? *Ann Surg, 241*(6), 861-869; discussion 869-871.

Stoppa, R. E., Rives, J. L., Warlaumont, C. R., Palot, J. P., Verhaeghe, P. J., & Delattre, J. F. (1984). The use of Dacron in the repair of hernias of the groin. *Surg Clin North Am, 64*(2), 269-285.

Stringer, M. D., Higgins, M., Capps, S. N., & Holmes, S. J. (1991). Irreducible inguinal hernia. *Br J Surg, 78*(4), 504-505.

Sugarbaker, P. H. (1985). Peritoneal approach to prosthetic mesh repair of paraostomy hernias. *Ann Surg, 201*(3), 344-346.

Tackett, L. D., Breuer, C. K., Luks, F. I., Caldamone, A. A., Breuer, J. G., DeLuca, F. G., et al. (1999). Incidence of contralateral inguinal hernia: a prospective analysis. *J Pediatr Surg, 34*(5), 684-687; discussion 687-688.

Taylor, C., Layani, L., Liew, V., Ghusn, M., Crampton, N., & White, S. (2008). Laparoscopic inguinal hernia repair without mesh fixation, early results of a large randomised clinical trial. *Surg Endosc, 22*(3), 757-762.

Telem, D. A., Schiano, T., & Divino, C. M. (2010). Complicated hernia presentation in patients with advanced cirrhosis and refractory ascites: management and outcome. *Surgery, 148*(3), 538-543.

Toy, F. K., Bailey, R. W., Carey, S., Chappuis, C. W., Gagner, M., Josephs, L. G., et al. (1998). Prospective, multicenter study of laparoscopic ventral hernioplasty. Preliminary results. *Surg Endosc, 12*(7), 955-959.

van 't Riet, M., Steyerberg, E. W., Nellensteyn, J., Bonjer, H. J., & Jeekel, J. (2002). Meta-analysis of techniques for closure of midline abdominal incisions. *Br J Surg, 89*(11), 1350-1356.

van Veen, R. N., van Wessem, K. J., Halm, J. A., Simons, M. P., Plaisier, P. W., Jeekel, J., et al. (2007). Patent processus vaginalis in the adult as a risk factor for the occurrence of indirect inguinal hernia. *Surg Endosc, 21*(2), 202-205.

van Wessem, K. J., Simons, M. P., Plaisier, P. W., & Lange, J. F. (2003). The etiology of indirect inguinal hernias: congenital and/or acquired? *Hernia, 7*(2), 76-79.

Ventral Hernia Working, G., Breuing, K., Butler, C. E., Ferzoco, S., Franz, M., Hultman, C. S., et al. (2010). Incisional ventral hernias: review of the literature and recommendations regarding the grading and technique of repair. *Surgery, 148*(3), 544-558.

Watson, S. D., Saye, W., & Hollier, P. A. (1993). Combined laparoscopic incarcerated herniorrhaphy and small bowel resection. *Surg Laparosc Endosc, 3*(2), 106-108.

Ziprin, P., Prabhudesai, S. G., Abrahams, S., & Chadwick, S. J. (2008). Transabdominal preperitoneal laparoscopic approach for the treatment of sportsman's hernia. *J Laparoendosc Adv Surg Tech A, 18*(5), 669-672.

11

Laparoscopic Incisional Hernia Repair

Anita Kurmann and Guido Beldi
Department of Visceral Surgery and Medicine, Bern University Hospital
University of Bern, Bern
Switzerland

1. Introduction

An incisional hernia (Fig 1.) is defined as any abdominal wall gap with or without a bulge in the area of a postoperative scar perceptible or palpable by clinical examination or imaging [1]. Incisional hernia is a common long-term complication following abdominal surgery and is estimated to occur in 11-23% [2, 3]. Risk factors for incisional hernia are male gender, body mass index, cancer, and previous laparotomy [4, 5].

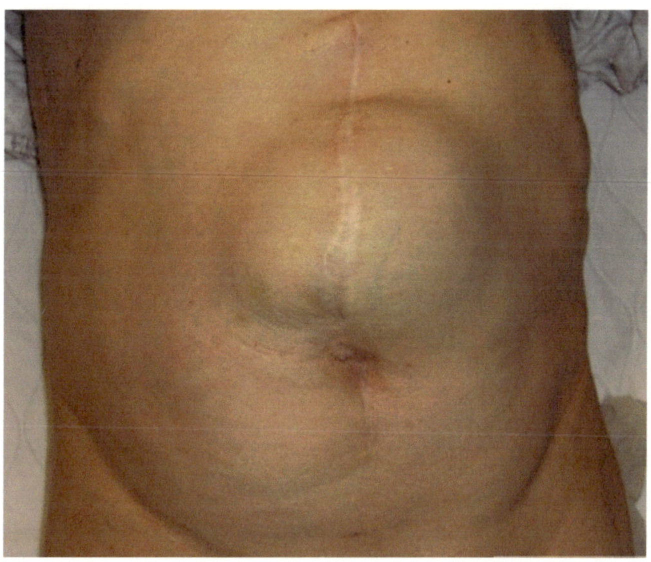

Fig. 1. Clinical presentation of a patient with a large incisional hernia

Conventional hernia repair with tissue approximation was associated with a recurrence rate of 60%. Theodore Billroths vision was the source of changes in hernia repair. Billroth told to his pupil Cerny: "If we could artificially produce tissues of the density and toughness of fascia and tendon the secret of the radical cure of hernia would be discovered". This statement appeard in the classic Beiträge zur Chirurgie in 1987. Francic C. Usher introduced 1957 a polypropylene based prosthesis to bridge the hernia defect and to reinforce the abdominal wall without tension [6]. With the implantation of prosthesis the recurrence rate in hernia repair was downsized [7].

Incisional hernia can be repaired by open or by laparoscopic approach and prosthetic meshes are nowadays implanted in most procedures. The use of laparoscopy for the treatment of incisional hernia was first reported in 1993 by LeBlanc and Booth [8]. With the introduction of modern two-layered mesh, laparoscopic incisional hernia repair has become an accepted therapeutic option. Feasibility and safety of laparoscopic incisional hernia repair has been shown in various randomized controlled trials.

2. Incisional hernia classification

Developing a good classification for incisional hernias is much more difficult than for groin hernias or for primary abdominal wall hernias because of their great diversity. The classification as established and published by the consensus meeting of the European Hernia Society held in Ghent, Belgium, 2008, (Tab 1.) comprises a division of subgroups for incisional hernia, including localization, width, and length of the hernia [9]. The use of the classification of the European Hernia Society is nowadays recommended. The analysis of subgroups may define patients with high risk for recurrences and may lead to specific treatment options. This classification is applicable in laparoscopic and open incisional hernia repair.

<table>
<tr><th colspan="4">EHS
Incisional Hernia Classification</th></tr>
<tr><td rowspan="5">Midline</td><td>subxiphoidal</td><td>M1</td><td></td></tr>
<tr><td>epigastric</td><td>M2</td><td></td></tr>
<tr><td>umbilical</td><td>M3</td><td></td></tr>
<tr><td>infraumbilical</td><td>M4</td><td></td></tr>
<tr><td>suprapubic</td><td>M5</td><td></td></tr>
<tr><td rowspan="4">Lateral</td><td>subcostal</td><td>L1</td><td></td></tr>
<tr><td>flank</td><td>L2</td><td></td></tr>
<tr><td>iliac</td><td>L3</td><td></td></tr>
<tr><td>lumbar</td><td>L4</td><td></td></tr>
<tr><td colspan="2">Recurrent incisional hernia?</td><td colspan="2">Yes O No O</td></tr>
<tr><td>length:</td><td>cm</td><td>width:</td><td>cm</td></tr>
<tr><td>Width
cm</td><td>W1
<4cm
O</td><td>W2
≥4-10cm
O</td><td>W3
≥10cm
O</td></tr>
</table>

Table 1. European Hernia Society classification for incisional abdominal wall hernia

3. Symptoms

A swelling or protrusion with or without abdominal pain can be observed in a patient with an incisional hernia when the patient sits up or coughs. In large incisional hernia peristaltic bowel movements can be observed through a thin skin, sometimes already accompanied with signs of a skin infection. Incisional hernias may occur along the full length of the incision with one or multiple hernial orifices. Incarceration is the main complication of an incisional hernia [10] and occurs in 1-3% of all hernias. Signs of incarceration are acute pain and vomiting. Clinically there is a tense, tender irreducible hernia. In these cases an emergency hernia repair is mandatory. Emergency hernia repair can also be performed by laparoscopy with an additional mini-laparotomy if bowel resection is necessary.
Incisional hernia can be diagnosed by physical examination. Additional ultrasound or CT-scan examination are recommended in cases of uncertainty (Fig 2).

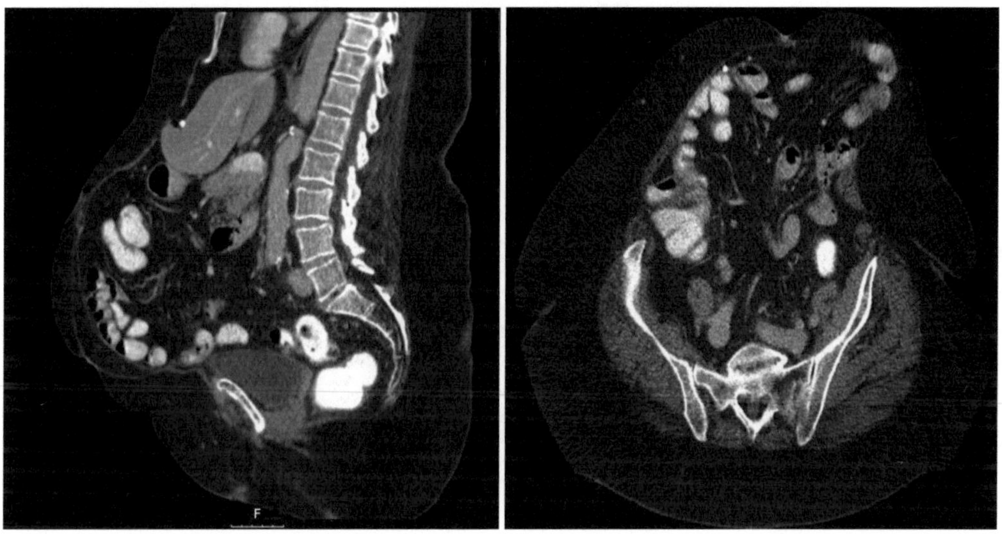

Fig. 2. CT-Scan of a patient with a large incisional hernia. The hernia contains small and large bowel.

4. Surgical technique of laparoscopic hernia repair

We routinely use a 30° camera. Scissors and two graspers have to be prepared for laparoscopic hernia repair. The screen is placed at the opposite of the surgeon. The patient is placed in a supine position with both arms unabducted under general anesthesia. A single shot of antibiotics is given preoperatively. The site of trocar placing depends on the localization of the hernia. If the hernia is localized in the right hemiabdomen, the trocars should be placed on the left side. Using a limited open technique the pneumoperitoneum is established and the optical trocar is inserted, and under direct vision, a minimum of two additional trocars at a suitable distance from the hernial orifice are inserted. Alternatively the pneumoperitoneum can be established using a Verres-Needle. After establishing the pneumoperitoneum at 12mmHg a diagnostic laparoscopy is performed. Adhesions between the omentum or intestine with the anterior wall surrounding the hernial orifice are divided, and the content of the hernia is reduced completely (Fig. 3). Adhesiolysis has to be performed with scissors and without electocoagulation under direct vision to avoid bowel lesions. In cases of incarceration the necrotic tissue has to be resected. If there is not enough working space or the trocars are not correctly placed an additional trocar can be helpful.

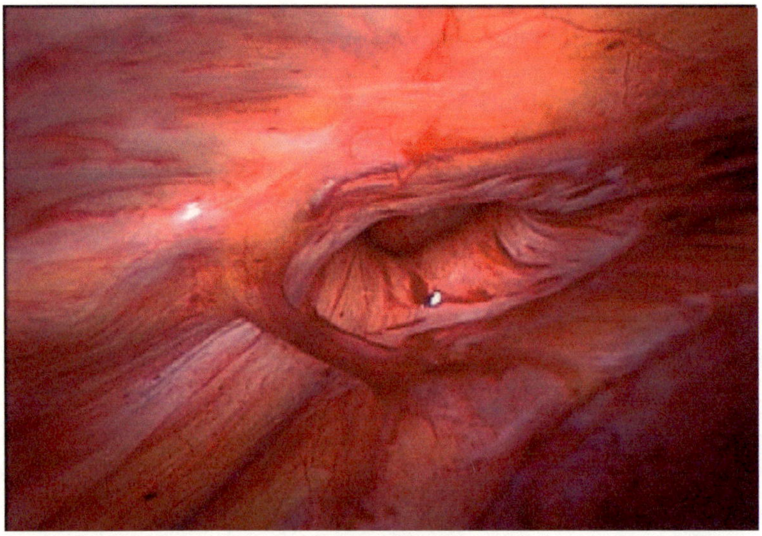

Fig. 3. Intraoperative laparoscopic view of the hernial orifice

In general, the hernial sac is left in situ. After completion of adhesiolysis, the pneumoperitoneum is released, the maximal longitudinal and horizontal hernia diameter is measured and marked on the skin (Fig. 4). An appropriate sized mesh is tailored in order to

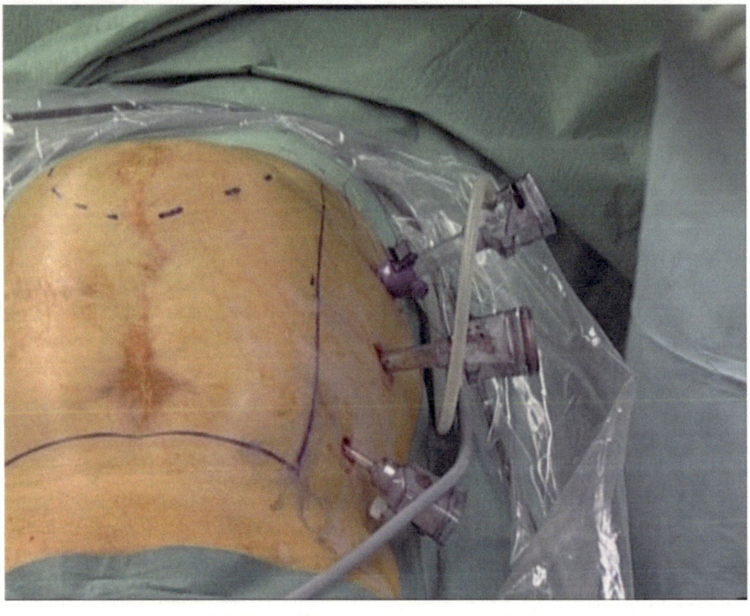

Fig. 4. Patient with an incisional hernia in the upper part of the scar. The hernia and the size of the mesh is marked on the patients skin.

overlap the hernia margins by at least 5 cm on each side. In addition, the mesh should overlap the full length of the incision of the primary operation. Non absorbable monofilament sutures are placed in 2-3 cm intervals along the mesh margin. The mesh is rolled up and inserted into the abdomen through a 12mm trocar.
Then the mesh is rolled up and introduced into the abdominal cavity. After the mesh is positioned correctly in the abdominal cavity, the suture ties are pulled through the abdominal wall with a suture passer and the threats are knotted smoothly with the knots buried in the subcutaneous tissue after reduction of the intraabdominal pressure to 8mmHg. We use titanium tackers that are applied between the sutures every 1 to 2 cm between the sutures and around the hernial orifice (Fig 5). If the skin is necrotic or to enhance cosmetic results in large incisional hernia an additional open cutaneous excision is recommended.

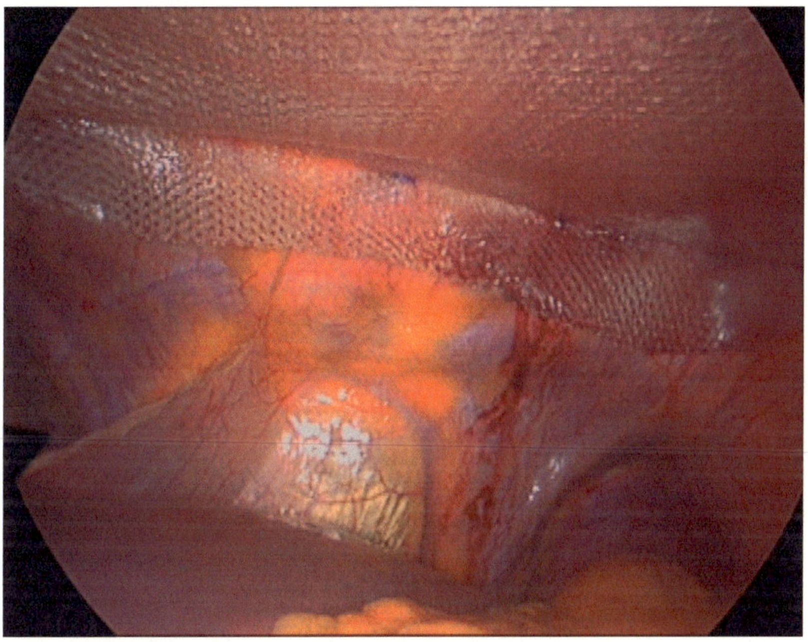

Fig. 5. Intraoperative laparoscopic view after Mesh implantation.

5. Patient selection

5.1 General considerations

In general we plan the laparoscopic approach for all patients with incisional hernia. Contraindications for laparoscopic hernia repair are the presence of anesthetic (severe pulmonary disease) or technical contraindications (eviscerated organs) or patients unwilling to undergo laparoscopic surgery.

5.2 Large incisional hernia

In our institution we prospectively evaluated 125 with a hernia diameter ≥5cm among 428 patients undergoing incisional hernia repair. We demonstrated that laparoscopic repair of large incisional hernias is technical feasible and associated with less SSI and shorter hospital stay but a comparable recurrence rate as open hernia repair (Table 2) [11].

	Lap. group n = 69	Open group n = 56	*P*-Value
SSI	4 (5.8)	16 (26.8)	0.006
Intestinal fistula	0 (0)	1 (1.8)	n.s.
Hospital stay (days)*	6 (1-23)	7 (1-67)	0.014
Recurrence	11 (15.9)	10 (17.9)	n.s.
Return to work (weeks)	3 (0-50)	6 (0-28)	n.s.
Pain at follow-up (VAS)	0.6 (0-6)	0.5 (0-5)	n.s.

Values in parentheses are percentages unless indicated otherwise. * Values are median (range).

Table 2. Results of outcome_parameters of large incisional hernia repair

5.3 Incisional hernia after liver transplantation

We showed that laparoscopic incisional hernia repair is feasible and safe even in patients under immunosuppressive therapy [12].

6. Postoperative outcome

6.1 Conversion to open surgery

The conversion rate to open surgery depends on the surgeons experience, the surgical skills, and intraoperative complications such as bowel lesions or bleeding. In the literature conversion to open surgery is mostly due to adhesions, with an overall conversion rate of 10-15% [12, 13]. However, complete adhesiolysis is very important especially in large incisional hernia to gain enough place for the mesh fixation and therefore to minimize the recurrence rate.

6.2 Operation time

There is a wide range in duration of the operation comparing laparoscopic and open incisional hernia repair. Most studies revealed that operation time in laparoscopic incisional hernia repair is longer compared to open surgery [12-14]. However, there was always a statistically difference in all these studies. Longer operation time can be explained with the learning curve in laparoscopy. Furthermore the fixation technique of the mesh can be time consuming especially in large incisional hernia repair. On the other hand there are some studies with no difference or even a shorter operation time in laparoscopic surgery [15, 16].

6.3 Sugical site infections

The definition of Surgical site infections (SSIs) according to the criteria developed by the Centers for Disease Control and Prevention include every SSI up to 30 days after the operation [17]. Infections are categorized as incisional (superficial or deep) infections or organ–space infections. Superficial SSIs involve only skin and subcutaneous tissue and exclude stitch abscesses. Deep SSIs involve deeper soft tissues at the site of incision. Organ–

space SSIs are defined as infections in any organ or space. In laparoscopic incisional hernia repair the incidence of SSI is low. In a meta-analysis of 8 randomized controlled trials Forbes et al. showed a significant reduced risk of surgical site infections in laparoscopic incisional hernia repair compared to open surgery [18]. The extensive tissue dissection which is associated with the open approach explains the significant higher infection rate in open surgery. Mostly SSIs in laparoscopic surgery are superficial and can be treated conservatively. Mesh removal due to an surgical site infection is very rare [19].

6.4 Enterotomy

In general the mortality rate of laparoscopic incisional hernia repair is low with 0.05% [8]. The most serious complication during laparoscopic incisional hernia repair is enterotomy [8]. Enterotomy occurs during adhesiolysis or as a burning lesion with the electorcauter. Therefore we avoid electrocauterisation during adhesiolysis to prevent bowel lesions and perforation. The incidence of intraoperative bowel injuries has been reported to be 1.78% [20] A recognized enterotomy during the operation is associated with a mortality rate of 1.7% [20]. However, if the enterotomy is not recognized during the operation the mortality rate is increased up to 7.7% [20]. Enterotomy can be repaired by laparoscopic or open approach with similar outcome result [20].

6.5 Enterocutaneous fistula

Enterocutaneous fistula after intraperitoneal non-resorbable mesh implantation was first reported in by Kaufman et al. in 1981 [21]. An overview of the current literature shows that enterocutaneous fistula after incisional hernia repair is a rare complication and occurs in up to 1% [22]. There was no association of enterocutaneous fistula if the omentum was placed between the mesh and bowel or not. In cases of enterocutaneous fistula the mesh has to be resected partially around the fistula. Complete mesh removal is very rare and depends on the surgeons experience [23]

6.6 Pain

Lomanto et al. showed that there is no difference in the amount of pain comparing laparoscopic and open hernia repair at 24 and 48 hours postoperatively [24]. However, patients undergoing laparoscopic repair had significantly less pain at 72 hours compared to open surgery allowing earlier discharge and return to work [24].

The threshold for chronic pain is set at three months postoperatively according to the International Association for the Study of Pain [25]. There is no meta-analysis investigating chronic pain after laparoscopic incisional hernia repair. Postoperative pain after mesh fixation with transfascial sutures is likely due to nerve irritation or entrapmen [26]. There is a randomized controlled trial investigating pain comparing two different techniques of mesh fixation [26]. Postoperative pain following suture fixation was significantly higher at 6 weeks postoperatively and two patients suffered from nerve irritation at sites of sutures. However, after 6 months, no difference was seen between the two groups. Pain after mesh fixation with transfascial sutures is likely due to nerve irritation or entrapment and the relatively small distance between individual sutures used in this study. The significant reduction of pain between 6 weeks and 6 months post operation in these patients could be in response to desensitisation of entrapped nerve fibres or in response to resolution of local inflammation [26]. Asencio et al. showed in their study that 22% of the laparoscopic group and 7% of the open group reported significantly pain three months after the operation [13]. But all were pain free one year after the operation [13] . Therefore when pain persists a surgical revisions due to nerve irritation is not recommended earlier than 6 months. Alternatively a postoperative local injection of bupivacaine and steroids or removal of the offending suture is recommended [27].

6.7 Recurrence rate

Recurrence rate is one of the most important long-term outcome parameters in laparoscopic incisional hernia repair. Forbes et al. showed in their meta-analysis no difference in the recurrence rate between laparoscopic and open incisional hernia repair [18]. The pooled recurrence rate in the laparoscopic group was 3.4% and in the open group 3.5% in this study. Such a low recurrence rate after either laparoscopic and open repair can be explained with a relatively short follow-up and the small size of the hernias [18]. A follow-up of at least three years is mandatory to evaluate correctly the real incidence of incisional hernia due to the fact that incisional hernia can occur up to 5 years after the operation. With such a long-term follow-up the incidence of recurrence has been reported to be up to 15-20% in laparoscopic and open repair [11, 13].

Two technical details can minimize the recurrence rate. First a sufficient overlap of the mesh and second the mesh fixation. We showed a significant decrease in horizontal mesh size after tack fixation (mean difference -3.1% ±3.9%) versus fixation using sutures (-0.1% ±2.3%; p=0.018) [26]. Mean vertical mesh size was not significantly different between the two groups: tack fixation -2.8% ±6.1%, suture fixation -0.7% ±4.1% (p=0.16). Mean mesh area in the tack fixation group was -12% and in the suture fixation group -2.9% at 6 months post operatively when compared to post-op day 2 (p=0.061) [26]. Therefore a sufficient mesh-overlap of the hernial orifice is mandatory in order to reduce recurrence rate.

Typical locations for hernia recurrences due to the mesh shrinkage are at the margin of the mesh as shown in Fig. 6. Because the risk to gain a second incisional hernia or a recurrent hernia along the full length of the incision, it is recommended to cover the whole length of the incision during the first operation.

6.8 Seroma formation

The retained hernia sac is responsible for seroma formation. Seroma formation is classified as a complication if it lasts more than 6 weeks after the operation. A randomized controlled trial of Olmi et al. showed an incidence of seroma formation of 7% [15]. In most cases no intervention is necessary. In cases of symptoms or if the seroma lasts longer than 8 weeks a drainage is recommended. Potentially a compression dressing over a period of 7 days may prevent seroma formation.

6.9 Hospitalisation time

Forbes et al. showed in their meta-analysis that duration of hospital stay is significantly shorter in laparoscopic incisional hernia repair compared to open surgery [18]. Less amount of pain [24] and a significantly lower rate of surgical site infections in laparoscopic repair [18] are reflected in a shorter hospital stay. Influence of shorter hospital stay on overall costs in laparoscopic hernia repair is discussed below.

6.10 Costs

On the one hand operative costs of laparoscopic incisional hernia repair compared to open surgery are significantly higher due to expensive surgical tools in laparoscopy. On the other hand in hospital costs are significantly lower in laparoscopic surgery due to shorter hospital stay, lower infection rate and less postoperative pain. However, laparoscopic incisional hernia repair is associated with significant lower overall costs. Therefore laparoscopic incisional hernia repair is cost effective [15, 28].

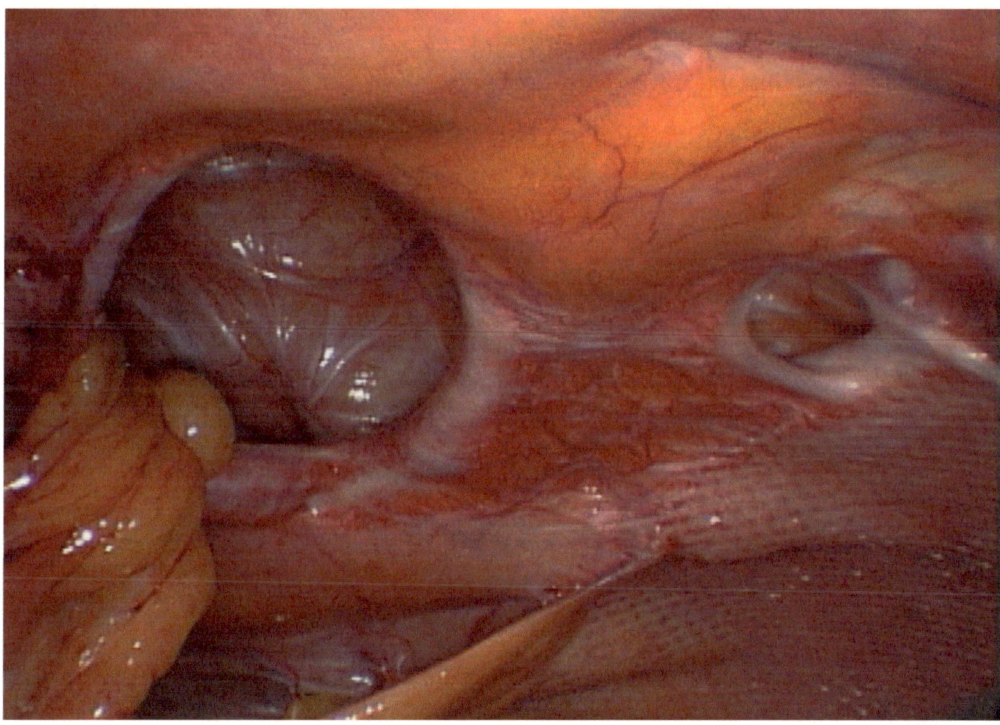

Fig. 6. Intraoperative laparoscopic view of a recurrent hernia along the incision at the edge of the mesh.

7. Conclusion

In conclusion laparoscopic incisional hernia repair is feasible and safe. Reduced SSI and reduced hospital stay are the major short term advantages associated with laparoscopy most likely as a consequence of reduced wound size [18, 27]. Recurrence rate are comparable in laparoscopic and open incisional hernia repair [18].

8. References

[1] M. Korenkov and E. Neugebauer. (2001). Comments on the letter from S. Petersen and K. Ludwig concerning our paper "Classification and surgical treatment of the incisional hernia. Results of expert meeting." Langenbeck's Arch Surg 386:65-73. *Langenbecks Arch Surg,* Vol. 386, No. 4, pp.310-311,

[2] K. Cassar and A. Munro. (2002). Surgical treatment of incisional hernia. *Br J Surg,* Vol. 89, No. 5, pp.534-545,

[3] M. Mudge and L. E. Hughes. (1985). Incisional hernia: a 10 year prospective study of incidence and attitudes. *Br J Surg,* Vol. 72, No. 1, pp.70-71,

[4] J. Hoer, G. Lawong, U. Klinge and V. Schumpelick. (2002). [Factors influencing the development of incisional hernia. A retrospective study of 2,983 laparotomy patients over a period of 10 years]. *Chirurg,* Vol. 73, No. 5, pp.474-480,

[5] L. T. Sorensen, U. B. Hemmingsen, L. T. Kirkeby, F. Kallehave and L. N. Jorgensen. (2005). Smoking is a risk factor for incisional hernia. *Arch Surg,* Vol. 140, No. 2, pp.119-123,

[6] F. C. Usher. (1962). Hernia repair with Marlex mesh. An analysis of 541 cases. *Arch Surg,* Vol. 84, No. pp.325-328,

[7] V. Schumpelick, J. Conze and U. Klinge. (1996). [Preperitoneal mesh-plasty in incisional hernia repair. A comparative retrospective study of 272 operated incisional hernias]. *Chirurg,* Vol. 67, No. 10, pp.1028-1035,

[8] K. A. LeBlanc. (2005). Incisional hernia repair: laparoscopic techniques. *World J Surg,* Vol. 29, No. 8, pp.1073-1079,

[9] F. E. Muysoms, M. Miserez, F. Berrevoet, G. Campanelli, G. G. Champault, E. Chelala, U. A. Dietz, H. H. Eker, I. El Nakadi, P. Hauters, M. Hidalgo Pascual, A. Hoeferlin, U. Klinge, A. Montgomery, R. K. Simmermacher, M. P. Simons, M. Smietanski, C. Sommeling, T. Tollens, T. Vierendeels and A. Kingsnorth. (2009). Classification of primary and incisional abdominal wall hernias. *Hernia,* Vol. 13, No. 4, pp.407-414,

[10] J. Nieuwenhuizen, G. H. van Ramshorst, J. G. Ten Brinke, T. de Wit, E. van der Harst, W. C. Hop, J. Jeekel and J. F. Lange. (2011). The use of mesh in acute hernia: frequency and outcome in 99 cases. *Hernia,* Vol. No.

[11] A. Kurmann, E. Visth, D. Candinas and G. Beldi. (2011). Long-term follow-up of open and laparoscopic repair of large incisional hernias. *World J Surg,* Vol. 35, No. 2, pp.297-301,

[12] A. Kurmann, G. Beldi, S. A. Vorburger, C. A. Seiler and D. Candinas. (2010). Laparoscopic incisional hernia repair is feasible and safe after liver transplantation. *Surg Endosc,* Vol. 24, No. 6, pp.1451-1455,

[13] F. Asencio, J. Aguilo, S. Peiro, J. Carbo, R. Ferri, F. Caro and M. Ahmad. (2009). Open randomized clinical trial of laparoscopic versus open incisional hernia repair. *Surg Endosc,* Vol. 23, No. 7, pp.1441-1448,
[14] U. Barbaros, O. Asoglu, R. Seven, Y. Erbil, A. Dinccag, U. Deveci, S. Ozarmagan and S. Mercan. (2007). The comparison of laparoscopic and open ventral hernia repairs: a prospective randomized study. *Hernia,* Vol. 11, No. 1, pp.51-56,
[15] S. Olmi, A. Scaini, G. C. Cesana, L. Erba and E. Croce. (2007). Laparoscopic versus open incisional hernia repair: an open randomized controlled study. *Surg Endosc,* Vol. 21, No. 4, pp. 555-559,
[16] M. C. Misra, V. K. Bansal, M. P. Kulkarni and D. K. Pawar. (2006). Comparison of laparoscopic and open repair of incisional and primary ventral hernia: results of a prospective randomized study. *Surg Endosc,* Vol. 20, No. 12, pp.1839-1845,
[17] (2004). National Nosocomial Infections Surveillance (NNIS) System Report, data summary from January 1992 through June 2004, issued October 2004. *Am J Infect Control,* Vol. 32, No. 8, pp.470-485,
[18] S. S. Forbes, C. Eskicioglu, R. S. McLeod and A. Okrainec. (2009). Meta-analysis of randomized controlled trials comparing open and laparoscopic ventral and incisional hernia repair with mesh. *Br J Surg,* Vol. 96, No. 8, pp.851-858,
[19] U. A. Dietz, L. Spor and C. T. Germer. (2011). [Management of mesh-related infections.]. *Chirurg,* Vol. 82, No. 3, pp.208-217,
[20] K. A. LeBlanc, M. J. Elieson and J. M. Corder, 3rd. (2007). Enterotomy and mortality rates of laparoscopic incisional and ventral hernia repair: a review of the literature. *Jsls,* Vol. 11, No. 4, pp.408-414,
[21] Z. Kaufman, M. Engelberg and M. Zager. (1981). Fecal fistula: a late complication of Marlex mesh repair. *Dis Colon Rectum,* Vol. 24, No. 7, pp.543-544,
[22] W. W. Vrijland, J. Jeekel, E. W. Steyerberg, P. T. Den Hoed and H. J. Bonjer. (2000). Intraperitoneal polypropylene mesh repair of incisional hernia is not associated with enterocutaneous fistula. *Br J Surg,* Vol. 87, No. 3, pp.348-352,
[23] S. Stremitzer, T. Bachleitner-Hofmann, B. Gradl, M. Gruenbeck, B. Bachleitner-Hofmann, M. Mittlboeck and M. Bergmann. (2010). Mesh graft infection following abdominal hernia repair: risk factor evaluation and strategies of mesh graft preservation. A retrospective analysis of 476 operations. *World J Surg,* Vol. 34, No. 7, pp.1702-1709,
[24] D. Lomanto, S. G. Iyer, A. Shabbir and W. K. Cheah. (2006). Laparoscopic versus open ventral hernia mesh repair: a prospective study. *Surg Endosc,* Vol. 20, No. 7, pp. 1030-1035,
[25] (1986). Classification of chronic pain. Descriptions of chronic pain syndromes and definitions of pain terms. Prepared by the International Association for the Study of Pain, Subcommittee on Taxonomy. *Pain Suppl,* Vol. 3, No. pp.S1-226,
[26] G. Beldi, M. Wagner, L. E. Bruegger, A. Kurmann and D. Candinas. (2010). Mesh shrinkage and pain in laparoscopic ventral hernia repair: a randomized clinical trial comparing suture versus tack mesh fixation. *Surg Endosc,* Vol. 25, No. 3, pp.749-755,

[27] M. S. Sajid, S. A. Bokhari, A. S. Mallick, E. Cheek and M. K. Baig. (2009). Laparoscopic versus open repair of incisional/ventral hernia: a meta-analysis. *Am J Surg,* Vol. 197, No. 1, pp.64-72,

[28] G. Beldi, R. Ipaktchi, M. Wagner, B. Gloor and D. Candinas. (2006). Laparoscopic ventral hernia repair is safe and cost effective. *Surg Endosc,* Vol. 20, No. 1, pp. 92-95,

Part 5

Laparoscopic Solid Organ Surgery

12

Spleen Preserving Surgery and Related Laparoscopic Techniques

Lianxin Liu, Dalong Yin and Hongchi Jiang
*Department of Hepatic Surgery,
The First Affiliated Hospital of Harbin Medical University, Key Laboratory of Hepatosplenic Surgery, Ministry of Education, Harbin, Heilongjiang Province
P.R. China*

1. Introduction

"The spleen" whose weight once thought to have been hindering the speed of runners to its role in cleansing process as its absence could result in the loss of laughing ability was called the "mysteriipleniorganon". Its biological function has been elusive for thousand of years and also had been assumed to have no vitality in life. It's been centuries since its existence has been under tremendous perusal and it wasn't until mid-twelfth century when the concept of blood purifying function was emphasized. In early 1900, however, numerous experiments have concluded its role in the host defense and immune function. Spleen surgery dates back to 1549. Zaccaelli carried out the first splenectomy in this year. In 1952, King and Schumaker reported the overwhelming postsplenectomy infection (OPSI) in children with hereditary spherocytosis who had undergone splenectomies, which caused a wide concern on the potential function of the spleen.

2. Splenic function

Immunity

The spleen richly contains T cells, B cells, K cells, macrophages/monocytes, natural killer cells, killer cells, lymphokine-activated killer (LAK) cells, dendritic cells and so forth, and in conjunction with a variety of immune factors to makes in vivo immune response. Tuftsin is a tetrapeptide produced by the spleen to stimulatepha- gocytosis through the activation of neutrophils, it is a typical anti-tumor substance in the spleen, and can reflect the spleen function. Spleen tyrosine kinase (SYK) is a non-receptor tyrosine kinase, initially expressed in the spleen hematopoietic cells. SYK plays an important role in the Fc-mediated phagocytosis, B cell receptor signal transduction, cytokine secretion, and integrin-mediated signal transduction.

Barrier function

Weiss first proposed in 1986 that there is a blood-spleen barrier (BSB) between the artery and vein in the spleen, which is similar to blood-brain barrier and can filter Plasmodium falciparum-infected red blood cells. Jiang and Zhu et al respectively made their study on rat spleens and set up the concept and architecture of the BSB: The blood-spleen barrier (BSB) is located in the marginal zone of the spleen, which lies at the periphery of the white pulp;

This is a biological barrier containing sinus-lining endothelial cells, basement membrane, macrophages, reticular cells, reticular fibers (reticular tissue), and collagen fibers.

Endocrine function

As an important immune organ, the spleen also has an endocrine function, and is an important part of the immuno–neuro–endocrine modulation system in the body. Normal spleen may secrete erythropoietin, colony-stimulating factor, thyroid–stimulating hormone, gonadotropin, growth hormone, etc.

Through the nineteenth and twentieth century splenectomy had been successfully performed for trauma and hypersplenism. It was observed that the patients recovered to their usual pursuits but the life-long probability of the infection, augmented rate of long-term thromboembolic complications, enhanced arteriosclerosis, and late coronary artery disease could not be ignored and the long-term survival seemed skeptic. It's obvious that the knowledge of spleen function is getting more apparent and deep. Its importance in the host defense and immune function is absolutely undisputed. So the surgeons and researchers came up with the notion of preserving the spleen. To the matter of fact this conception didn't go in vain as it has been established now that that the preservation of at least 25% of the splenic parenchyma ensures an adequate short and long-term splenic function.

The anatomy of the spleen and its surrounding structures is indispensible. At the spleen hilum, all the vascular structures enter and divide to the related poles. Sometimes in patients the vessels divide into three branches thus any injury at the pedicle can result in the ischemia to the part supplied by the other branches(figure 1). Since, there is an ample amount of blood flow through the spleen. So, if the flow is interrupted to the part not being dissected "reperfusion injury" should be well thought-out. If the crisis is in the superior or inferior pole the dissection is not to difficult compared to the crisis at the hilum. The hilum also has the pancreatic tail landing on it; therefore, the activities at the hilum must be with care and precision so as not to injure pancreas. While draining the abscess there is an increased risk of the content to leak and reach the peritoneal cavity that is probable to cause sepsis around. Before starting the dissection of the splenic tissue, its abdominal adherence should be resected with care and after the surgery the remenant spleen should be place carefully to the left upper quadrantto avoid rotation, which further can re-open the cut surface and vessels. The size, location of cysts, abscess, hemangioma and trauma plays an essential role in the decision for choosing the best-suited technique.

Spleen injury scale

At present, there are dozens of methods for spleen injury scaling. Main methods include Schackford Grade V (1981), Feliciano Grade V(1985), Gall & Scheele Grade IV(1986), Uranus Grade V(1990), American Association for the Surgery of Trauma(AAST, 1994 Revision) Grade V, and Patcher Grade IV(1998) and so on. These methods have different characteristics, but sometimes cannot effectively guide clinical work and operation. The 6th National Symposium on Spleen Surgery of China held in September 2000 in Tianjin adopted the spleen injury scale criteria as below. Grade I: subcapsular splenic rupture whose length ≤ 5.0cm & depth ≤ 1.0cm shown in the surgery. Grade II: the length of the spleen laceration≥5.0cm & depth ≥ 1.0cm, but the splenic hilum is not involved, or segmental splenic vessels are injured. Grade III: splenic rupture involves into splenic hilum, or partial spleen is broken apart, or spleen trabecular vessels are injured. Grade IV: extensive rupture exists in the spleen, or there is an injury in splenic pedicle, and main veins and arteries. Such scaling method helps to quickly determine the injury condition, but cannot cover all damages; so there is a need to make a revision and improvement according to actual situation in clinical work to adjust the treatment.

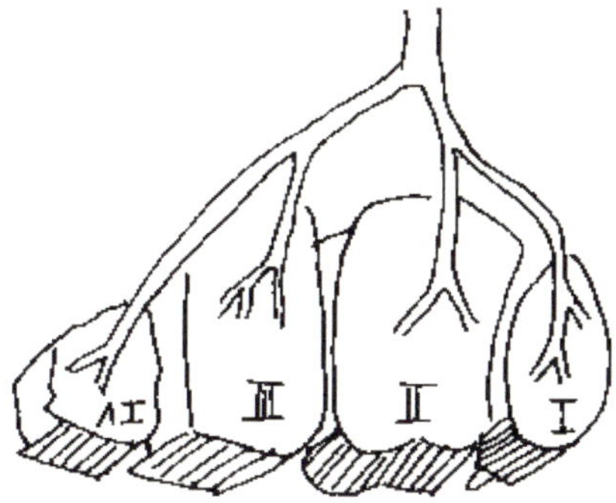

a)

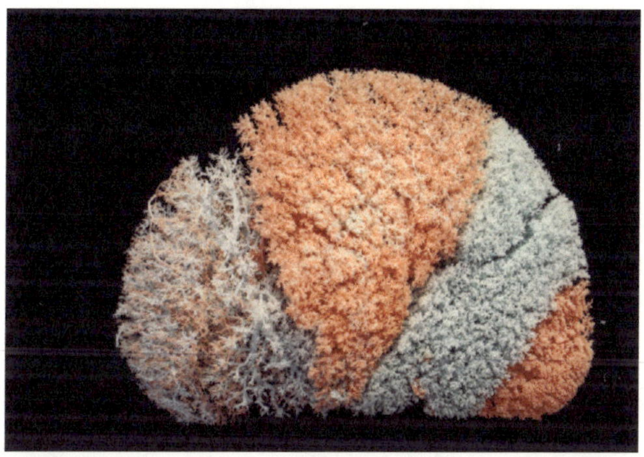

b)

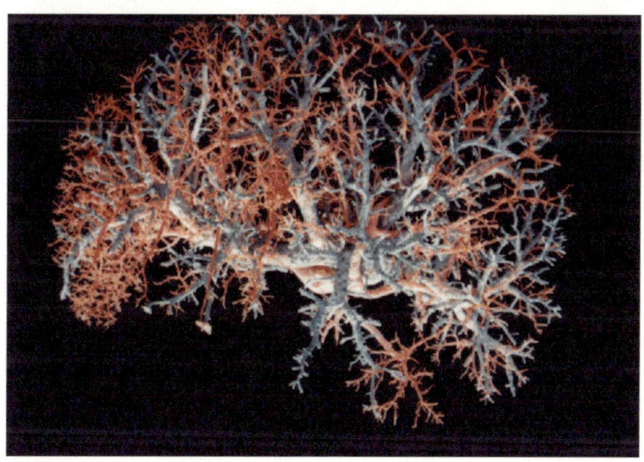

c)

Fig. 1. a) spleen artery is divided four branches into different segment , b) the anatomic basis of preseving spleen , c) model of spleen vessels

The spleen preserving surgeries of course was the remedy for many complications but with the open nature of surgery came handful of post operative complication like infection, delayed healing which at times altered the well being of the patients and "yes" the recovery. It's evident that the spleen preserving surgeries have been evolving through decades (figure2). It's apparent that the advents of novel laparoscopic techniques have opened new gates to the spleen preserving surgeries. The dawn of nineteenth century could see the concept of laparoscopic partial splenectomy blooming and by late nineties many centers around the world adapted it as a routine procedure. Surgery is an evolving science and in recent times there are several pioneering techniques that have minimized the technical flaws and surgical outcomes.

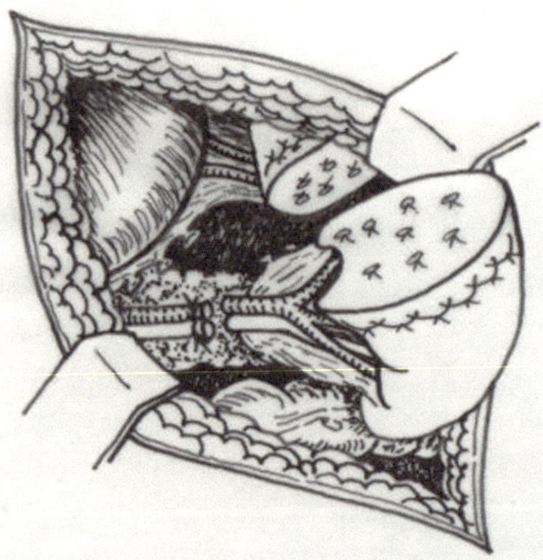

a)

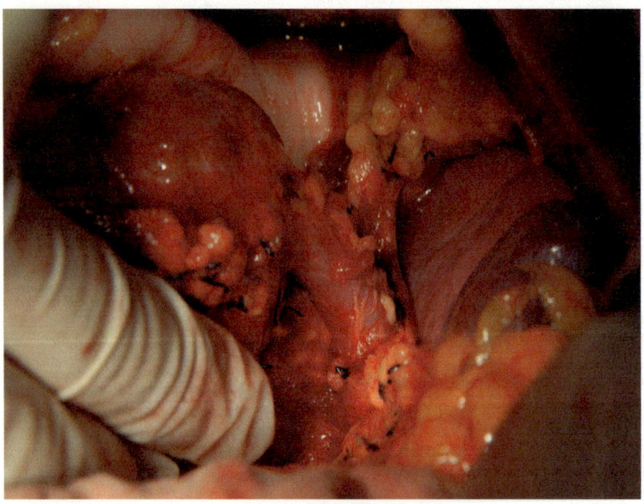

b)

Fig. 2. a) remnant spleen section after partial splenectomy , b)conservation of the spleen with distal pancreatetomy

3. Laparoscopic surgery in spleen-preserving surgery

Carroll et al reported the laparoscopic splenectomy for the first time in 1992. Since then, the laparoscopic surgery has extended to the traditional fields covered by laparotomy, e.g. spleen adhesion, splenorrhaphy, artery ligation, partial splenectomy and the like, and has been combined with such new techniques as LigaSure, splenic arterial embolization, CUSA, radiofrequency ablation, thus adding a new vitality to the spleen-preserving surgery. The laparoscopic spleen-preserving surgery is somehow difficult, time-consuming, and costly. However, when compared to laparotomy, this surgery has more advantages, for example, clear operative field, minimal invasion, rapid recovery, and short hospital stay.

Laparoscopic inspection: To determine the extent and scope for splenic injuries or lesions; to understand injuries or lesions in the surrounding tissues or organs of spleen; to judge the extent for the bleeding area and vascular injuries; to carry out the pathological examination for the spleen or the surrounding tissues and organs under direct vision biopsy.

The laparoscopic spleen-preserving surgery has the following indications: Grade I-II splenic injuries with hemodynamic and vital sign stability; local benign lesions in the spleen, e.g. splenic cyst, splenichemangioma, echinococcosis, and etc.; hypersplenia, e.g. portal vein hypertension, hereditary spherocytosis and etc.; perisplenic tumors, e.g. pancreatic tumor, gastric cancer and etc.; splenic congenital diseases, e.g. splenectopia, accessory spleen and so on. Contraindications: Grade IVsplenic injuries; severe portal hypertension; splenomeglia; severe coagulopathy.

The spleen-preserving surgery is similar to the laparotomy:

1. For Grade I spleen injuries, the bleeding can be controlled by electric coagulation, biological glue, fibrin and the like. For Grade II spleen injuries, the following methods are adopted: splenorrhaphy, partialsplenectomy, splenic artery ligation and the like. For Grade III spleen injuries, the following methods are adopted: partialsplenectomy, and splenic artery ligation etc.
2. For splenic benign lesions, the laparoscopic resection is conducted.
3. For hypersplenia, the laparoscopic partial splenectomy is conducted.
4. The spleen can be conserved through laparoscopic resection for perisplenic tumors.
5. For splenectopia, the laparoscopic fixation can be conducted. For accessory spleen, the laparoscopic resection can be conducted.

In the laparoscopic spleen-preserving surgery, the complications include hemorrhage, visceral injury, infection, splenic vein thrombosis and so on.

The laparoscopic spleen-preserving surgery is still in trial stage, and its efficacy is uncertain. Clinically, we should not blindly pursue new technology ignoring its efficacy; instead, we should never forget the damage control principles for splenic surgery, always save life first, and then deal with the injury.

In the current study, the spleen function is not very clear, but we begin to know it can play an important role in human body. Spleen-preserving surgeries have been widely implemented. Moreover, the extensive laparoscopic application has brought new opportunities, making the future splenic surgery more scientific and reasonable.

4. Techniques

The laparoscopic surgery is classically done via four ports (trocars) through the abdominal wall viz.12mm left umbilical trocar, 5mm trocar positioned 5cm distal to the xiphoid process and slightly to the right of the midline, a 12 mm trocar positioned below the left costal arch on the mammillary line and a 12mm trocar positioned below the left costal arch on the anterior axillary linea. The surgery by this technique is quite efficient owing to the excellent view of abdominal anatomical landmarks. The resection is very clean and efficient with outstanding hemostasis from the cut surfaces. The 12 mm left umbilical trocar sometimes is replaced by 15mm ones for the introduction of the linear staplers. Surgical adhesives and meshes can be equally used with perfection if required. The surgery with spleen is technically challenging, thus, the electro cautery must be used efficiently with minimizing over use, because its overuse can cause the destruction of splenic parenchyma. The manipulation of the instruments should be with care at the pedicle, which may permanently disrupt the blood flow to the remenant spleen. The camera must be used in conjunction with the operator's maneuvers. The electro cautery can control the hemorrhage to some extent but if the cut surface becomes large then many surgeries are probable of becoming total. The eschar of electrocautery is a clinical concern as it may disrupt after surgery and cause future complications. The eschars at the hilum are more prone to disrupt because of the pressure in the blood vessels and rotation. The control of the suction is equally important as it may sometimes disturb the meshes and eschar.

The use of harmonic scalpel has improved the lapraroscopic surgery, and because of the greater precision near the vital structures it has bought wonders to the spleen preserving surgeries. It has become an important tool in the surgical armamentarium. It doesn't produce noxious smoke plume, which makes the surgeons view even clearer. It also has the additional benefit of minimal, if any, lateral thermal tissue damage that reduces the postoperative sepsis and necrosis. It causes minimal charring and desiccation. The reduced need for ligatures has contributed to the excellent recovery. There is no escharformation, which makes this technique very advantageous as it clearly prevents its disruption, thus preventing postoperative hemorrhage. The introduction of high definition cameras has made the surgeries more vivid.

There is also a new widely adapted plasma scalpel and its use provides excellent results. Its use has the benefit of giving a better precision, which makes this technique highly promising. The comfort and ease with which it dissects the tissues is overwhelming. It nearly gives the surgeon a blood less view of the surgery field. It causes minimum scarring and has the advantage of faster healing which reduces the operating room time. Using plasma scalpel minimizes the instrument changes that are good aspects for surgeons to consider.

Radiofrequency (RF) ablation has recently evolved as a boon to the surgical world. It has advantage over other techniques because it makes the surgery merely bloodless; hence lesser post-operative complication, sepsis, and minimal hospital stay. Recently it was stated that RF is used to coagualate not the tumor itself, but a thin zone of normal organ parenchyma surrounding it, in order to achieve near bloodless division of the parenchyma. However, only case reports and small series have been reported regarding RF-assisted partial splenectomy. It is already successful on liver, brain and lungs and needs more effort, trial and expertise corresponding spleen. The preservation of splenic parenchyma is the requisite in spleen preserving surgeries and hemorrhage is yet another factor governing the success of surgery. The use of laparoscope already has minimized the bleeding, scar, pain and hospital stay and when used in symbiosis with RF ablation will undoubtedly bring better outcome to spleen preserving surgeries.

The argon beam coagulator has good effect on solid organ surfaces such as the spleen. Smoke is minimal as argon gas surrounds the target site. In a laparoscopic adaptation, 5 and

10mm diameter (disposable) probes are employed. It provides an optimum hemostasis. Argon beam coagulator uses a no-touch technique, and the stream of argon gas, as it conducts the electrical energy, simultaneously has a" blast" effect on the target tissues, momentarily blowing away blood, fluid, and debris for more efficient coagulation. The electrical generator is inexpensive but the electrode tips are relatively expensive, requiring frequent replacement. However, the efficacy of the argon beam coagulator, with its potential for a reduction of operating room time and its efficient achievement of (otherwise tedious) hemostasis, may negate these expenses.

The laparoscopic techniques have bought about essential changes in the surgery and have given a different vision and most importantly precision. The innovative robotic technologies at some centers are used in conjunction with laparoscopy. The use of robotic cameras have added the function of zoom in and zoom out and the 180 degree view have provided surgeons with the desired angle to see splenic pedicle and surrounding landmarks. Robotic cauteries, cameras can also be used with joysticks and voice activation so in delicate moments like achieving hemostasis during pedicle dissection, The surgeons just have to give a command to get the exact view thus saving time manpower and with ease. There are many centers using the davinci system to perform procedures asdelicate as splenectomies. Although, it will need more trial for this technique to be worldwide adopted.

Not only the tools to obtain optimum results during the surgeries are evolving but also the laparoscopic surgery have also evolved. The minimal invasive is on a path of becoming even more minimal. The technique like SILS (single incision laparoscopic surgery) has bought revolution in the laparoscopic world. There are many literatures world wide showing the use of SILS for partial splenectomies. This technique in particular draws lot of attention owing to the fact that it's used through single trocar introduced through a small umbilical incision. From a single port three to four instruments as camera, scalpel, suction can be introduced and operated. The instruments have a multiple operating and viewing angles so the surgery doesn't need many ports. The tips of the instruments are available with multiple degree of rotation, which is the basic tenet of SILS. Partial splenectomies can be done with intricate surgical maneuvers made easy. The reduced operating room time and the nearly invisible scar also improve the pain, hospital stay and post operative complications.

During the laparoscopic surgeries there are many instances where accidents causes oozing of blood and a condition of momentary panic because of either the unsuccessful clamping of vessels or the spillage of resected spleen from the bag and also due to the deprived view of the surgical site. The new idea of HALS (hand assisted laparoscopic surgery) prevents momentary panic and also is an efficient and clever choice. In HALS there is a umbilical incision where lap pad is fixed through which gloved hands are introduced into the abdomen to improve depth perception, regain tactile sensation, aid in tissue extraction, and reduce operative time. There are two to three additional incisions for the trocars. The other hand operates the scalpel and suction. This technique can be considered as the hybrid of laparoscopic and open surgery. The surgery as delicate as spleen has a major hemostatic and technical issues. The direct introductions of hands in conjunction with the advanced laparoscopic instruments have yielded good results. For instance, the panic due to the uncontrolled hemorrhage can be stopped directly with the hands and the spleen remnant in case spillage can easily be obtained. The exact texture of the spleen can be felt and the desired amount retraction can be perfectly attained and not to forget the other hands actively dissecting through the laparoscopic ports. In this technique lap pads are used so that minimal incision is enough to introduce the hand in the abdominal cavity.

5. Discussion

As the splenic function mentioned above is better understood, spleen surgeries have developed from the early stage of random splenectomy to the second stage of non-selective spleen preserving, and to today's stage of selective spleen preserving. The concept of spleen preserving has become gradually popular, and various procedures to preserve the spleen have been widely applied which has achieved aoptimal result. Current spleen- preserving methods are mainly as follows:

1. Hemostasismethods, which involve hemostatic materials (such as gelatin sponge, fibrin tissue adhesive), radiofrequency ablation, argon beam coagulator and other technical equipment.
2. Suture repair for ruptured spleen.
3. Partial splenectomy.
4. Spleen autotransplantation.
5. Selective arterial embolization.

Partial splenectomies can be successfully performed for complication like splenic cyst, splenichemangioma, splenic mass, blunt traumas and splenic cysts. Proper hemostasis and uninterrupted view of the surgical site has always been a surgical concern. With the advent of laparoscopic techniques many flaws have been obviated which makes partial splenectomies more justifiable. The laparoscopic spleen surgeries, which once started with classical four trocarsand electrocautery have evolved to have come long way. The assistance of better HD cameras with robotic zoom in and zoom out function have given the surgeons the most uninterrupted clear view of the surgical site which has bought the ease in locating a structure and active hemostasis. The cameras once used by the fellow operator can now be operated with voice commands and joysticks of the surgeon. The 180degree rotations of the cameras have made the view extremely vivid circumventing accidents. The electro cautery had drawbacks like the eschar formation that have been eliminated with the development of harmonic and plasma scalpels. The harmonic and plasma scalpel and uses of laser prevents escharformation, which prevents postoperative disruption and bleeding. These scalpels works with better precision near the vital structures as the pedicle of spleen. There is minimal thermal tissue damage, which is pivotal for postoperative recovery. The uses of ligatures have become least and the charring and dissication have been minimized. The postoperative healing, pain have also been greatly minimized with lesser hospital stay. A surgeon should choose a specific way depending on experience, overall cost and the simplicity in manipulating instruments. The robotic instruments, the use of harmonic and plasma scalpels in other instance needs a constant technical assistance. Robotic instruments are cumbersome and needs constant upgrading and high cost of compatible instruments prevents worldwide adoption. There is also an operative time delay when using robotics and it needs special training to surgeons.

Laser in the other hand has the advantage of checking blood loss, sealing the most small blood vessels, ability to work in relatively dry field which facilitates visibility, minimum tissue trauma less pain, edema (due to sealing of nerve endings and lymphatics) decreases chance of malignant cells to spread, scarring due to precision and most importantly decreases stenosis which is appropriate for splenic hemangiomas. The use of laser needs a surgical technologist (ST) at all times as its failure during the surgery can cause panic. Strict safety precautions must be enforced, eye protection for patients and all personnel in the room is mandatory for most lasers and flammable prep solutions and other flammable liquids should not be used in the area where the laser is used. All dry materials in or near the operative field must be dampened with saline or water that makes the process more tedious.

The argon beam coagulator has its advantages of its own in giving a competent hemostasis with its "blast effect" which blows away the debris and coagulated blood for excellent hemostasis. It has very good results for splenic abscess as it has a large oozing surface. The major concern in this technique is the potential of gas embolism during the laparoscopic surgery. So the ultrasonography and ECG is constantly needed to check if the embolism has reached the heart and lungs to prevent further damages.

The minimal invasive surgery has become more minimal with SILS. The cameras,suction and cutting shears all fit through one trocar. The single port for the trocar has laparosonic cutting shears (LCS) and the cameras also have all round vision, which makes this method promising. It has single small incision, therefore less invasive and traumatic. Like every technique has its advantage and disadvantages. SILS is not very efficient if the tumor size is large. It is a good option only for the spleens with normal size or only slightly enlarged. Because of the single small incision the macerated spleen is liable to spillage. In case of sudden bleeding it is difficult to control the hemostasis and still needs ergonomic improvement. The fulcrum effect should be minimized to make this technique better so robotic zoom in and zoom out cameras can be a good replacement. The hybrid technique as HALS has eliminated many shortcomings from the laparoscopic surgery. Since, one hand is inside the abdominal cavity it gives perfect retraction and uninterrupted view. The margin of tumor can be felt so dissection margin can be precise without hampering the normal spleen parenchyma. The bleeding site can be actively clamped with just a move of a finger. The splenic parenchyma is frail and the use of hands directly to retract can certainly circumvent bleeding and improper traction. There are many instances in spleen preserving surgeries when the macerated spleen within the bag gets spilled in the abdominal cavity so its recovery is quicker as the spleen gets implanted very soon. This technique can be very efficient in blunt trauma cases when laparotomy is urgently required. The camera in the other hand can work in conjunction with the hand to explore the abdominal cavity. This technique is irrespective of the size of spleen because even the bigger spleen can be handled with care and taken out without spillage and optimum safety. The pitfalls of HALS are the air leakage from the lap pads and the hands getting tired in 20% of the surgeons.

6. Conclusion

A laparoscopic spleen preserving surgery as aforementioned is a technically demanding procedure. The spleen parenchyma is frail and the tears or the parenchymal bleeding can occur. Thus, from a surgeon's point of view it requires exquisite care and control to avoid parenchymal rupture and cell spillage. There are many techniques available to do the same procedure in a logical and proficient way. The surgeons must be familiar with all the details and complications before choosing for one. Every technique has a virtue of its own over the other, so it is vital to discriminate techniques to choose the ideal one. The need of the laparoscopic surgery must be understood with the operative time and cost in mind. The postoperative outcome is the most important part of perioperative care and in the abdominal surgeries as spleen; adhesion is serious complication that affects the motility of abdominal structures later on. The complication as eschar formation, which may disrupt postoperatively is capable of causing bleeding. Thus, the technique that offers minimum adherence, eschar formation, sepsis, and necrosis should be employed.

7. References

[1] Barbaros U, Dinççağ A. Single incision laparoscopic splenectomy: the first two cases. J Gastrointest Surg. 2009;13(8):1520-3.
[2] Carrara S, Arcidiacono PG, Albarello L, et al. Endoscopic ultrasound-guided application of a new internally gas-cooled radiofrequency ablation probe in the liver and spleen of an animal model: a preliminary study. Endoscopy. 2008;40(9):759-63.
[3] Targarona EM, Espert JJ, Balagué C, et al. Residual Splenic Function After Laparoscopic Splenectomy. Arch Surg. 1998;133(1):56-60.
[4] Ghuliani D, Agarwal S, Thomas S, et al. Giant cavernous haemangioma of the spleen presenting as massive splenomegaly and treated by partial splenectomy. Singapore Med J. 2008;49(12) : e356.
[5] Ball, Kay. Lasers:ThePerioperative Challenge, ed III. Mosby, 1995. 86-120.
[6] Standards of Perioperative Clinical Practice in Laser Medicine and Surgery, www.aslms.org/health/standards_perioperative.html
[7] Troust, D, et al. Surgical Laser Properties and Their Tissue Interaction.Mosby Year Book, 1992. 131-162
[8] Robotics and Technology. Wikipedia, Nov 2006, http://en.wikipedia.org/wiki/ robotic_surgery.
[9] Hermes Intelligent Operating Room®, www.trueforce.com/medical_ robotics/medical_robotics_ companies_hermes.htm
[10] Kaul, Sanjeev. Laparoscopic and Robotic Radical Prostectomy.eMedicine,Feb 28, 2005, www.emedicine.com/med/topic3723.htm
[11] Lanfranco, Anthony, et al. Robotic Surgery. Annals of Surgery, 2004, 239:14
[12] Harmonic Scalpel®. Gateway Products Information and Ultrasonic Cutting and Coagulation Devices. Johnson & Johnson, 2001-2006, Ethicon Endosurgery,Inc, www.harmonicscalpel.com
[13] Harmonic Scalpel®. Intermedix International Experts, Inc, www. armonicscalpelrepaircenter. com/harmonic.html
[14] Link, W. J. A Plasma Scalpel: Comparison of Tissue Damage and Wound Healing With Electrosurgical and Steel Scalpels. Arch Surg, 1976,111(4):392-397,
[15] Marino, Ignazio RA. New Option for Patients Facing Liver ResectionSurgery. 2006 Plasma Surgical Limited, www.plasmasurgical.com/article-Marino.htm
[16] Jiang HC, Sun B, Qiao HQ, et al. Clinical application of serial operations with preserving spleen. World J Gastroenterol. 2001,7(6):876-9.
[17] Reger,T. B., Janhke, M. E. Robotic Cardiac Surgery. AORN J, 2003,77:182

13

Laparoscopic Gastropexy for the Treatment of Wandering Spleen With or Without Gastric Volvulus

Caroline Francois-Fiquet[1], Yohann Renard[2], Claude Avisse[2], Hugues Ludot[3], Mohamed Belouadah[1] and Marie-Laurence Poli-merol[1]

[1]Department of Pediatric Surgery
[2]Department of Anatomy
[3]Department of Anesthesiology
American Memorial Hospital CHU REIMS / REIMS University of Medicine
France

1. Introduction

Wandering spleen is a rare condition. This congenital or acquired pathology is found in children and adults alike. It is characterized by a hypermobile spleen causing in some cases splenic torsion with ischemia.
We will successively look at the anatomy, etiologies, epidemiology, clinical pictures, additional imaging examinations and surgical possibilities for this pathology.

2. Anatomy

Wandering spleen is caused by failed fusion of the dorsal peritoneum, or absence or abnormal development of its suspensory ligaments that hold the spleen in its normal position in the left upper quadrant of the abdomen.
The splenic ligaments are the gastrosplenic, splenorenal (splenopancreatic), splenophrenic, splenocolic ligaments. (Couinaud, 1963)
Embryologically, the splenic ligaments develop in the coeliac artery territory, from the primitive dorsal mesentery (mesogastrium), which is responsible for the formation of peritoneum, the greater omentum and the several peritoneal folds. However, developmental anomalies or variations may take place. These variations in the embryologic development of the spleen's primary supporting ligaments could explain the wandering spleen.
These ligaments may be absent, may be too long or too short, too wide or too narrow, or abnormally fused.

3. Etiology

Wandering spleen can be a congenital or acquired condition.

3.1 Congenital form

Wandering spleen is in most cases a randomly distributed birth defect but in some cases it can be part of a syndrome.

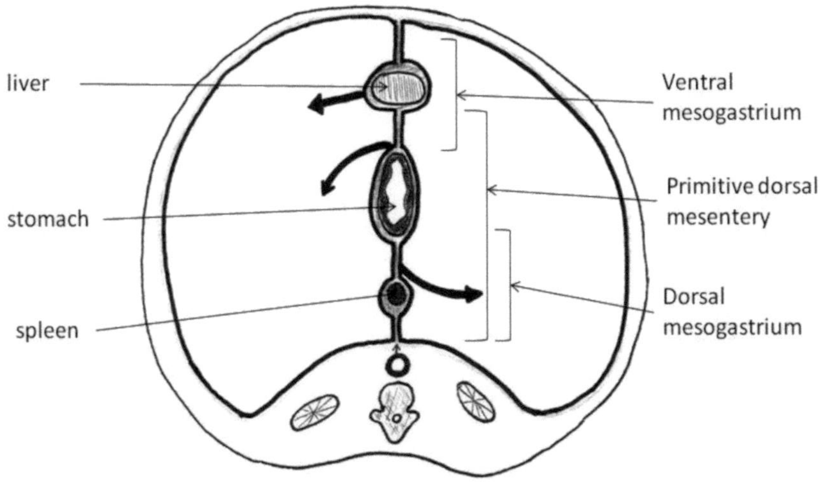

Fig. 1. Transverse section. Development of peritoneal reflexions of spleen during primitive embryonic stage. Coeliac artery territory.

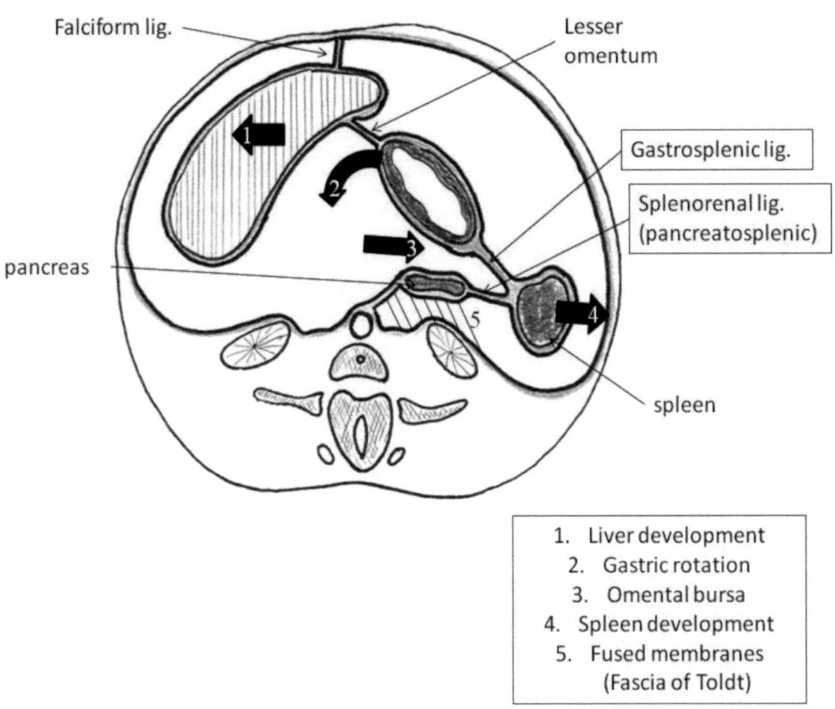

Fig. 2. Transverse section. Peritoneal reflexions of spleen are developed from dorsal mesogastrium (primitive dorsal mesentery).

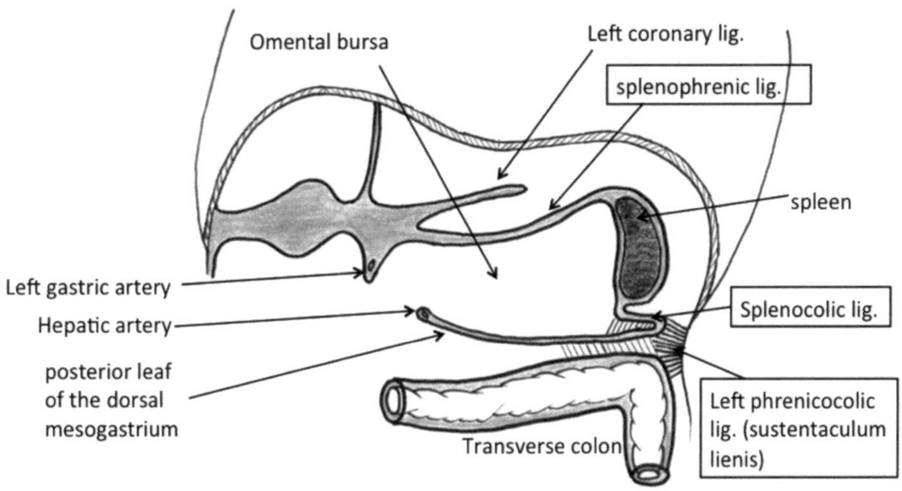

Fig. 3. Frontal section showing the formation of splenocolic ligament and phrenicocolic ligament

3.1.1 Association

3.1.1.1 Congenital diaphragmatic hernia

The first case of wandering spleen associated to congenital diaphragmatic hernia (CDH) was described in the literature in 1940 by Bohrer. Several cases have been reported since then (Yasuda et al, 2010; Fiquet-François et al, 2010; Yilmaz et al, 2008; De Foer et al, 1994). The diagnosis of both pathologies can occur at the same time or the diagnosis of wandering spleen can be secondary to CDH. With CDH wandering spleen can be a result of an abnormal or absence of retroperitoneal fixation. Based on these data, all patients with CDH should be considered as potential candidates for wandering spleen.

3.1.1.2 Omphalocele

Yilmaz reported the unusual case of wandering spleen associated to omphalocele. (Yilmaz et al, 2008) As a possible cause for this association they listed defects on the abdominal walls through which the organs were protruding, resulting in a restriction of the stomach and spleen normal rotation or inefficient fusion after the rotation has been completed

3.1.2 Familial wandering spleen

Ben Ely described the first case of familial wandering spleen with two sisters diagnosed at a 3-year interval. (Ben Ely et al, 2008)

3.2 Acquired form

3.2.1 Postoperative (subtotal splenectomy)

Even if these data are not found in the literature, our multicenter study (Fiquet-François et al, 2010) reported 4 cases of wandering spleen post subtotal splenectomy. They were in fact excluded from the study that only focused on congenital forms. These cases are quite interesting and probably unveil a technical defect. When the subtotal splenectomy involves resection of the upper pole of the spleen, with the section of suspensory ligaments, promoting acquired wandering spleen. To avoid this type of complications it is preferable to preserve the upper pole of the spleen and promote resection of the lower pole. It is important to bring up the possibility of wandering spleen in case of sudden or chronic abdominal pain in a patient having a history of subtotal splenectomy.

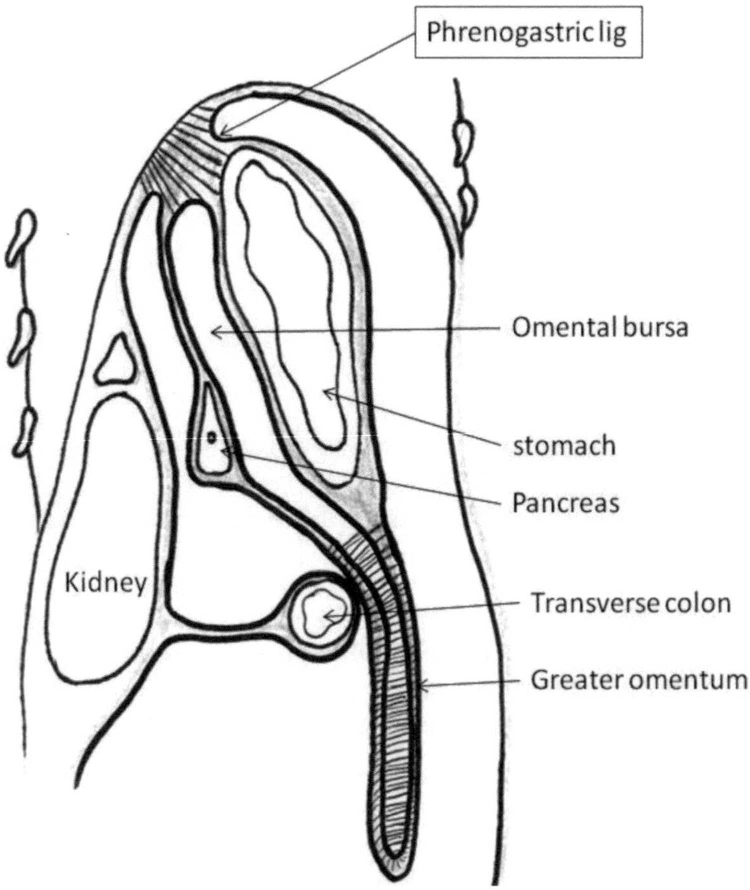

Fig. 4. Sagittal section showing the Phrenogastric ligament. This ligament prolonge the splenophrenic ligament to the right, and this splenophrenic ligament is an extension of the splenorenal ligament.

3.2.2 Traumatic diaphragmatic hernia

As discussed above, CDH can be associated to wandering spleen; in fact traumatic diaphragmatic hernia can also generate acquired wandering spleen.

3.2.3 Malarial infection

Malarial infection has not been clearly validated as responsible for the onset of secondary wandering spleen, but it can clearly trigger the pathology, asymptomatic until then.

Cripps described the case of a patient who had a malarial infection at the age of 5 and the CT-Scan done at the time validated a normally located spleen. (Cripps et al, 2010) However at the age of 18 she developed clinical symptoms and the diagnosis concluded to wandering spleen that could have resulted from a congenital fusion anomaly or attenuation of the patient's suspensory ligaments caused by her previous malarial infection and splenomegaly. However we can wonder if the malarial splenomegaly did not simply unveil an underlying congenital abnormality.

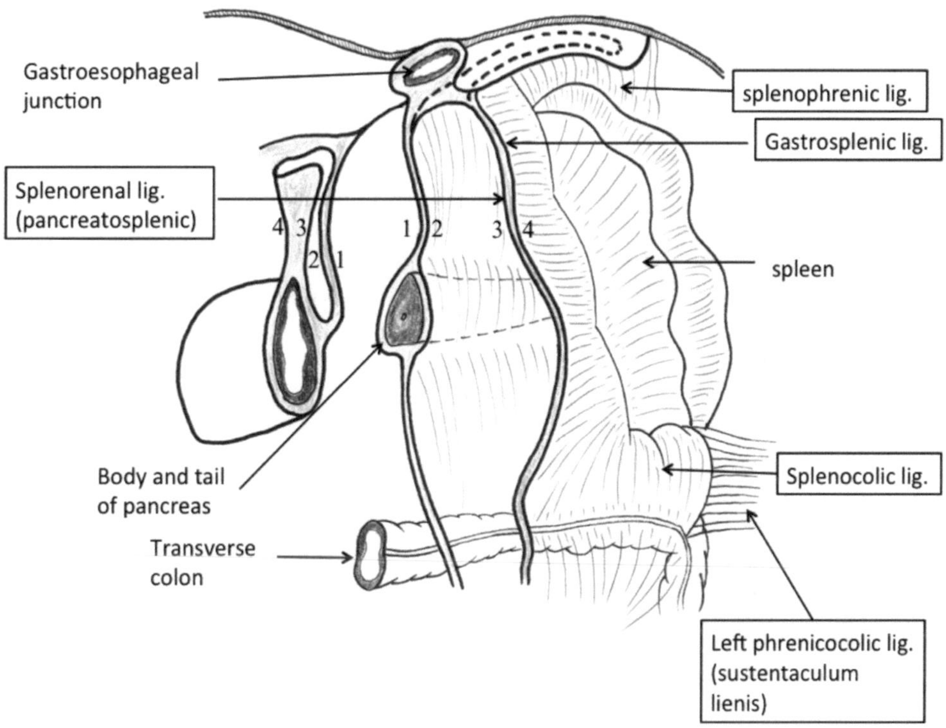

Fig. 5. Frontal view. Peritoneal attachments of spleen. Stomach is retracted to the right

4. Epidemiology

The incidence of wandering spleen is uncertain and difficult to assess. The diagnosis is often made following complications. The incidence of this pathology is probably dramatically underestimated.

Romero and Barksdale evaluated the peak incidence for wandering spleen between the age of 20 and 40 (Romero & Barksdale, 2003; Lin et al, 2005). Generally, 70–80% of the reported cases occur in women of childbearing age. (Steinberg et al, 2002) Hormonal changes and fluctuations explain this female predominance in adults. Furthermore the literature has reported that potentially predisposing elements in this population include multiparity and abdominal laxity thought to be secondary to pregnancy-induced hormonal effects on the abdominal wall. (S. Zarrintan et al, 2007) Ghazeeri et al (Ghazeeri et al, 2010) reported the case of splenic torsion on wandering spleen in a pregnant woman in her twelfth week of twin pregnancy.

This pathology is also found in children seemingly affecting more boys than girls (Allen & Andrews, 1989; François-Fiquet et al, 2009; Fiquet-François et al, 2010). This condition can occur very early on as seen in neonatal cases (Balliu et al, 2004; Fiquet-François et al, 2010, Arleo et al, 2010). During the first years of life the sex ratio is probably reversed. (Brown et al, 2003)

5. Clinical pictures

The diagnosis of wandering spleen is extremely difficult since it is such a rare condition and is clinically non-specific. In our recent multicenter study in children (Fiquet-François et al, 2010), we reported that the abdominal pain is at the forefront of all symptoms (93 % of cases), and its severity brings 86% of all cases to Emergency Room care. Furthermore, in 57% of all cases it was their first symptomatic episode of this type. The pain location is clinically non-specific: diffuse, periumbilical, left side, pelvis, left hypochondrium… Vomiting can be associated in 57% of cases. None of the diagnoses of wandering spleen were based on clinical evidence only. Even if the diagnosis cannot solely be based on clinical observations, it is important to note that the clinical presentation for wandering spleen can be either acute or chronic pain (Fiquet-François et al, 2010). The acute clinical pictures require emergency surgery because of the high risk of ischemia.

5.1 The acute clinical picture

The acute clinical picture can show two types of presentations: splenic torsion but also gastric volvulus, associated or not to splenic torsion.

5.1.1 Splenic torsion

This is the main complication of wandering spleen, it usually reveals this abnormality. Pain is at the forefront of the symptoms. Splenic torsion is an emergency situation as it can quickly lead to irreversible splenic ischemia. In our series (François-Fiquet et al, 2010), 6 patients (43%) had splenectomy for splenic ischemia, but the torsion can complicate up to 65% of pediatrics cases (Romero & Barksdale, 2003).

5.1.2 Gastric volvulus +/- associated to splenic torsion

The clinical picture groups together painful symptoms associated to high occlusion with vomiting. In some cases patients can be in a real state of shock.

Gastric volvulus associated to wandering spleen is a rare condition, and its quick clinical improvement with a simple medical treatment often delays the diagnosis and access to proper surgical care (Fiquet-François et al, 2010; François-Fiquet 2009; Spector & Chappell, 2000; Qazi & Awadalla, 2004). The semiological difficulty is quite real when faced with complex clinical pictures associating gastric volvulus, wandering spleen and even in some cases a diaphragmatic hernia (Liu & Lau, 2007).

The combination of wandering spleen and gastric volvulus should be explored by additional imaging exams, and requires a quick and adapted therapeutic care.

5.2 Chronic clinical picture

Between 39% and 43% of children treated for wandering spleen had already presented similar symptoms. (Brown et al, 2003; Fiquet-François et al, 2010). Most often these children had been complaining about non-systematic recurrent but inconsistent abdominal pain for

the past months (even several years). Some children were even hospitalized several times before making a proper diagnosis. This is mostly due to the quick clinical improvement when the child was lying down (Fiquet-François et al, 2010; François-Fiquet et al, 2009).
The chronic clinical picture once again underlines the difficulty in making a proper diagnosis when faced with an atypical clinical picture.

6. Additional imaging examinations

Additional imaging examinations are key elements for the diagnostic evaluation of wandering spleen. The diagnosis cannot be made on non-specific clinical symptoms only.

6.1 Abdominal sonogram

An abdominal sonogram is the current diagnostic modality of choice for wandering spleen since it can validate the diagnosis without using radiation. (Fiquet-François et al, 2010; Brown et al, 2003; Di Crosta et al, 2009; Karmazyn et al, 2005).
It is essential to ask the radiologists to correctly evaluate the location and viability of the spleen when faced with gastric volvulus, but also dull abdominal pain.

6.2 CT-scan and abdominal magnetic resonance imaging

The efficacy of contrast enhanced CT-scan imaging has been validated and can be quite helpful in an emergency situation since it is not radiologist dependent and might sometimes be faster to access. Thus, it remains a perfect choice for acute pictures such as diagnostic evaluation of splenic torsion associated to a wandering spleen with a high risk of ischemia. It is the whorled appearance of the splenic vessels and surrounding fat that is considered pathognomonic of that condition. (Gomez et al, 2006). However even if this examination is well indicated in adults, CT-scan should remain a last-resort examination in children because of radiation exposure (Ben et al, 2006; Marinaccio et al, 2005). Abdominal magnetic resonance imaging (MRI) (Fig 7-8-9), since it does not require any anesthesia seems to be a good alternative to CT-scan for adults or older children with chronic pain. However, because it is not available in all clinical settings, it can limit its indications. It can also be recommended for uncomplicated chronic types.

6.3 Dynamic sonogram

Dynamic sonogram (on the side, standing up) is a simple examination that can help define the splenic ptosis and be relevant for chronic and hard-to-identify cases. It is also properly indicated for follow-up and monitoring exams.

6.4 Plain abdomen radiography

Plain abdomen radiography is still useful as first-line imaging examination. It allows for a quick diagnosis of gastric volvulus (Fig 10).
A well-designed imaging check-up can usually validate the diagnosis. But in some cases the diagnosis will only be validated during surgery.

7. Complications of wandering spleen

Splenic ischemia is the main complication of wandering spleen. It justifies in itself emergency therapeutic care. Gastric volvulus is a well-known complication of wandering spleen; however its incidence is lower than splenic torsion. Sometimes there can be a pancreatitis and gastric outlet obstruction via direct external compression (sanchez et al, 2010) or even a pancreatic tail infarction (Dirican et al, 2009)

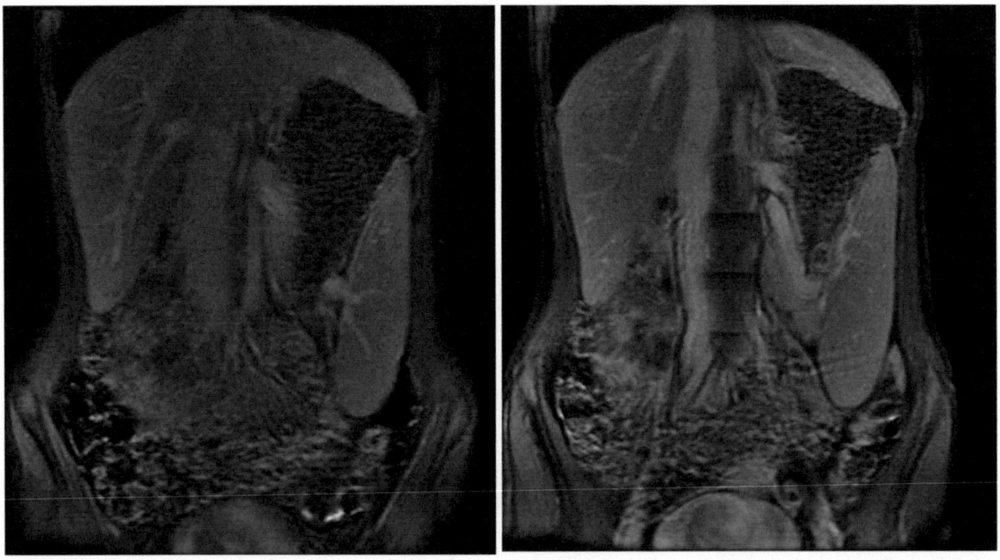

(a) (b)

Fig. 7. a-b Magnetic resonance imaging abdominal frontal view. Spleen in a low position below the stomach, long pedicle, good vascularization

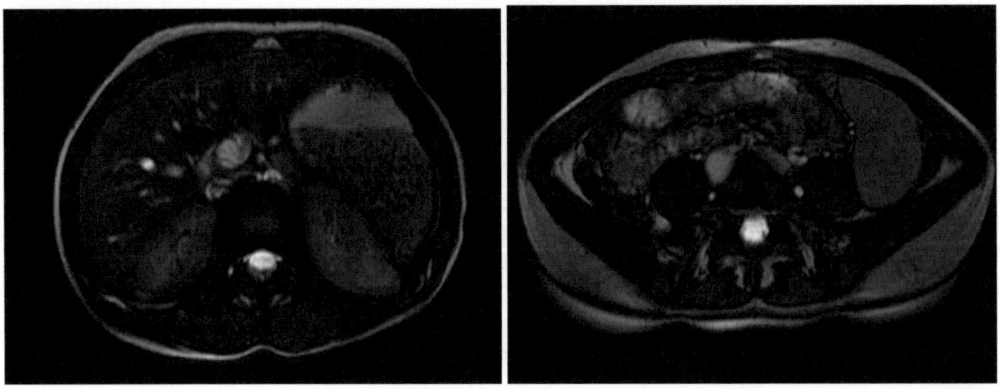

(a) (b)

Fig. 8. Magnetic resonance imaging abdominal transversal view. a : not visible on a view going through both kidneys and b : well-vascularized spleen still visible in the left iliac fossa

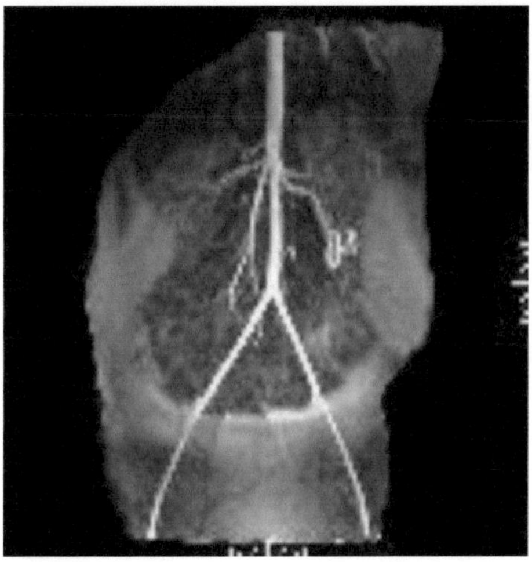

Fig. 9. Magnetic resonance imaging abdominal frontal view. Long pedicle, good vascularization

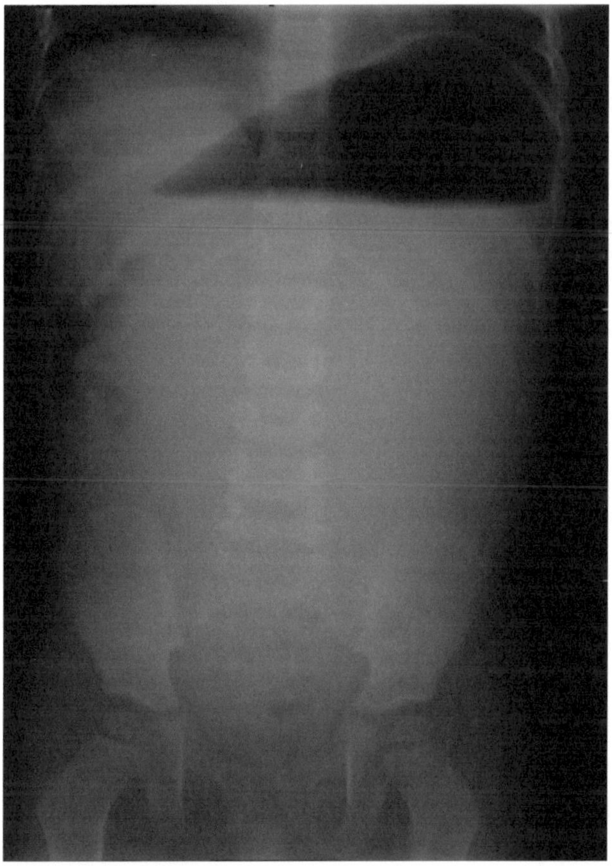

Fig. 10. Plain Abdomen: gastric volvulus

8. Surgery

Surgery is the only option to guarantee the viability of the spleen; however it should not trigger any secondary ischemia. Its objective will be to restore the spleen in its anatomical position as close to normal as possible to avoid the dangling effect of the spleen at the end of its pedicle.

8.1 States of art

Surgery is the appropriate therapeutic choice, but many different approaches are available: laparoscopic surgery, laparotomy, splenopexy, gastropexy, and splenectomy.

8.1.1 Surgical approaches

In the literature, we found that in 49% of the cases the diagnosis was made during surgery (Brown et al, 2003). In this context, laparoscopic surgery is the procedure of choice. It allows for an etiological diagnosis, a good evaluation of the surgical situation while offering several therapeutic possibilities: splenectomy (Carmona et al, 2010), splenopexy (Hirose et al, 1998; Kleiner et al, 2006), gastropexy (François-Fiquet et al, 2009; Fiquet-François et al, 2010) or even a combination of several techniques such as gastropexy and splenopexy (Okazaki et al, 2010)

The choice for classic open surgery or laparoscopic surgery varies according to the different surgical teams. When there is no history of abdominal surgery, laparoscopic procedure seems to be the procedure of choice.

The risk of gastric perforation is an argument for laparotomy as the procedure of choice in case of gastric volvulus, but it does not seem to be a limiting factor for an experienced laparoscopic technician. (Mayo et al, 2001) The surgical treatment should only take place after medical treatment has been administered. The gastric suction avoids the risk of spontaneous or laparoscopy-induced gastric perforation.

8.1.2 Surgical procedures

Nowadays, it is commonly accepted to try and preserve the spleen, when viable, during the procedure, to avoid post-splenectomy infectious complications.

It is necessary to be aware of this rare clinical pathology in order to avoid delaying surgical care, which could lead to splenic ischemia or even gastric ischemia.

Nevertheless, splenic ischemia after torsion is quite common and the rate varies from 43% to 65% of cases according to the series (Fiquet-François 2010; Romero et al, 2003).

Splenectomy will be the gold standard for major splenic ischemia, when there is splenic necrosis after torsion repair and the spleen is no longer viable.

Faced with a viable or almost viable spleen, the surgery should aim for splenic conservation. The surgery should focus on a fixation technique that will:

- reposition the spleen properly in order to avoid any further risks of torsion. The goal is to reconstruct the best possible physiological anatomy with surgical fixation.
- but also avoid gastric volvulus complication. This is why it is also recommended, as a preventive measure, to perform a gastropexy on patients with a wandering spleen in order to avoid any risk of developing a gastric volvulus. (Spector & Chappell, 2000; Soleimani et al, 2007)
- while limiting spleen manipulation that could be responsible for secondary splenic ischemia. (Fiquet-François et al, 2010)

Taking all these elements into account we have proposed an approach by Laparoscopic Assisted Gastropexy (LAG)

8.2 Procedure: LAG laparoscopic assisted gastropexy

This technique can be used in adults and children alike and in both cases of congenital or acquired wandering spleen. It can be done as an emergency procedure in case of splenic ischemia or scheduled for uncomplicated chronic cases.

8.2.1 Installation

After gastric tube decompression (in case of gastric volvulus), the patient is positioned supine on the surgical table.

A general anesthetic technique completed by bilateral Transversus Abdominis Plane Block (TAPB) to allow for eviction curare substances.

Tracheal tube and positive pressure ventilation with O2-air (0.5,0.5) was used. The nitrous oxide is formally cons indicated. (intestinal dilatation)

In children, the surgeon and assistant are at the right of the child. The laparoscopy column is placed at the level of the patient's left shoulder. (Fig 11) In adults, the French lover position allows for the surgeon's assistant to be perfectly positioned for this procedure.

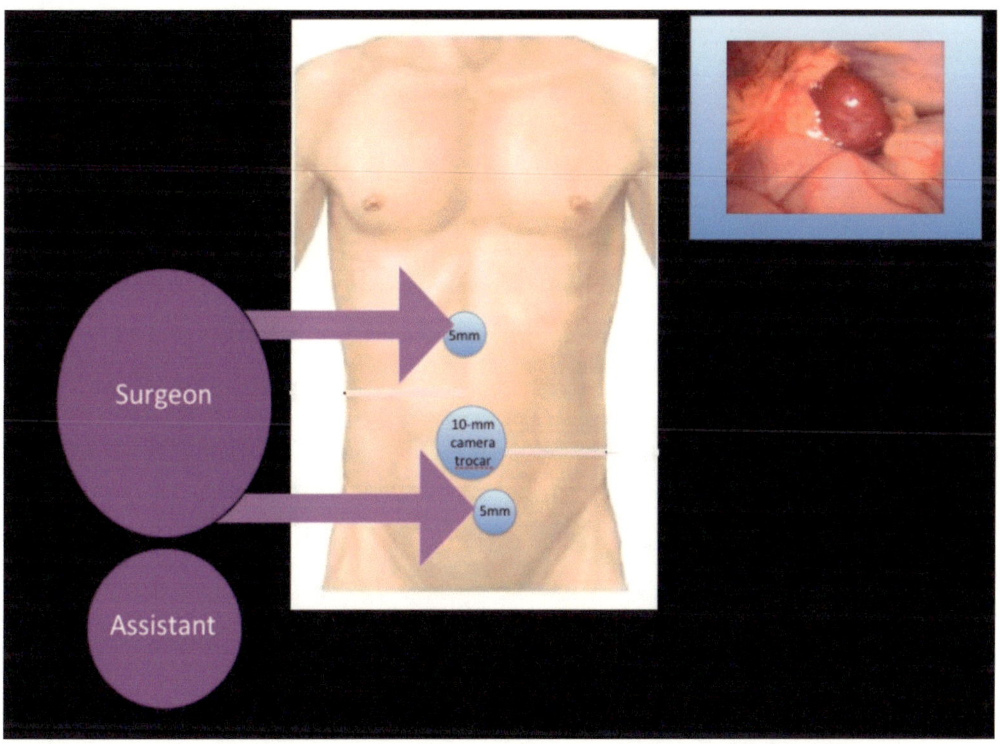

Fig. 11. Diagram presenting the positions of: the patient, trocar entry sites, surgeon, surgeon's assistant and laparoscopic column.

8.2.2 Procedure

A 10-mm camera trocar was inserted in the sub-umbilical region using open laparoscopy.
A laparoscope (0° degree) was inserted through the umbilical port.
2 additional working ports (5mm) were inserted: below and above the umbilicus. A third port can be inserted if necessary.
Laparoscopic exploration validated:

- the abnormal location of the spleen located in the lower left quadrant (in most of cases) and its lack of supportive ligaments,
- the vascularization of the spleen with or without ischemia, the aspect of the stomach. Normal or associated to gastric volvulus. In most of cases,during surgey we do not find the gastric volvulus identified by abdominal X-rays, it became devolvulated non-ischemic. However there is evidence of gastric distension with flaccid wall.

If the spleen is completely ischemic after de-torsion, we proposed a splenectomy.
Faced with splenic viability, we decided to perform a gastropexy. (Fig 12)

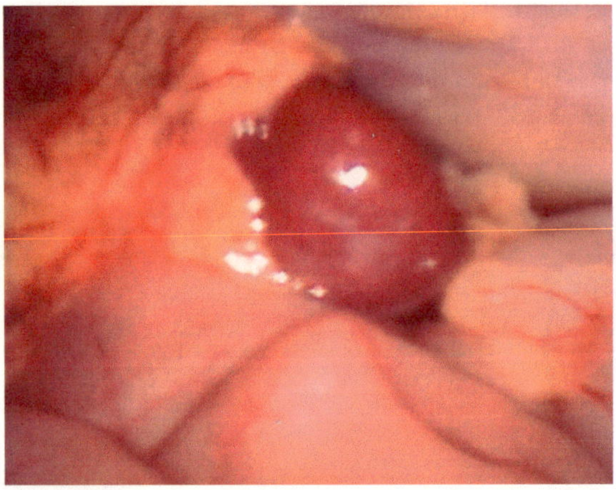

Fig. 12. Well-vascularized spleen in the left iliac fossa

The spleen was then moved freely from its abnormal location (left iliac fossa) to its normal one (sub-diaphragmatic). (Fig 13)

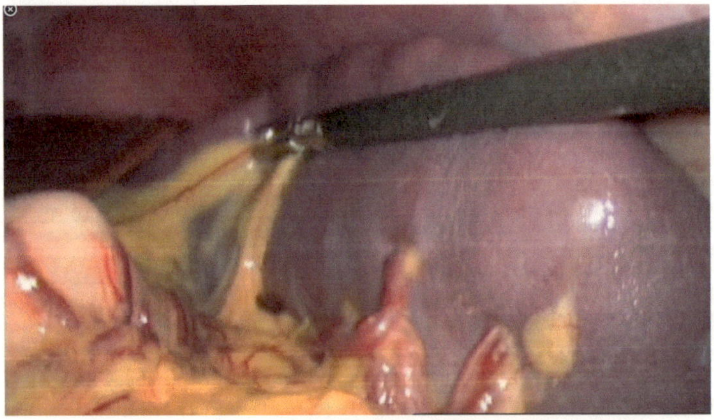

Fig. 13. Repositioning the spleen at the level of the right hypochondrium

We created an extra peritoneal pocket. We performed a parietal peritoneal posterolateral incision, opposite the large gastric curve, up to the diaphragm (7 cm). (Fig 14)

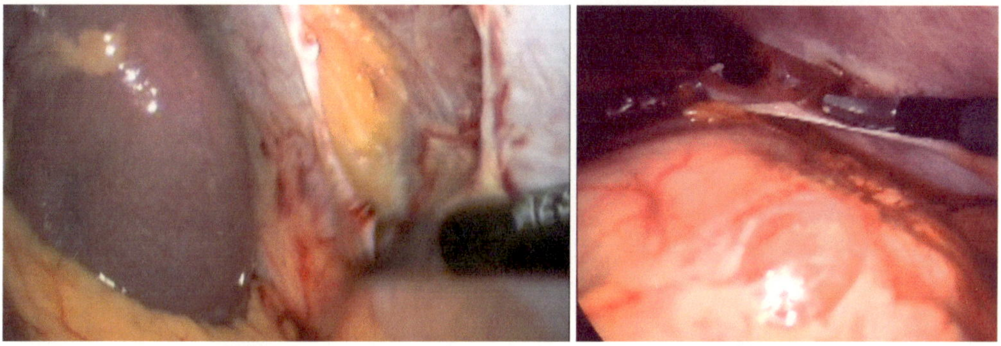

(a) (b)

Fig. 14. a - b Parietal peritoneal posterolateral incision

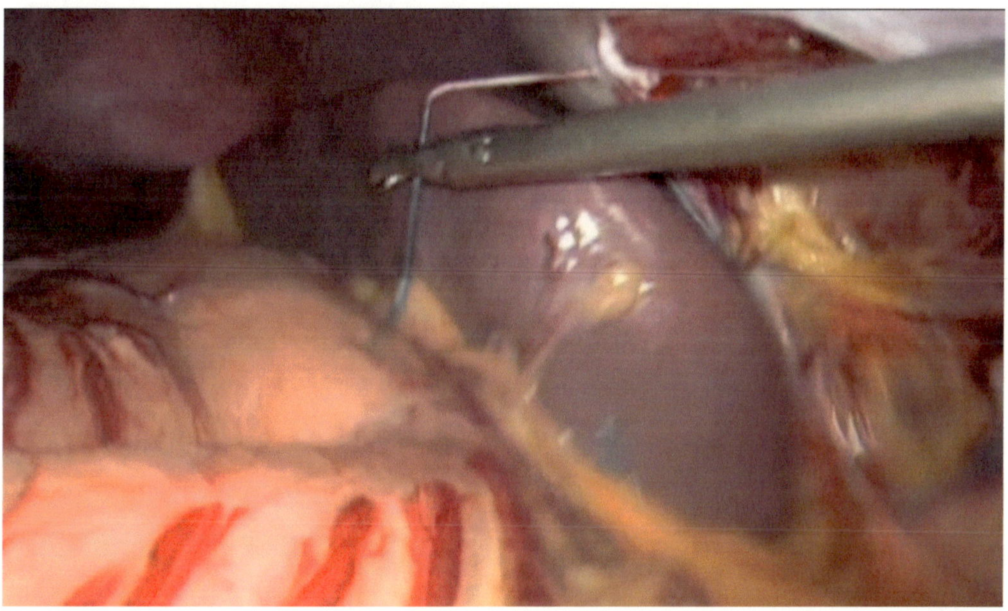

Fig. 15. Gastropexy by suturing the peritoneal wall to the greater curvature of the stomach

We proceeded to the gastropexy. (Fig 18) We fixed the anterior stomach lining with sutures (Mersuture® 3/0; Johnson and Johnson, Somerville, NJ) on the free anterior peritoneum (Fig 15), in two planes. (Fig 16-17-18)

This suture can be done in separate stitches sutures or by two surgeons.

No drain was inserted. The nasogastric tube was removed at the end of the procedure.

Carbon dioxide gas was expelled, trocars removed, and incisions were are closed.

It is essential in case of splenectomy to ensure vaccination (pneumococcal, meningococcal, and haemophilus) and prescribe the usual antibiotic course post-splenectomy. In case of conservative splenic management, in spite of some signs of splenic suffering, it can be useful in the immediate postoperative period to vaccinate as a precaution. Then, at 1-month postoperative and according to imaging controls (Doppler sonogram or contrast CT-Scan) showing the lack of spleen viability, an antibiotic course will be started.

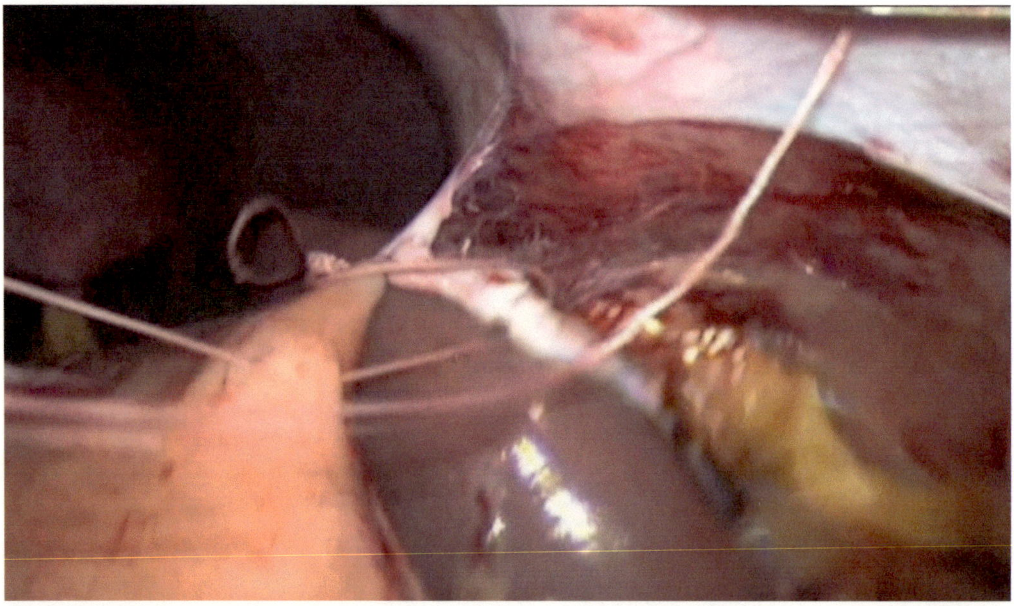

Fig. 16. Gastropexy posterior wall suture done by one surgeon

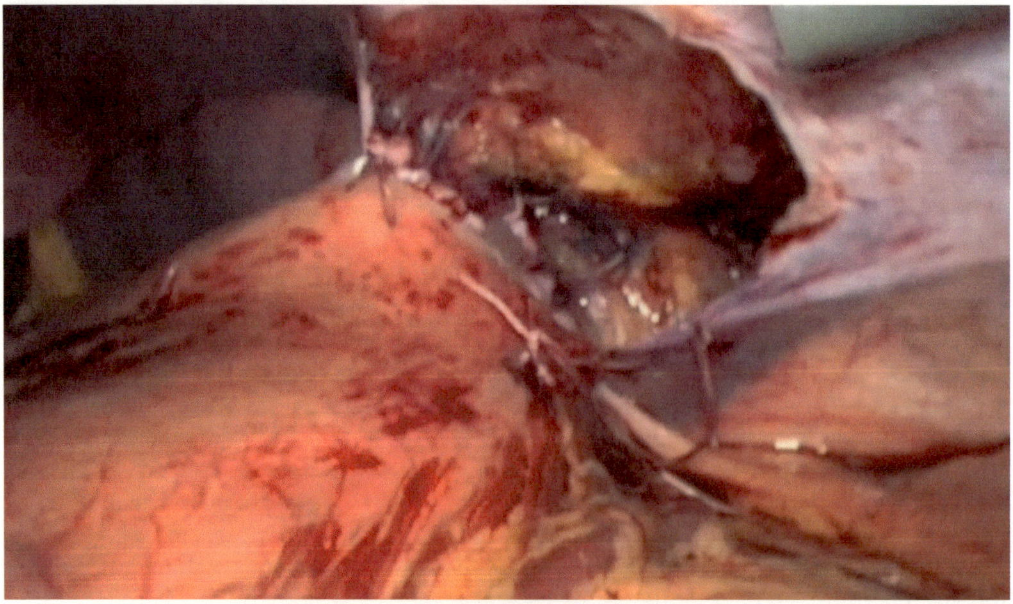

Fig. 17. Final aspect of the posterior plane of the gastropexy

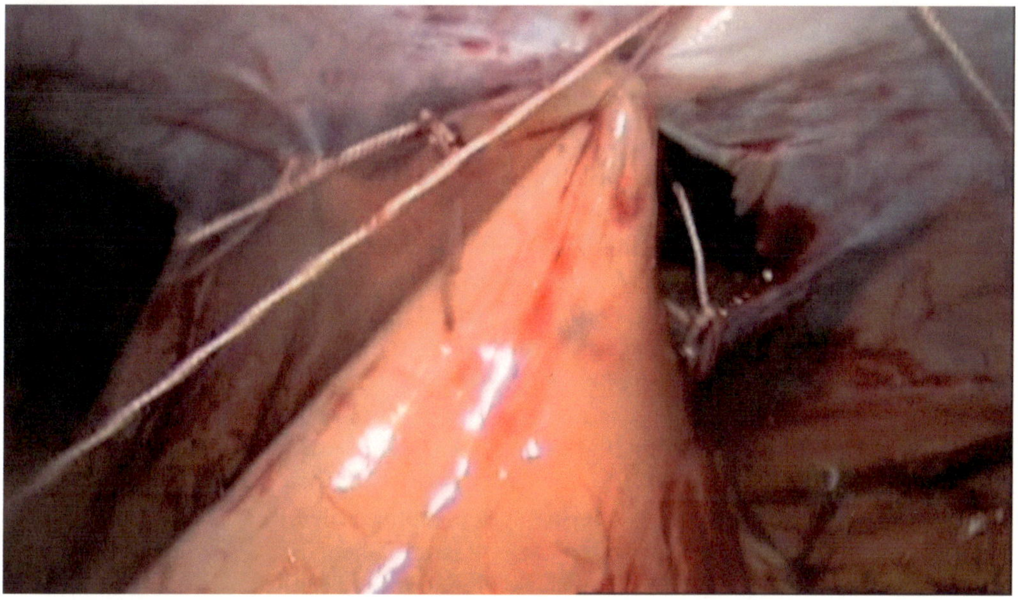

Fig. 18. Suture of the anterior plane (peritoneal-gastric) of the gastropexy

8.2.3 Postoperative care

The patient can drink on the day of the surgery after the legal delays post- anesthesia.
Eating can be started at D1. The patient will be kept laying down on this back the first 24 hours in order to limit shoulder pain.
The convalescence will last 10 days. The patient will be asked to stop all sport activities from 1 to 3 months according to patient's age, clinical picture and type of sports.

8.2.4 Follow-up and monitoring imaging examination

Children will be seen again for a surgical consultation at M1, M4, M10, M24 and postoperative follow-up then again every 3 years until adulthood. Doppler and dynamic sonograms (on the side, standing up) are the key examinations for this follow-up. They can assess the vascularization and viability of the spleen but also make sure the sutures are adequate and discard any residual ptosis.
If there is a doubt on splenic vascularization, a contrast CT-Scan will be proposed.

9. Conclusion

The diagnosis of wandering spleen is extremely difficult to establish because it is such a rare condition and is clinically nonspecific.
Early diagnosis and surgical care are the best guarantees for preserving the spleen. Additional imaging examinations, especially abdominal sonogram as the imaging examination of choice, can help establish a diagnosis when faced with an abnormal location of the spleen. Splenopexy and gastropexy are two surgical fixation approaches aiming to maintain the viable spleen in place.
The results of the gastropexy procedures seem encouraging, but faced with such a small number of cases, no conclusion can be established. Gastropexy seems to avoid the risk of

gastric volvulus by restoring the best possible physiological anatomy while preserving the spleen by lack of manipulation.

10. References

Allen, KB., Andrews, G. (1989). Pediatric wandering spleen. The case for splenopexy: Review of 35 reported cases in the literature, *J Pediatr Surg* 24: 432–435.

Arleo, EK., Kovanlikaya, A., Mennitt, K., Acharya, S., Brill, PW. (2010). Multimodality imaging of a neonatal wandering spleen, *Clin Imaging* 34.(4): 302-5.

Balliu, PR., Bregante, J., Pérez-Velasco, MC., Fiol, M., Galiana, C., Herrera, M., Mulet, J. (2004). Splenic haemorrhage in a newborn as the first manifestation of wandering spleen syndrome, *J Pediatr Surg* 39.(2): 240-2.

Ben Ely, A., Zissin, R., Copel, L. Vasserman, M., Hertz, M., Gottlieb, P., Gayer, G. (2006). The wandering spleen: CT findings and possible pitfalls in diagnosis, *Clin Radiol* 61: 954-8.

Bohrer, JV. (1940). Torsion of a wandering spleen : complicated by diaphragmatic hernia, *Ann Surg.* 111.(3): 416-26.

Brown, C., Virgilio, G., Vazquez, D. (2003). Wandering spleen and its complications in children: A case series and review of the literature, *J Pediatr Surg* 38: 1676–1679.

Carmona, J., Lugo Vicente, H. (2010). Laparoscopic splenectomy for infarcted splenoptosis in a child: a case report, *Bol Asoc Med P R* 102.(2): 47-9.

Cavazos, S., Ratzer, ER., Fenoglio, ME. (2004). Laparoscopic management of the wandering spleen, *J Laparoendosc Adv Surg Tech A* 14: 227–229.

Couinaud, C. (1963). Anatomie de l'abdomen. Tome 1. Edition Doin. Paris.

Cripps, M., Svahn, J. (2010). Hand-assisted laparoscopy for wandering spleen, *Surg Endosc.* 25.(1): 312.

De Foer, B., Breysem, L., Smet, MH., Baert, AL. (1994). Late-onset Bochdalek hernia with a rare postoperative complication: case report. *Pediatr Radiol.* 24.(4):306-7

Di Crosta, I., Inserra, A., Gil, CP., Pisani, M., Ponticelli, A. (2009). Abdominal pain and wandering spleen in young children: the importance of an early diagnosis, *J Pediatr Surg* 44: 1446-9.

Dirican, A., Burak, I., Ara, C., Unal, B., Ozgor, D., Meydanli, MM. (2009). Torsion of wandering spleen, *Bratisl Lek Listy* 110.(11): 723-5.

François-Fiquet, C., Belouadah, M., Chauvet, P., Lefebvre, F., Lefort,G., Poli-Merol, ML. (2009). Laparoscopic gastropexy for the treatment of gastric volvulus associated with wandering spleen, *J Laparoendosc Adv Surg Tech* 19: 137-9.

Fiquet-Francois, C., Belouadah, M., Ludot, H., Defauw, B., Mcheik, JN., Bonnet, JP., Kanmegne, CU., Weil, D., Coupry, L., Fremont, B., Becmeur, F., Lacreuse, I., Montupet, P., Rahal, E., Botto, N., Cheikhelard, A., Sarnacki, S., Petit, T., Poli Merol, ML. (2010). Wandering spleen in children: multicenter retrospective study, *Journal of Pediatric Surgery* 45.(7): 1519–1524.

Ghazeeri, G., Nassar, AH., Taher, AT., Musallam, KM., Jamali, FR. (2010). The wanderer At 12 weeks' gestation, the patient presented with abdominal pain and a palpable mass, *Am J Obstet Gynecol* 202.(6): 662 e1.

Gomez, D., Patel, R., Rahman, SH., Guthrie, JA., Menon, KV. (2006). Torsion Of A Wandering Spleen Associated With Congenital Malrotation Of The Gastrointestinal Tract, *The Internet Journal of Radiology*. Volume 5

Hirose, R., Kitano, S., Bando, T., Ueda, Y., Sato, K., Yoshida, T., Suenobu, S., Kawano, T., Izumi, T. (1998). Laparoscopic splenopexy for pediatric wandering spleen, *J Pediatr Surg* 33: 1571-3.

Karmazyn, B., Steinberg, R., Gayer, G., Grozovski, S., Freud, E., Kornreich, L. (2005). Wandering spleen—the challenge of ultrasound diagnosis: report of 7 cases, *J Clin Ultrasound* 33: 433-8.

Kleiner, O., Newman, N., Cohen, Z. (2006). Pediatric wandering spleen successfully treated by laparoscopic splenopexy, *J Laparo- endosc Adv Surg Tech A* 16: 328–330.

Lacreuse, I., Moog, R., Kauffmann, I., Méfat, L., Bailey, C., Becmeur, F. (2007). Laparoscopic splenopexy for a wandering spleen in a child, J *Laparoendosc Adv Surg Tech A* 17: 255–257.

Lin, CH., Wu, SF., Lin, WC., Chen, AC. (2005). Wandering spleen with torsion and gastric volvulus, *J Formos Med Assoc* 104: 755–758.

Liu, HT., Lau, KK. (2007). Wandering spleen: an unusual association with gastric volvulus, *AJR Am J Roentgenol*. 188.(4): 328-30.

Lu, CC., Chen, HH., Hsieh, MJ. (2004). Wandering spleen presenting as gastric outlet obstruction after repair of traumatic diaphragmatic hernia, *J Trauma* 56.(2): 431-2.

Marinaccio, F., Caldarulo, E., Nobili, M., Magistro, D., Marinaccio, M. (2005). Uncommon etiology of acute abdomen in pediatric age: the torsion of spleen, *G Chir* 26: 34-6.

Mayo, A., Erez, I., Lazar, L., Rathaus, V., Konen, O., Freud, E. (2001). Volvulus of the stomach in childhood: The spectrum of the disease, *Pediatr Emerg Care* 17: 344–348.

Okazaki, T., Ohata, R., Miyano, G., J.Lane, G., Takahashi, T. (2010). Laparoscopic splenopexy and gastropexy for wandering spleen associated with gastric volvulus, *Pediatr Surg Int* 26.(10): 1053-5.

Qazi, A., Awadalla, S. (2004). Wandering spleen: a rare cause of mesenteroaxial gastric volvulus, *Pediatr Surg Int* 20: 878-80.

Romero, J., Barksdale, E. (2003). Wandering spleen: A rare cause of abdominal pain, *Pediatr Emerg Care* 19: 412–414.

Sanchez, R., Lobert, P., Herman, R., O'Malley, R., Mychaliska, G. (2010). Wandering spleen causing gastric outlet obstruction and pancreatitis, *Pediatr Radiol*. 40.(Suppl 1): S89-91.

Soleimani, M., Mehrabi, A., Kashfi, A., Fonouni, H., Büchler, MW., Kraus, TW. (2007). Surgical treatment of patients with wandering spleen: Report of six cases with a review of the literature, *Surg Today* 37: 261–269.

Spector, JM., Chappell, J. (2000). Gastric volvulus associated with wandering spleen in a child, *J Pediatr Surg* 35: 641-2.

Steinberg, R., Karmazyn, B., Dlugy, E., Freud, E., Horev, G., Zer, M. (2002). Clinical presentation of wandering spleen, *J Pediatr Surg* 10: E30.

Yasuda, H., Inoue, M., Uchida, K., Otake, K., Koike, Y., Fujikawa, H., Miki, C., Kusunoki, M. (2010). Wandering spleen causing intestinal obstruction after repair of congenital diaphragmatic hernia, *Eur J Pediatr Surg* 20.(2): 121-3.

Yilmaz, O., Genc, A., Ozcan, T., Aygoren, RS., Taneli, C. (2008). Unusual association of omphalocele and wandering spleen, *Eur Surg Res* 41.(4): 331-3.

Part 6

Miscellaneous Laparoscopic Procedures

14

Laparoscopic Approach to Abdominal Sepsis

José Sebastião Santos, Carlos A.M. Donadelli, Rafael Kemp,
Alberto Facury Gaspar and Wilson Salgado Jr.
Medical School, University of São Paulo, Ribeirão Preto, São Paulo
Brazil

1. Introduction

Diagnostic laparoscopy (DL) was introduced in surgical practice at the beginning of the 20th century but its use was limited for about 80 years. During the second half of the 20th century, laparoscopic access started to be used as a diagnostic resource in the traumatic and non-traumatic acute abdomen (Llanio & Sarle, 1956). Over the last decades, with the advent of new video systems, with the development of laparoscopic instruments and the improved visualization of the entire abdominal cavity, DL achieved an excellent level (Geis & Kim, 1995). Within this context of progress, DL started to be successfully used in critically ill patients in intensive care units, with a diagnostic accuracy of 96% and with no significant changes in hemodynamic parameters during the procedure (Brandt et al., 1993; Forde & Treat, 1992).

The easy identification of the types of organic fluids, the resources for the aspiration of pus, blood, bile and the intestinal content and the increased surgical experience have contributed to the therapeutic success of laparoscopy in an acute abdomen of surgical cause (Boyd & Nord, 1992; Cueto et al., 1997; Easter et al., 1992; Geis & Kim, 1995).

With growing reports of its therapeutic efficacy, laparoscopy quickly became the preferential route of access for the treatment of acute cholecystitis (Z'graggen et al., 1995; Colonval et al., 1997) and was also standardized for the treatment of acute appendicitis, adnexial diseases, and perforated gastric or duodenal ulcers (Branicki, 2002; Sauerland et al., 2006). It also represents an alternative access route for the exploration of the the bile ducts (Tagorona et al., 1995), necrosectomy and drainage of collection in acute pancreatitis (Pamoukian & Gagner, 2001).

There is a growing use of laparoscopy in peritonitis secondary to the perforation of diverticular disease of the colons as an option for cavity washing and drainage, and for the resection of the segment involved, especially in elective procedures (Tonelli et al., 2009; Chatzimavroudis et al.,2009). Selected cases of intestinal obstruction or perforation with early intervention before the installation of sepsis or of circulatory shock can also benefit from a laparoscopic access (Branicki, 2002).

2. Laparoscopy in peritonitis

Although DL represents a standard procedure for critically ill patients with an acute abdomen (Pecoraro et al., 2001), there is controversy about its therapeutic use in the presence of sepsis and of hemodynamic repercussions. The insufflation of CO_2 into the peritoneal cavity reduces the peritoneal immunity mediated by macrophages, with lower production of inflammatory cytokines (IL-1, IL-6, TNF-α). However, laparoscopic surgery is associated with a lower systemic inflammatory response compared to open surgery (Buunen et al., 2004). Studies of the effect of laparoscopy in an animal model of severe peritonitis have obtained conflicting results (Bloechle et al., 1998; Gurtner et al., 1995; Salgado Jr et al., 2008; Wichterman et al., 1979).

There is experimental evidence that pneumoperitoneum predisposes to bacterial translocation and increases the systemic inflammatory response (Bloechle et al., 1998), but other studies have not confirmed this finding (Gurtner et al., 1995; Wichterman et al., 1979).

In a model of peritonitis induced by bacterial inoculation in rats subjected to laparoscopy, elevation of the abdominal wall and laparotomy, the changes of the peritoneal immune system in response to the abdominal infection were lower in the group treated by laparoscopy (Targarona et al., 2006). In a similar study, the number of bacterial colonies obtained in the peritoneal fluid, the rates of positive blood cultures and the peritoneal levels of IL-1 and IL-6 were significantly lower after 24 and 72 hs in the groups subjected to laparoscopy. CO_2 did not appear to influence bacterial growth (Balague et al., 1999)

The incidence of bacteremia due to *B. fragilis* and *E. faecalis* was lower in secondary experimental bacterial peritonitis submitted to washing of the cavity by laparoscopy compared to laparotomy even when the duration of peritonitis exceeded 3 hs, suggesting that laparoscopy produces a lower local trauma and preserves the intra-abdominal conditions (Linhares et al., 2001)

In an experimental rat model of severe bacterial peritonitis (Figure 1) it was demonstrated that antibiotic therapy and an early approach to the abdominal cavity by laparotomy or laparoscopy had similar effects on survival. The approach to the abdominal cavity by laparoscopy induces a greater elevation of the pro-inflammatory cytokines TNF-alpha and IL-6 compared to laparotomy, but when the procedures are associated with the use of broad spectrum antibiotic therapy (gentamicin and metronidazole) there is no difference between them (Salgado Jr et al., 2008).

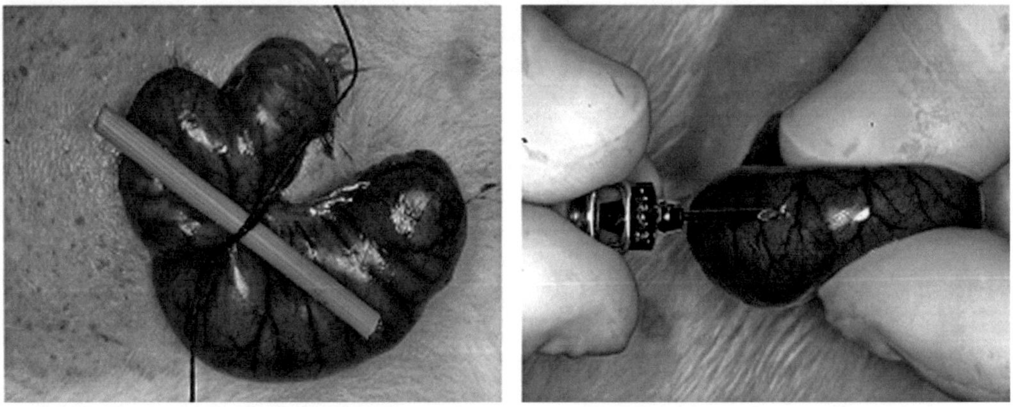

Fig. 1. Experimental model for bacterial peritonitis in rats. Cecal ligation against a rigid mold and 17 gauge needle puncture (Salgado Jr et al., 2008).

Pneumoperitoneum induces an increase in circulating endotoxin but the survival of animals treated by the laparoscopic route is greater than that of animals subjected to laparotomy,

indicating that the overall result of the laparoscopic method may be superior (Chatzimavroudis et al.,2009).
Today, hemodynamic instability is still a limiting factor regarding the use of laparoscopy. The lack of appropriate equipment and of a qualified team continues to be an absolute contraindication of the method. Abdominal distention poses additional risks and reduces the yield of this access route (Stefanidis et al., 2009).
The early use of laparoscopy in an acute abdomen is defended as an appropriate method to prevent a delay in obtaining a definitive diagnosis. Diagnostic laparoscopy within 48 h of hospital admission provided a definitive diagnosis in 90% of cases and modified the clinical diagnosis in 30% of them. A significant portion of patients (83%) were submitted to the laparoscopic procedure as the final treatment of their conditions, with a 7% rate of conversion to open surgery. Peritonitis was present in 180 patients and there was one postoperative death involving a patient with a perforated gastric neoplasia (Golash & Willson, 2005).
An etiologic diagnosis of a non-traumatic acute abdomen by laparoscopy was obtained in 98.6% of cases. The surgical treatment was performed by the laparoscopic route in 75% of the patients and by laparotomy directed by the laparoscopic diagnosis in 13%. Due to a diagnostic error in 2 cases of intestinal obstruction in patients with no abdominal surgery, in this situation the authors recommend laparotomy or investigation by means of other exams (Kirshtein et al., 2003).
The 2005 Consensus of the European Association of Endoscopic Surgery recommends the use of all non-surgical diagnostic means in order to obtain the etiologic diagnosis in patients with a non-traumatic acute abdomen. If the etiology is not detected, DL should be indicated. A perforated peptic ulcer, appendicitis, acute cholecystitis and pelvic inflammatory disease should be treated by the laparoscopic route. The benefits regarding other etiologies have not been sufficiently clarified (Sauerland et al., 2006).

3. Laparoscopy in nonspecific abdominal pain and abdominal sepsis

Nonspecific acute abdominal pain is characterized by a duration of less than 7 days and by diagnostic uncertainty after basic clinical and laboratory evaluation. Under these circumstances, DL is useful for establishing the etiology by means of direct inspection of large areas of the surface of abdominal organs and for obtaining material for biopsy, culture and aspirate, with complementation by laparoscopic ultrasonography. In most cases it is also possible to perform a therapeutic intervention by the same route of access (Stefanidis et al., 2009).
The accuracy of DL ranges from 70 to 99% and its use reduces the time of hospitalization without interfering with morbidity when compared to expectant management of nonspecific abdominal pain (Cueta et al., 1998; Cueto et al., 1997; Decadt et al.,1999; Fahel et al., 1999; Gaita et al., 2002; Golash & Willson, 2005; Majewski, 2000; Navez et al., 1995; Ou & Rowbotham, 2000; Poulin et al., 2000; Sanna et al., 2003; So¨zu¨er et al., 2000; Stefa'nson et al., 1997).
DL is also useful in intensive care when the abdomen is the suspected source of sepsis, of systemic inflammatory response syndrome (SIRS) or multiple organ failure. DL can be used in critically ill patients who present abdominal pain with peritonism accompanied by some signs and symptoms of an inflammatory process, but still without an indication of laparotomy (Stefanidis et al., 2009).

DL can be performed by the bedside, a fact that avoids the risk associated with the transportation of intensive care patients. The contraindications of DL are the same as those for any laparoscopic intervention: hypercapnia, clotting disorder with no possibility of correction, mutliple previous abdrominal surgeries with adhesions, and abdominal surgery in the last 30 days. The use of pneumoperitoneum pressure of 8 to 12 mmHg is recommended, although some authors have used pressures of up to 15 mm Hg with no adverse consequences under these circumstances (Stefanidis et al., 2009).
The diagnostic accuracy of DL in intensive care patients is 90 to 100% (Almeida et al., 1995; Brandt et al., 1993; Brandt et al., 1994; Gagne et al., 2002; Hackert et al., 2003; Jaramillo et al., 2006; Kelly et al., 2000; Orlando & Crowell, 1997; Pecoraro et al., 2001; Walsh & Hoadley, 1998). These success rates are due to the more frequent abdominal diseases occurring in this population (acalculous acute cholecystitis and mesenteric ischemia). The method may fail to detect retroperitoneal processes such as pancreatitis (Stefanidis et al., 2009).
Several studies which evaluated the resolutive capacity of laparoscopy in different clinical situations are summarized in Table 1.

Clinical Setting	Study	N	Study type	Laparoscopy Resolution (%)	Morbidity (%)	Mortality (%)
Acute abdomen	Cueto et al., 1997	107	Review	87,9	14	4,6
Acute abdomen	Perri et al., 2002	221	Review	87%	3	0,5
Acute Abdomen	Golash & Willson, 2005	1320	Retrospective	83	0,9	0,07
ICU	Brandt et al., 1993	25	Clinical series (retrospective)		8	0
Perforated duodenal ulcer	Druart et al., 1997	100	Prospective	92	9	5
Acute Cholecystitis	Z'Graggen et al., 1995	103	Prospective	95,1	10,7	0
Acute Cholecystitis	Colonval et al. , 1997	221	Retrospective	90	13,5	0,9
Small Bowel Obstruction	Kirshtein et al., 2003	44	Retrospective	52	6,4	4,5
Diverticular disease	Torenvliet et al., 2010	231	Review	95,7%	10,4	1,7

Table 1. Evidence for the use of laparoscopy for diagnosis and for some therapeutic purposes in clinical practice.

4. Laparoscopy in acute appendicitis

Appropriate clinical history and physical examination are sufficient for the correct diagnosis of acute appendicitis with typical clinical presentation, a context within which imaging exams are of little value. Computed tomography (CT) is the most valuable exam when there is a diagnostic doubt in acute appendicitis and its complications. CT has 94 to 98%

sensitivity, 83 to 100% specificity and 93 to 96% accuracy and can reduce the number of unnecessary laparoscopiess and laparotomies (Spirit et al., 2010).
Appendectomy by the laparoscopic route yields better results than treatment by laparotomy, especially in patients with disease in the gangrenous phase or with perforation and localized peritonitis. There are isolated reports of the limitation of laparoscopic appendectomy in patients with diffuse peritonitis due to the difficulty in cleaning the peritoneal cavity, the debris and the infected secretion, whereas most reports emphasize the resources of laparoscopic surgery in terms of providing a view of the peritoneal cavity and its recesses, with similar or even more satisfactory conditions for washing the peritoneal cavity compared to laparotomy (Saeurland et al., 2006).
For acute appendicitis, the laparoscopic approach reduces the levels of infection of the surgical wound and favors a more rapid return to habitual activities for the patient compared to laparotomy. Women of reproductive age benefit more from laparoscopy, but other groups also experience this advantage. Laparoscopic treatment of acute appendicitis is also recommended in cases of perforation and contamination of the cavity (Saeurland et al., 2006).
A cohort study was conducted at various academic and private medical centers in the United States to compare laparoscopy and laparotomy for appendectomy. There was no difference in mortality between groups and the group subjected to laparoscopy had a lower incidence of infection of the surgical wound and of episodes of sepsis. The group subjected to laparotomy had a lower incidence of abdominal abscesses and, according to the authors, the approaches yielded similar results (Hemmila et al., 2010).
Among the advantages of the laparoscopic method are the possibility of complete inspection of the abdominal cavity, the preservation of the appendix when normal, and the opportunity to also treat by the laparoscopic route or by guided laparotomy other inflammatory processes or processes of varied characteristics detected on the occasion of inspection (Saeurland et al.,2006).

5. Laparoscopy in abdominal sepsis due to affections of the small bowel (mesenteric ischemia, intestinal obstruction and incarcerated hernias)

Peritonitis secondary to obstruction or ischemia of the small bowel is infrequent. According to the most recent consensus about obstructive intestinal processes, conservative treatment may be maintained for up to 72 hours as long as there is no evidence of strangulation or incarceration. After 3 days of expectant treatment, whether or not these signs are present, surgical exploration is obligatory (Catena et al., 2011).
Some evidence supports the use of the laparoscopic route in the lysis of abdominal adhesions and in the treatment of incarcerated hernias before the onset of necrosis and perforation of the intestinal loops. After the occurrence of these events, most authors recommend surgery by laparotomy (Saeurland et al., 2006).
The lysis of adhesions by laparotomy, the universally accepted route of access for this situation, leads to the later formation of new adhesions, to recurrent intestinal obstruction and to a new laparotomy in 10 to 30% of cases (Landercasper et al., 1993).
In animal models, laparoscopy showed a lower incidence and a smaller number of adhesions, as well as a less severe obstructive situation compared to open surgery. Thus, the laparoscopic approach, when viable, can be considered to prevent obstruction due to adhesions (Tittel et al., 2001). Other clinical and experimental studies have also shown

evidence of a lesser formation of adhesions at the surgical site and on the abdominal wall when laparoscopy is used (Gadallah et al., 2001; Gamal et al., 2001).

The lysis of adhesions by the laparoscopic route has several theoretical advantages over open surgery: 1) less intense postoperative pain, 2) more rapid resolution of the ileum, 3) shorter hospitalization, 4) earlier return to daily activities, 5) lower incidence of complications of the surgical wound, and 6) a reduced formation of postoperative adhesions (Nagle et al., 2004). However, no randomized and controlled studies comparing adhesion lysis by the laparoscopic and open route were detected. Thus, the indications and the results of the less invasive procedure continue to be unclear (Catena et al., 2011).

Today laparoscopy should be reserved for well selected cases, with the use of an open technique for the initiation of pneumoperitoneum, preferentially in the upper left quadrant of the abdomen. It is preferable to use it in case of a first obstructive episode and also when a single or a few adhesions are predicted (for example, when the previous surgery was an appendectomy). A high rate of conversion is expected and the risk of damage to bowel is higher compared to surgery by laparotomy. Findings of a bowel segment larger than 4 cm, of multiple adhesions and of findings compatible with malignant neoplasias supports the option for conversion (Catena et al., 2011).

The extent of release of adhesions is a matter of debate and divides the opinion of authors between the option for lysis of all adhesions in the cavity in an attempt to prevent a new obstructive event or sufficient release for the resolution of obstruction (Scott-Coombes et al., 2003).

Treatment of abdominal wall hernias by laparoscopy has progressed considerably over the last decades and in general this is considered to be the access route of choice in an elective situation. However, it is not possible to transfer the knowledge acquired with this practice to urgency situations such as incarceration, strangulation and bowel injury with contamination of the cavity and infection. There are isolated reports of favorable results for properly selected cases treated by experienced surgeons (Saeurland et al., 2006).

The contribution of laparoscopy to mesenteric ischemia is small. For this situation, DL is less precise than angiography and CT and has not proved to be able to reduce the number of unnecessary laparotomies. DL can detect ischemia when present but cannot rule out this diagnosis when the intestinal loops have a normal appearance upon laparoscopy (Saeurland et al., 2006).

6. Laparoscopy in peritonitis due to gynecological causes

Gynecological affections should always be part of the clinical reasoning in the evaluation of abdominal pain in women. The more frequent causes of abdominal and pelvic pain are ectopic pregnancy, salpingo-oophoritis, pelvic adhesions, endometriosis, and ovarian cysts. In contrast to abdominal processes, CT is less valuable in these conditions. Transvaginal and conventional ultrasonography with a pregnancy test for women of reproductive age are part of the initial evaluation. DL is superior to all other tests and can correct the preoperative diagnosis in up to 40% of cases (Saeurland et al., 2006).

7. Laparoscopy in trauma

DL has been indicated for victims of trauma with suspected intra-abdominal injuries in order to reduce the rate of non-therapeutic laparotomies with their morbidity, mortality and costs. The indications of DL include the suspicion of intra-abdominal injury maintained after an initial negative workup in closed traumas, stab wounds with proven or possible penetration of the cavity, gun-shot wounds with a possible intra-abdominal course, a diagnosis of diaphragm perforation in penetrating wounds of the thoraco-abdominal region, and the creation of a pericardiac transdiaphragmatic window to rule out heart injury (Stefanidis et al., 2009).

Absolute contraindications of DL are hemodynamic instability due to hemorrhagic shock or evisceration, and the relative contraindications include peritonitis, known or obvious intra-abdominal injury, posterior penetrating trauma with a high probability of intestinal injury and, of course, the lack of experienced professionals and of appropriate equipment (Stefanidis et al., 2009).

The accuracy of DL in defining the need for laparotomy ranges from 75 to 100%. In a review, DL prevented non-therapeutic laparotomy in 17 to 89% (median: 57%) of traumatized patients. The procedure involved a 6% rate of false-positive results (0-44%). In addition to providing an etiologic diagnosis, laparoscopy permits the appropriate treatment of intracavity injuries in up to 83% of cases (Hori, 2008).

A review of 37 studies including more than 1900 patients revealed a rate of DL complication of 1% (Villavicencio & Aucar, 1999). More recent reviews have revealed even lower rates close to zero. Intraoperative complications may occur during the creation of the pneumoperitoneum, the introduction of trochars, the occurrence of pneumothorax during inspection due to an unidentified diaphragmatic injury, during the perforation of hollow viscera, the laceration of solid viscera, during gas dissection in the subcutaneous layer of the peritoneum and vascular injuries (more frequently of the epigastric or epiploic arteries) (Hori, 2008).

8. Laparoscopy in the perforation of diverticular disease of the colon

Perforation of diverticular colon disease, generally in the sigmoid colon, with localized contamination of the abdominal cavity can be treated with antibiotics during the early stages, but abscesses larger than 5 cm must be approached surgically. Sigmoidectomy is indicated in patients who have suffered at least 2 crises of diverticulitis and in patients younger than 50 years who have suffered only one episode (Saeurland et al.,2006). Even within an urgency context, this surgery can be performed by the laparoscopic route with a surgical time and results comparable to those of laparotomy and has been performed with a conversion rate of 10% (Tonelli et al., 2009).

Over the last few years, there has been an increased use of peritoneal washing and drainage of the cavity by the laparoscopic route without resection, allied to antibiotic treatment during the episode of peritonitis secondary to diverticular perforation. Definite treatment by colectomy can be performed in an elective manner after the resolution of the inflammatory process (Saeurland et al., 2006; Tonelli et al., 2009).

In a systematic literature review of 231 cases of acute diverticulitis with purulent peritonitis treated in this manner, abdominal sepsis was effectively controlled in 95.7% of the patients. Mortality was 1.7%, morbidity was 10.4% and 1.7% of the patients required a stoma. A long recurrence-free period of time was observed in the patients not subjected to colon resection, and later elective resection of the segment involved by the laparoscopic route was possible in most cases (Toorenvliet et al., 2010).

Although most studies are retrospective, this conservative approach has a clear advantage. However, there is a consensus on the fact that laparoscopic washing and drainage is not recommended for cases of fecal peritonitis, and the results are unsatisfactory for cases of formation of an abscess in the pelvis. Several prospective and randomized studies are being conducted in order to better define in which clinical situations this approach should be indicated (Toorenvliet et al., 2010).

9. Conclusion

Access by laparoscopy seems to be of advantage over laparotomy as a diagnostic and therapeutic method in the approach to peritonitis and sepsis of abdominal origin by involving a lower surgical trauma, by providing a good field of view of the peritoneal cavity and by permitting to obtain tissue and fluid samples under direct vision. The rate of unnecessary laparotomies can be reduced when laparoscopy is used for a diagnostic and therapeutic approach in cases of acute abdomen, even in the presence of peritonitis or sepsis of abdominal origin.

In the management of peritonitis by laparoscopy, the inflammatory response is milder compared to management by laparotomy. The elevation of inflammatory cytokines is moderate and macrophages present a better basal immunologic performance. In contrast to what occurs with laparotomy, the acute phase of the inflammatory response associated with perioperative sepsis is attenuated during laparoscopy, and the immune function seems to be better preserved after the latter.

Despite the doubts about the feasibility and efficiency of laparoscopy compared to laparotomy for the approach to peritonitis, minimally invasive surgery is gaining acceptance among surgeons, especially regarding patients with abdominal sepsis.

10. Acknowledgments

Financial support: Fundação Waldemar Barnsley Pessoa

11. References

Almeida J, Sleeman D, Sosa JL, Puente I, McKenney M & MartinL. (1995). Acalculous cholecystitis: the use of diagnostic laparoscopy. *J Laparoendosc Surg,* Vol. 5, pp. (227–231).

Balague C, Targarona EM, Pujol M, Fillela X, Espert JJ & Trias M. (1999). Peritoneal response to a septic challenge comparison between open laparotomy, pneumoperitoneum laparoscopy, and wall lift laparoscopy. *Surg Endosc,* Vol.13, pp. (792–796).

Bloechle C, Emmermann A, Strate T, Scheurlen UJ,Schneider C, Achilles E, Wolf M, Mack D, Zornig C & Broelsch CE (1998). Laparoscopic versus open repair of gastric perforation and abdominal lavage of associated peritonitis in pigs. *Surg Endosc,* Vol. 12, pp. (212–218).

Boyd WP Jr & Nord HJ (2000). Diagnostic Laparoscopy. *Endoscopy,* Vol. 32, No.2, pp. (153-158)

Brandt CP, Priebe PP & Eckhauser ML. (1993). Diagnostic laparoscopy in the intensive care patient. Avoiding the nontherapeutic laparotomy. *Surg Endosc* , Vol. 7, No.3, pp. (168-172).

Brandt CP, Priebe PP, & Jacobs DG. (1994). Value of laparoscopy in trauma ICU patients with suspected acute acalculous cholecystitis. *Surg Endosc*, Vol. 8, pp.(361–364).

Branicki FJ. Abdominal Emergencies: Diagnostic and Therapeutic Laparoscopy (2002). *Surgical Infections*, Vol. 3, No.3, pp. (269-282).

Buunen M, Gholghesaei M, ET, Veldkamp R, Meijer DW, Bonjer HJ & Bouvy ND. (2004). Stress response to laparoscopic surgery. *Surg Endosc*, Vol.18. pp. (1022-1028).

Catena F, Di Saverio S, Kelly MD, Biffi WL, Ansaloni L, Mandalá V, Velmahos GC, Sartelli M, Tugnoli G, Lupo M, Mandalá S, Pinna AD, Sugarbaker PH, Van Goor H, Moore EE & Jeekel J. (2011). Bologna Guidelines for Diagnosis and Management of Adhesive Small Bowel Obstruction (ASBO): 2010 Evidence Based Guidelines of the World Society of Emergency Surgery. *World Journal of Emergency Surgery*, Vol. 21, pp. (6.5).

Chatzimavroudis G, Pavlidis TE, Koutelidakis I, Giamarrelos-Borboulis EJ, Atmatzidis S, Kountopoulo U, Marikis G & Atmatzidis Kl. (2009).CO2 Pneumoperitonium Prolongs survival in an animal model of peritonitis compared to laparotomy. *Journal of Surgical Research*, Vol. 152, pp. (69–75).

Colonval P, Navez B, Cambier E, Richir C, de Pierpont B, Scohy JJ & Guiot P. (1997). Is laparoscopic cholecystectomy effective and reliable in acute cholecystitis? Results of a prospective study of 221 pathologically documented cases. *Arch Chir*, Vol. 51, No. 7, pp. (689-696).

Cuesta MA, Eijsbouts QA, Gordijn RV, Borgstein PJ & De Jong D. (1998). Diagnostic laparoscopy in patients with an acute abdomen of uncertain etiology. *Surg Endosc*, Vol. 12, pp. (915–917).

Cueto J, Díaz O, Garteiz D, Rodríguez M & Weber A. (1997). The efficacy of laparoscopic surgery in the diagnosis and treatment of peritoniotis. *Surg Endosc*, Vol. 11, pp. (366-370).

Decadt B, Sussman L, Lewis MP, Secker A, Cohen L, Rogers C, Patel A & Rhodes M. (1999). Randomized clinical trial of early laparoscopy in the management of acute nonspecific abdominal pain. *Br J Surg*, Vol. 86, pp. (1383–1386).

Easter DW, Cuschieri A, Nathanson LK & Lavelle-Jones M. (1992). The utility of diagnostic laparoscopy for abdominal disorders. Audit of 120 patients. *Arch Surg*, Vol. 127, No. 4, pp. (379-383)

Fahel E, Amaral PC, Filho EM, Ettinger JE, Souza EL, Fortes MF, Alca^tara RS, Regis AB, Neto MP, Sousa MM, Fogagnoli WG, Cunha AG, Castro MM & Santana PA Jr. (1999). Nontraumatic acute abdomen: videolaparoscopic approach. *JSLS*, Vol. 3, pp. (187–192).

Forde KA & Treat MR. (1992). The role of peritoneoscopy (laparoscopy) in the evaluation of the acute abdomen in critically ill patients. *Surg Endosc*, Vol. 6, No.5, pp. (219-221).

Gadallah MF, Torres-Rivera C, Ramdeen G, Myrick S, Habashi S & Andrews G. (2001). Relationship between intraperitoneal bleeding, adhesions, and peritoneal dialysis catheter failure: a method of prevention. *Adv Perit Dial*, Vol. 17, pp.(127-129).

Gagne´ DJ, Malay MB, Hogle NJ & Fowler DL. (2002). Bedside diagnostic minilaparoscopy in the intensive care patient. *Surgery*, Vol. 131, pp.(491–496).

Gaita´n H, Angel E, Sa´nchez J, Go´mez I, Sa´nchez L & Agudelo C. (2002).Laparoscopic diagnosis of acute lower abdominal pain in women of reproductive age. *Int J Gynaecol Obstet*, Vol. 76, pp. (149–158).

Gamal EM, Metzger P, Szabo G, Brath E, Peto K, Olah A, Kiss J, Furka I & Mikó I. (2001). The influence of intraoperative complications on adhesion formation during laparoscopic and conventional cholecystectomy in an animal model. *Surg Endosc*, Vol. 15, pp.(873-877).

Geis WP & Kim HC. (1995).Use of laparoscopy in the diagnosis and treatment of patients with surgical abdominal sepsis. *Surg Endosc,* Vol.9, pp. (178–182).

Golash V, Willson PD. Early laparoscopy as a routine procedure in the management of acute abdominal pain: a review of 1,320 patients. *Surg Endosc*. 2005;19(7):882–885

Gurtner GC, Robertson CS, Chung SCS, Ling TKW, Ip SM & Li AKC (1995). Effect of carbon dioxide pneumoperitoneum on bacteraemia and endotoxaemia in an animal model of peritonitis. *Br J Surg*, Vol. 82, pp. (844–848).

Hackert T, Kienle P, Weitz J, Werner J, Szabo G, Hagl S, Bu¨chlerMW & Schmidt J. (2003). Accuracy of diagnostic laparoscopy for early diagnosis of abdominal complications after cardiac surgery. *Surg Endosc*, Vol.17, pp. (1671–1674)

Hemmila MR, Birkmeyer NJ, Arbabi S, Osborne NH, Wahl WL & Dimick JB. (2010). Introduction to Propensity Scores. A case study on the comparative effectiveness of laparoscopic vs open appendectomy. *Archives of Surgery*, Vol. 145, No. 10, pp. (939-945).

Hori Y. (2008). SAGES Guidelines Committee. Diagnostic laparoscopy guidelines: This guideline was prepared by the SAGES Guidelines Committee and reviewed and approved by the Board of Governors of the Society of American Gastrointestinal and Endoscopic Surgeons (SAGES). *Surg Endosc*. Vol. 22, No. 5, pp. (1353-1383).

Jaramillo EJ, Trevino JM, Berghoff KR & Franklin ME Jr. (2006). Bedside diagnostic laparoscopy in the intensive care unit: a 13-year experience. *JSLS*, Vol.10, pp. (155–159).

Kelly JJ, Puyana JC, Callery MP, Yood SM, Sandor A & Litwin DE. (2000). The feasibility and accuracy of diagnostic laparoscopy in the septic ICU patient. *Surg Endosc*, Vol. 14, pp. (617–621).

Kirshtein B, Roy-Shapira A, Lantsberg L, Mandel S, Avinoach E & Mizrahi S. (2003). The use of laparoscopy in abdominal emergencies. *Surg Endosc*, Vol. 17, pp. (1118–1124).

Landercasper J, Cogbill TH, Merry WH, Stolle RT & Strutt PJ. (1993). Long-term outcome after hospitalization for small-bowel obstruction. *Arch Surg*, Vol. 128, pp.(765-770).

Linhares L, Jeanpierre H, Borie F, Fingerhut A & Millat B. (2001). Lavage by laparoscopy fares better than lavage by laparotomy: experimental evidence. *Surg Endosc*, Vol. 15, No. 1, pp. (85–89).

Llanio R & Sarle H. (1956). Interet de La peritoneoscope chez politraumatises. *Marseille Chirurg*, Vol. 8, pp. (82-86).

M. L. Druart, R. Van Hee, J. Etienne, G. B. Cadie`re, J. F. Gigot, M. Legrand, J. M. Limbosch, B. Navez, M. Tugilimana, E. Van Vyve, L. Vereecken,3 E & Wibin, J. P. (1997). Yvergneaux Laparoscopic repair of perforated duodenal ulcer. A prospective multicenter clinical trial. *Surgical Endoscopy*, Vol. 11, pp. (1017–1020)

Majewski W. (2000). Diagnostic laparoscopy for the acute abdomen and trauma. *Surg Endosc*, Vol. 14, pp. (930–937).

Nagle A, Ujiki M, Denham W & Murayama K. (2004). Laparoscopic adhesiolysis for small bowel obstruction. *Am J Surg*, Vol. 187, No. 4, pp. (464-470).

Navez B, d'Udekem Y, Cambier E, Richir C, de Pierpont B & Guiot P. (1995). Laparoscopy for management of nontraumatic acute abdomen. *World J Surg*, Vol. 19, (382–386).

Orlando R III & Crowell KL. (1997). Laparoscopy in the critically ill. *Surg Endosc*, Vol. 11, pp. (1072–1074)

Ou CS & Rowbotham R. (2000). Laparoscopic diagnosis and treatmentof nontraumatic acute abdominal pain in women. *J Laparoendosc Adv Surg Tech A*, Vol.10, pp (41–45).

Pamoukian VN & Gagner M.(2001). Laparoscopic necrosectomy for acute necrotizing pancreatitis. *J Hepatobiliary Pancreatic Surg*, Vol. 8, No. 3, pp. (221-223).

Pecoraro AP, Cacchione RN, Sayad P, Williams ME & Ferzli GS. (2001). The routine use of diagnostic laparoscopy in the Intensive Care Unit. *Surg Endosc*, Vol. 15, pp. (638–641).

Perri SG, Altilia F, Pietrangeli F, Dalla Torre A, Gabbrielli F, Amendolara M, Nicita A, Nardi M Jr, Lotti R & Citone G. (2002). Laparoscopy in abdominal emergencies. Indications and limitations. *Chir Ital*, Vol. 54, No. 2, pp. (165-178).

Poulin EC, Schlachta CM & Mamazza J. (2000). Early laparoscopy to help diagnose acute nonspecific abdominal pain. *Lancet*, Vol. 355, pp. (861–863).

Salgado Jr W, Santos JS &Cunha FQ (2008) The effect of laparoscopic Access and antibiotics on the outcome of severe bacterial peritonitis in rats. *Journal of Laparoscopy and Advanced Surgery Techniques*, Vol.18, No.1, pp.(5-12).

Sanna A, Adani GL, Anania G & Donini A. (2003). The role of laparoscopy in patients with suspected peritonitis: experience of a single institution. *J Laparoendosc Adv Surg Tech A*, Vol.13, pp. (17–19).

Sauerland S, Agresta F, Bergamaschi R, Borzelino Z, Budzynski A, Champault G, Fingerhut A, Isla A, Johansson M, Lundorff P, Navez B, Saad S & Neugebauer EA. (2006). Laparoscopy for abdominal emergencies: evidence-based guidelines of the European Association for Endoscopic Surgery (EAES). *Surg Endosc*, Vol. 20, pp.(14-29).

Scott-Coombes Dm, Vinpond MN & Thompson JM. (1993). General surgeons attidues to the treatment and prevention of abdominal adhesions. *Annals of the Royal College of Surgeons of England*, Vol. 75, pp. (123-128).

So¨zu¨er EM, Bedirli A, Ulusal M, Kayhan E &Yilmaz Z. (2000). Laparoscopy for diagnosis and treatment of acute abdominal pain. *J Laparoendosc Adv Surg Tech A*, Vol. 10, pp. (203–207).

Spirt MJ. (2010). Complicated intra-abdominal infeccions: a focus on appendicitis and diverticulitis. *Postgrad Med*, Vol. 122, No.1, pp. (39-51).

Stefa´nsson T, Nyman R, Nilsson S, Ekbom A & Pa'hlman L. (1997). Diverticulitis of the sigmoid colon: a comparison of CT, colonic enema, and laparoscopy. *Acta Radiologica*, Vol. 38, pp. (313-319).

Stefanidis D, Richardson WS, Chang L, Earle DB & Fanelli RD. (2009). The role of diagnostic laparoscopy for acute abdominal conditions: an evidence based review. *Surg Endosc*, Vol. 23, pp. (16-23).

Targarona EM, Balagué C, Espert JJ, Pérez Ayuso RM, Ros E, Navarro S, Bordas J, Téres J, & Trias M. (1995). Laparoscopic treatment of acute biliary pancreatitis. *Int Surg* , Vol. 80, No. 4, pp. (365-368).

Targarona EM, Rodr´ıguez M, Camacho M, Balagué C, Gich I, Vila L & Trias M. (2006). Immediate peritoneal response to bacterial contamination during laparoscopic surgery. *Surg Endosc*, Vol. 20, No. 2, pp. (316–321).

Tittel A, Treutner KH, Titkova S, Ottinger A & Schumpelick V. (2001). Comparison of adhesion reformation after laparoscopic and conventional adhesiolysis in an animal model. Langenbeck's. *Arch Surg,* Vol. 386, pp. (141-145).

Tonelli F, Di Carlo V, Liscia G &Serventi A. (2009) Diverticular disease of the colon: diagnosis and treatment. Consensus Conference, 5th National Congress of the Italian Society of Academic Surgeons. *Ann Ital Chir,* Vol. 80, No.1, pp. (3-8).

Toorenvliet BR, Swank H, Schoones JW, Hamming JF & Bemelman WA. Laparoscopic peritoneal lavage for perforated colonic diverticulitis: a systematic review. *Coloretal disease,* Vol. 12, pp. (862-867).

Villavicencio, RT & Aucar, JA. (1999). Analysis of Laparoscopy in Trauma. Review. *Journal of the American College of Surgeons,* Vol. 189, No.1, pp. (11-20).

Walsh RM, Popovich MJ & Hoadley J. (1998). Bedside diagnostic laparoscopy and peritoneal lavage in the Intensive Care Unit. *Surg Endosc,* Vol. 12, pp.(1405–1409).

Wichterman KA, Chaudry IH & Baue AE (1979). Studies of peripheral glucose uptake during sepsis. *Arch Surg,* Vol. 114, pp (740–750).

Z'graggen K, Metzger A, Birrer S & Klaiber C (1995). Laparoscopic cholecystectomy as standard therapy in acute cholecystitis. A prospective study. *Chirurg,* Vol. 66, No.4, pp. (366-370).

15

Role of Endoscopy in Laparoscopic Procedures

Mohamed O. Othman, Mihir Patel and Timothy Woodward
Mayo Clinic Jacksonville
USA

1. Introduction

Endoscopy is a viable tool in the diagnosis and management of various gastrointestinal disorders. In this chapter we will discuss the role of Endoscopy in facilitating laparoscopic procedures. Endoscopy can be done before, during or after the laparoscopic procedures and can be an alternative management technique for laparoscopy. We will focus on the recent advances in the frontier and what the future holds.

2. Endoscopy prior to laparoscopy

2.1 Tattooing prior to laparoscopic resection

Accurate localization of the surgical site is crucial prior to laparoscopic resection. Flat colorectal polyps or cancer are often hard to localize by visualization of the colonic wall or even by palpation. Measuring the distance of the lesion from the anal verge or correlating with a barium enema is usually not accurate enough for localizing the segment prior to colonic resection. Intra-operative colonoscopy is accurate in localizing the lesions, but it might interfere with patient positioning or laparoscopic field by air insufflation; in addition to prolonging the procedure time looking for the lesion.

Endoscopic tattooing of the lesion prior to laparoscopic resection has proven to be accurate and efficient. Feingold et al in a retrospective study of 50 patients who underwent endoscopic tattooing prior to laparoscopic resection found that 88% of these lesions were accurately localized during the laparoscopic procedure; no complications were reported.[1]

Many agents have been studied for use in endoscopic tattooing. Methylene blue and indigo carmine can successfully stain the serosa. However, these agents disappear in few days, making it not suitable for endoscopic tattooing. [2,3] Indian ink, however, can stain the serosa for years making it the ideal agent for tattooing [4]. Indian ink should be sterilized and diluted prior to injection [5]. A prepackaged sterilized and already diluted Indian ink, SPOT® (GI Supply, Camp Hill, Pennsylvania, USA) is currently used by many endoscopists for endoscopic tattooing [6]. It is recommended to inject the tattoo in 3 circumferential sites distal to lesion in case one of these sites is on the mesenteric side of the colon [4] The long-term safety of Indian ink was evaluated in a study of 55 patients; no clinical complications such as fever, infection or abdominal pain were reported. There was mild chronic inflammation at the site of injection in 6 patients without clinical significance[7]. Intraperitoneal spillage of Indian ink can happen and it is usually without clinical significance. There are a few case reports of peritonitis or peritoneal abscess as a result of intraperitoneal spillage [8].

Preoperative endoscopic tattooing of pancreatic lesions prior to laparoscopic distal pancreatectomy has been recently reported [9]. This technique utilizes endoscopic ultrasound with the use of a fine needle for tattooing under endoscopic guidance. In a study of 36 patients who underwent laparoscopic distal pancreatictomy, 10 patients had preoperative endoscopic tattooing. Patients in the preoperative tattooing group had shorter operation times compared to the control group [10]. Figure 1 Illustrate tattooing of duodenal lesion prior to laparoscopic removal.

2.2 Endoscopic sphincterotomy prior to laparoscopic cholecystectomy

Common bile duct stones are found in 10% of patients undergoing elective cholecystectomy [11]. In these patients, management of common bile duct stones includes endoscopic sphincterotomy (ES) prior to or after laparoscopic cholecystectomy (LC) or LC with intraoperative common bile duct exploration. Many studies evaluated both approaches with controversial outcomes. A meta-analysis of 12 studies did not find any difference in mortality, morbidity or in the need for an additional procedure between both approaches [12]. However, a decision analysis published in 2008 suggested that LC with intraoperative bile duct exploration is superior to ES with LC [13]. Most likely, these controversial results could be explained by the difference in expertise among surgeons in performing laparoscopic common bile duct exploration. Recently, Intraoperative Endoscopic sphicnterotomy by Endoscopic Retrograde Cholangiopancreatography (ERCP) during LC was introduced as an alternative technique for the management of Choledocholithiasis. Enochsson et al. evaluated this technique in 37 patients with a 93.5% success rate and none of the patients developed post ERCP pancreatitis [14]. Intraoperative ERCP was compared to preoperative ERCP in patients with choledocholithiasis in a study by ElGeidie et al. The study included 198 patients and it did not find any difference in the morbidity or in the procedure time between the two approaches [15]. However, Intraoperative ERCP during LC has the advantage of being able to perform the procedure and surgery in a single stage procedure, making it an attractive option.

3. Endoscopy during laparoscopy (combined laparoscopic endoscopic procedure)

3.1 Laparoscopic monitored colonoscopic polypectomy (LMCP) to avoid segmental colon resection

The majority of large colonic polyps can be resected with colonoscopy. In few circumstances, patients are referred to laparascopic segmental colonic resection either because of the polyp size or because of the polyp location. Laparoscopic monitored colonoscopic polypectomy was suggested as a new technique which can reduce the number of segmental colonic resections. In this technique, the laparoscope can guide the endoscope to the site of the polyp and mobilize the colon to achieve easier polypectomy. This technique is particularly valuable in patients with angulated sigmoid colon from prior surgery and adhesion. This technique was evaluated in a study by Grunhagen et al in which 11 patients with difficult polypectomy were enrolled. Segmental colonic resection was avoided in 9 patients. No residual polyps were seen in the follow-up period [16]. Another trial included 47 patients who had LMCP and showed that 97% of the patients had a successful procedure without any complications[17]. In another trial from Germany that included 23 patients, LMCP was successful in 17 patients [18]. In all previously mentioned trials, there was minimal to no discomfort from the laparoscopic part of the procedure.

3.2 Endoscopy assisted laparoscopic wedge resection

Laparoscopic wedge resection is currently the standard of care for the removal of gastric submucosal tumor and in particular Gastrointestinal Stromal Tumor (GIST). Laparoscopic wedge resection is more feasible in tumors located at the anterior wall of the stomach Tumors located in the posterior wall of the stomach or the gastro-esophageal junctions were traditionally managed by surgery to ensure negative margins and to avoid excessive gastric resection. Endoscopy assisted laparoscopic wedge resection was successfully performed in gastric submucosal tumors located in the above mentioned area to spare open surgery. In this technique, endoscopy is used simultaneously during laparoscopy to localize the tumor and ensure negative margins. In a trial of 18 patients, this technique was proven successful with a single complication (perforation) in one case [19]. A new technique described by Hiki et al utilizes endoscopic submucosal dissection (ESD) of three-fourths of the circumference around the submucosal tumor followed by seromuscular dissection of the exact three-fourths of the circumference by laparoscopy then the tumor is removed by a laparoscopic stapling device [20]. This technique is successful regardless of the tumor location and the initial ESD done by endoscopy to ensure the exact margins of the tumor.

3.3 Combined colonoscopy and laparoscopy to close colonic perforation

Iatrogenic colonic perforation can be treated with segmental laparoscopic resection or with laparoscopic suturing [21]. A new technique was proposed to close iatrogenic colonic perforation with combined endoscopy and laparoscopy approach. This technique involves mucosal closure using endoscopic clips, serosal closure using laparoscopy and a leak test with air insufflations and water irrigation [22].

3.4 Combined laparoscopic-endoscopic approach for duodenal lesions

Endoscopic mucosal resection and endoscopic mucosal dissection of duodenal lesions is feasible [23]. However, it is complicated with higher rates of bleeding, perforation and tumor recurrence compared to EMR and ESD of colonic and stomach lesions [24]. Sakon et al described a new technique utilizing ESD of the margins of the duodenal lesion followed by laparoscopic resection. This promising technique was associated with less procedure time and minimal bleeding [25].

3.5 Laparoscopy assisted foreign body removal

Most of ingested foreign body can be removed endoscopically. In few instances, sharp foreign body can invade through the gastrointestinal wall to other organ and require surgical assistance. Lanitis et al described a case in which a patient ingested two sharp needles, one of them migrated to the liver and another one invaded into the abdominal wall. Combined endoscopy and laparoscopy technique was successful in removing both lesions [26]. Another case report described the removal of large dental bridge by the combined approach. The foreign body was snared by the endoscopy in the stomach but it could not pass through the overtube in the esophagus. Gastrostomy was done using laparoscope then the snared foreign body was delivered to a laparoscopy grasper through the gastrostomy

[27]. This technique has many advantages in difficult cases of foreign body removal. Endoscopy provides trans-illumination of the stomach and help to localize the foreign body for laparoscopic removal. In addition, laparoscopy provides the opportunity to clean the peritoneal spillage and ensure the closure of the abdominal wall [28].

4. Endoscopy after laparoscopy

4.1 Endoscopy in the treatment of bariatric surgery complications

Morbid obesity and its complications became an endemic problem in most developed countries [29]. Laparoscopic bariatric surgery has gained popularity in the field of surgical treatment of obesity. Laparoscopic gastric bypass and laparoscopic adjustable gastric banding account for more than 50% of bariatric surgeries performed worldwide [30]. Endoscopy is a useful tool in assessing complications of bariatric surgeries in addition to its role in the initial assessment of these patients prior to surgery.

Stomal stenosis is the one of the most frequent complications after Laparoscopic Roux en Y Gastric Bypass (RYGBP) [31]. Stomal stenosis occurs in 1-5% of patients undergoing Laparoscopic RYGBP [32-34]. Endoscopic dilation of the stomal stenosis has proven to be successful without the need of surgical revision. Ukleja et al performed endoscopic balloon dilation of the stomal stricture in 61 patients. Dilation was done in 1 to 5 sessions and it was successful in all patients without a need for surgical revision. However, the procedure was complicated by perforation in 2.2% of all dilations (3 patients) [35]. In another series by Go et al which included 38 patients with stomal stenosis after RYGBP, the success rate of endoscopic balloon dilation was 95% with a 3% complication rate [36]. Similar results were published by Peifer et al in their cohort of 43 patients, in which 2 endoscopic dilation sessions up to 15 mm were successful in 93% of the patients without any perforations[34].

Laparoscopic gastric banding (LGB) can be complicated with band erosion and band slippage in 1% and 4.9% of procedures performed, respectively [37]. Band erosion can be seen by endoscopy as a white ring in retroflexion in the stomach. Removal of the gastric band can be successfully done with endoscopy, especially if more than 50% of the band eroded through the wall of the stomach. Expectant management is advisable when less than 50% of the gastric band eroded through the stomach wall [38]. Successful removal of gastric bands was described in many case reports by cutting the thinnest part of the band using papillotome, mixed current Argon Plasma Coagulation or with scissors [39-41].

Choleithiasis and its related billiary complications are common after bariatric surgery [42]. Occasionally, the endoscopists will face the challenge of accessing the bypassed intestinal limb to the ampulla of vater in order to perform billiary procedures [43]. Many techniques have been described in order to access the ampulla of vater in this circumstance. Wright et al described their experience in 15 patients with RYGBP who underwent billiary interventions. Initially, forward-viewing colonoscope was used to explore the afferent limb to find the ampulla. Billiary cannulation with the use of the colonoscope was achieved in 2 patients. In the rest of the patients, a guidewire was left and duodenoscope was advanced over the guidewire to the ampulla. This technique was successful in two-thirds of the enrolled patients [44]. Another described technique includes the use of the double balloon enteroscopy for ERCP.The feasibility of this technique was illustrated in many case series with a success rate of 80-90% in cannulating the common bile duct (CBD) and a more than 60% success rate in performing therapeutic intervention of the biliary tract [45-47]. The use of double balloon enteroscopy offers the advantage of exploration of the afferent limb in less time;, however, the lack of elevator could be problematic in gaining deep access of the CBD, especially in patients with naive papilla. Another novel technique utilizes the creation of a gastrostomy tube by an interventional radiologist in the excluded part of the stomach followed by the use of an ERCP endoscope through the gastrostomy[48]. Although this technique enables the use of an ERCP endoscope, it requires delaying the ERCP until maturation of the gastrostomy tube. A new technique of laparoscopic-assisted ERCP was proven to be successful in RYGBP patients [49]. Initially, a laparoscopic examination is done, followed by identification of the stomach remnant to create gastrostomy as an access for the ERCP endoscope. The endoscope is inserted through trochar from the abdominal wall to the gastrostomy opening and then to the biliary tract. This technique was successful in 9 out of 10 patients included in the study by Lopes et al. These impressive results were confirmed by Bertin et al, in which successful biliary cannulation was achieved in 94% of 21 RYGBP patients who underwent laparoscopic assisted ERCP [50]. In conclusion, bariatric surgeries are increasing due to the obesity epidemic. Endoscopists will have a major role in either evaluating these patients prior to surgery or in treating post-surgical complications.

4.2 Endoscopy in treatment of post-surgical leaks and fistulas

Anastomotic leaks are one of the major complications after gastrointestinal surgery. After laparoscopic RYGBP, anastomotic leaks can develop in 0.3 to 8% of patients[51]. Traditionally these leaks were managed surgically. The introduction of self-expandable removable stents offered a less invasive approach for management of anastomotic leak. In a retrospective study that included 5 patients with anastomotic leak and one patient with chronic gastrocutaneous fistula; self-expandable plastic stent was successful in closing the leak in all 5 patients but not in the patient with the fistula [52]. In another retrospective study that included 11 patients with acute leak and 2 patients with chronic fistula as a complication of bariatric surgery, self-expandable removal stents (metal and plastic) were successful in healing the acute leak in 89% of patients and one of the two patients with chronic fistula [53]. A new endoscopic device named "over the scope clip(OSC)," which utilizes a combination of clip with grasper and large suction cap to ensure serosa to serosa closure, was recently introduced to clinical practice. The new system has been evaluated in 12 patients with post-operative leaks or fistula with successful closure in 10 patients [54]. Currently, this system is approved in Europe but is not yet available for clinical use in United States. The recently published experiences of the use of this new OSC in different applications such as leaks, fistula and perforation are extremely encouraging [54-57].

5. Endoscopy as an alternative to laparoscopy

The recent advances in therapeutic endoscopy opened a new frontier for endoscopists to manage complicated clinical scenarios that were only managed surgically in the past. In this section we are going to discuss a few examples of the use of endoscopy in these clinical scenarios where surgery is contraindicated or considered a more invasive approach.

5.1 Endoscopic gallbladder drainage

Cholecystectomy (mainly by laparoscopic approach) is the standard of care for management of acute cholecystitis. In high risk patients for surgery percutaneous cholecystostomy is advocated as a temporarizing measure [58]. However, this approach could be problematic in patients with coagulopathy or due to anatomical reasons. In addition, an indwelling catheter is predisposed to infection and it reduces the quality of life. Endoscopic transpapillary drainage was introduced as a more attractive approach in this subset of patients. The technique utilizes the ERCP endoscope to cannulate the billiary tree and the cystic duct followed by placement of cystic duct stent or a nasocholecystic catheter in the gallbladder [59, 60]. The outcome of this endoscopic approach was evaluated retrospectively in 35 surgically high-risk patients with acute cholecystitis. Nasocholecystic catheter was inserted in 21 patients, plastic stent in 6 patients and combined approach in 2 patients. The procedure was not successful in 6 of the 35 patients (17 %). Among the 29 patients with successful gallbladder drainage, 24 patients clinically improved within 3 days, while 4 patients died of septic complications. Although this technique was successful in 83 % of the patients, long-term follow-up showed a 20% relapse rate for acute pancreatitis which emphasizes the role of this approach as a bridge until the patient is surgically fit [61].

5.2 Endoscopic treatment of GERD

Endoscopic treatment of GERD has been an attractive topic for the last 15 years. Hope for a successful cure of GERD with endoscopy has been a rollercoaster. In this section we will briefly discuss various endoscopic modalities currently available for GERD treatment. One of the earliest devices to treat GERD by endoscopic approach is the "Stretta Device". This device uses thermal coaogulation of the mucosa of the lower esophageal sphincter (LES) in order to narrow the esophagus and prevent GERD. Although the device showed modest success, its clinical use was hindered by the higher rate of complications such as esophageal perforation and aspiration pneumonia. Currently this system is not commercially available [62, 63]. Other devices utilize suturing techniques to produce endoscopic plication of the LES in an effort to decrease GERD. There are more than five plicator devices available in the market. There are multiple cases series and non-randomized trials investigating the effectiveness of this technique. In summary, it showed a modest decrease in acid reflux but the procedure is lengthy and there is an increased risk of complication [64-66]. Based on the available data, it is premature to support incorporating these devices in clinical practice. A third technique that involves injecting bulking agents at the LES to prevent GERD has been recently introduced. The injected materials are either plexigal microsphere or ethylene vinyl alcohol (biodegradable microsphere) as in the Enteryx device. Although the technique is easy to use, the Enteryx device was recalled by the United States' Food and Drug Administration due to the associated complications such esophageal abscess, polymer migration and death [67-69]. Although many of the above mentioned results are disappointing, there are other devices currently being researched which could alter the current grim look for use of endoscopy in GERD.

5.3 Endoscopic myotomy for esophageal achalasia

Traditionally, the endoscopy role in achalasia was limited to endoscopic dilation and endoscopic injection of BOTOX [70]. A new technique involving creating a submucosal tunnel in the lower esophagus followed by advancing the endoscope in the new created space to the lower esophageal sphincter (LES) and electrocautery disruption of circular muscle of LES was proven feasible in an animal model [71]. This technique was proven successful in 17 patients with achalasia who underwent endoscopic myotomy in a tertiary referral center in Japan. Patients had significant improvement of their dysphagia and in the resting LES pressure. No major complications were reported [72]. The first case of endoscopic myotomy in the United States was reported in December 2010 by Stavropoulos et al; the procedure was successful with improvement in dysphagia in the follow-up period [73]. This technique has many advantages including the minimally invasive nature of the procedure, the lower incidence of reflux since only an incision of the circular muscle is done and the option of performing laparoscopic myotomy if needed. However, long-term data are not yet available for this new approach.

6. References

[1] Feingold, D.L., et al., *Safety and reliability of tattooing colorectal neoplasms prior to laparoscopic resection.* J Gastrointest Surg, 2004. 8(5): p. 543-6.

[2] Lane, K.L., et al., *Endoscopic tattoo agents in the colon. Tissue responses and clinical implications.* Am J Surg Pathol, 1996. 20(10): p. 1266-70.

[3] Price, N., et al., *Safety and efficacy of India ink and indocyanine green as colonic tattooing agents.* Gastrointest Endosc, 2000. 51(4 Pt 1): p. 438-42.

[4] Yeung, J.M., C. Maxwell-Armstrong, and A.G. Acheson, *Colonic tattooing in laparoscopic surgery - making the mark?* Colorectal Dis, 2009. 11(5): p. 527-30.

[5] Nizam, R., et al., *Colonic tattooing with India ink: benefits, risks, and alternatives.* Am J Gastroenterol, 1996. 91(9): p. 1804-8.

[6] Askin, M.P., et al., *Tattoo of colonic neoplasms in 113 patients with a new sterile carbon compound.* Gastrointest Endosc, 2002. 56(3): p. 339-42.

[7] Shatz, B.A., et al., *Long-term safety of India ink tattoos in the colon.* Gastrointest Endosc, 1997. 45(2): p. 153-6.

[8] Singh, S., et al., *Complication after pre-operative India ink tattooing in a colonic lesion.* Dig Surg, 2006. 23(5-6): p. 303.

[9] Lennon, A.M., et al., *EUS-guided tattooing before laparoscopic distal pancreatic resection (with video).* Gastrointest Endosc, 2010. 72(5): p. 1089-94.

[10] Newman, N.A., et al., *Preoperative endoscopic tattooing of pancreatic body and tail lesions decreases operative time for laparoscopic distal pancreatectomy.* Surgery, 2010. 148(2): p. 371-7.

[11] Vezakis, A., et al., *Intraoperative cholangiography during laparoscopic cholecystectomy.* Surg Endosc, 2000. 14(12): p. 1118-22.

[12] Clayton, E.S., et al., *Meta-analysis of endoscopy and surgery versus surgery alone for common bile duct stones with the gallbladder in situ.* Br J Surg, 2006. 93(10): p. 1185-91.

[13] Kharbutli, B. and V. Velanovich, *Management of preoperatively suspected choledocholithiasis: a decision analysis.* J Gastrointest Surg, 2008. 12(11): p. 1973-80.

[14] Enochsson, L., et al., *Intraoperative endoscopic retrograde cholangiopancreatography (ERCP) to remove common bile duct stones during routine laparoscopic cholecystectomy does not prolong hospitalization: a 2-year experience.* Surg Endosc, 2004. 18(3): p. 367-71.

[15] ElGeidie, A.A., G.K. ElEbidy, and Y.M. Naeem, *Preoperative versus intraoperative endoscopic sphincterotomy for management of common bile duct stones.* Surg Endosc, 2011. 25(4): p. 1230-7.

[16] Grunhagen, D.J., et al., *Laparoscopic-monitored colonoscopic polypectomy: a multimodality method to avoid segmental colon resection.* Colorectal Dis, 2010.

[17] Franklin, M.E., Jr., et al., *Laparoscopic-assisted colonoscopic polypectomy: the Texas Endosurgery Institute experience.* Dis Colon Rectum, 2000. 43(9): p. 1246-9.

[18] Ommer, A., et al., *[Laparoscopic-assisted colonoscopic polypectomy--indications and results].* Zentralbl Chir, 2003. 128(3): p. 195-8.

[19] Ludwig, K., et al., *Laparoscopic-endoscopic rendezvous resection of gastric tumors.* Surg Endosc, 2002. 16(11): p. 1561-5.

[20] Hiki, N., et al., *Laparoscopic and endoscopic cooperative surgery for gastrointestinal stromal tumor dissection.* Surg Endosc, 2008. 22(7): p. 1729-35.

[21] Coimbra, C., et al., *Laparoscopic repair of colonoscopic perforation: a new standard?* Surg Endosc, 2010.

[22] Senadhi, V., et al., *Combined colonoscopy and laparoscopy to close a colonic perforation.* Endoscopy, 2010. 42 Suppl 2: p. E213-4.

[23] Alexander, S., et al., *EMR of large, sessile, sporadic nonampullary duodenal adenomas: technical aspects and long-term outcome (with videos).* Gastrointest Endosc, 2009. 69(1): p. 66-73.

[24] Abbass, R., J. Rigaux, and F.H. Al-Kawas, *Nonampullary duodenal polyps: characteristics and endoscopic management.* Gastrointest Endosc, 2010. 71(4): p. 754-9.

[25] Sakon, M., et al., *A novel combined laparoscopic-endoscopic cooperative approach for duodenal lesions.* J Laparoendosc Adv Surg Tech A, 2010. 20(6): p. 555-8.

[26] Lanitis, S., et al., *Combined laparoscopic and endoscopic approach for the management of two ingested sewing needles: one migrated into the liver and one stuck in the duodenum.* J Laparoendosc Adv Surg Tech A, 2007. 17(3): p. 311-4.

[27] Olson, J.A., Jr., L.B. Weinstock, and L.M. Brunt, *Combined endoscopic and laparoscopic approach to remove a sharp gastric foreign body.* Gastrointest Endosc, 2000. 51(4 Pt 1): p. 500-2.

[28] Iafrati, M.D., et al., *A novel approach to the removal of sharp foreign bodies from the stomach using a combined endoscopic and laparoscopic technique.* Gastrointest Endosc, 1996. 43(1): p. 67-70.

[29] Padwal, R., S.K. Li, and D.C. Lau, *Long-term pharmacotherapy for obesity and overweight.* Cochrane Database Syst Rev, 2004(3): p. CD004094.

[30] Buchwald, H. and S.E. Williams, *Bariatric surgery worldwide 2003.* Obes Surg, 2004. 14(9): p. 1157-64.

[31] Podnos, Y.D., et al., *Complications after laparoscopic gastric bypass: a review of 3464 cases.* Arch Surg, 2003. 138(9): p. 957-61.

[32] Msika, S., *[Surgery for morbid obesity: 2. Complications. Results of a Technologic Evaluation by the ANAES].* J Chir (Paris), 2003. 140(1): p. 4-21.

[33] Kothari, S.N., et al., *Excellent laparoscopic gastric bypass outcomes can be achieved at a community-based training hospital with moderate case volume.* Ann Surg, 2010. 252(1): p. 43-9.

[34] Peifer, K.J., et al., *Successful endoscopic management of gastrojejunal anastomotic strictures after Roux-en-Y gastric bypass.* Gastrointest Endosc, 2007. 66(2): p. 248-52.

[35] Ukleja, A., et al., *Outcome of endoscopic balloon dilation of strictures after laparoscopic gastric bypass.* Surg Endosc, 2008. 22(8): p. 1746-50.

[36] Go, M.R., et al., *Endoscopic management of stomal stenosis after Roux-en-Y gastric bypass.* Surg Endosc, 2004. 18(1): p. 56-9.

[37] Singhal, R., et al., *Band slippage and erosion after laparoscopic gastric banding: a meta-analysis.* Surg Endosc, 2010. 24(12): p. 2980-6.

[38] Neto, M.P., et al., *Endoscopic removal of eroded adjustable gastric band: lessons learned after 5 years and 78 cases.* Surg Obes Relat Dis, 2010. 6(4): p. 423-7.

[39] Meyenberger, C., C. Gubler, and P.M. Hengstler, *Endoscopic management of a penetrated gastric band.* Gastrointest Endosc, 2004. 60(3): p. 480-1.
[40] De Palma, G.D., et al., *Endoscopic management of intragastric penetrated adjustable gastric band for morbid obesity.* World J Gastroenterol, 2006. 12(25): p. 4098-100.
[41] Weiss, H., et al., *Gastroscopic band removal after intragastric migration of adjustable gastric band: a new minimal invasive technique.* Obes Surg, 2000. 10(2): p. 167-70.
[42] Caruana, J.A., et al., *Incidence of symptomatic gallstones after gastric bypass: is prophylactic treatment really necessary?* Surg Obes Relat Dis, 2005. 1(6): p. 564-7; discussion 567-8.
[43] Lopes, T.L. and T.H. Baron, *Endoscopic retrograde cholangiopancreatography in patients with Roux-en-Y anatomy.* J Hepatobiliary Pancreat Sci, 2010.
[44] Wright, B.E., O.W. Cass, and M.L. Freeman, *ERCP in patients with long-limb Roux-en-Y gastrojejunostomy and intact papilla.* Gastrointest Endosc, 2002. 56(2): p. 225-32.
[45] Monkemuller, K., et al., *ERCP with the double balloon enteroscope in patients with Roux-en-Y anastomosis.* Surg Endosc, 2009. 23(9): p. 1961-7.
[46] Parlak, E., et al., *Endoscopic retrograde cholangiography by double balloon enteroscopy in patients with Roux-en-Y hepaticojejunostomy.* Surg Endosc, 2010. 24(2): p. 466-70.
[47] Moreels, T.G., et al., *Diagnostic and therapeutic double-balloon enteroscopy after small bowel Roux-en-Y reconstructive surgery.* Digestion, 2009. 80(3): p. 141-7.
[48] Martinez, J., et al., *Endoscopic retrograde cholangiopancreatography and gastroduodenoscopy after Roux-en-Y gastric bypass.* Surg Endosc, 2006. 20(10): p. 1548-50.
[49] Lopes, T.L., R.H. Clements, and C.M. Wilcox, *Laparoscopy-assisted ERCP: experience of a high-volume bariatric surgery center (with video).* Gastrointest Endosc, 2009. 70(6): p. 1254-9.
[50] Bertin, P.M., K. Singh, and M.E. Arregui, *Laparoscopic transgastric endoscopic retrograde cholangiopancreatography (ERCP) after gastric bypass: case series and a description of technique.* Surg Endosc, 2011.
[51] Baker, R.S., et al., *The science of stapling and leaks.* Obes Surg, 2004. 14(10): p. 1290-8.
[52] Edwards, C.A., et al., *Management of anastomotic leaks after Roux-en-Y bypass using self-expanding polyester stents.* Surg Obes Relat Dis, 2008. 4(5): p. 594-9; discussion 599-600.
[53] Eubanks, S., et al., *Use of endoscopic stents to treat anastomotic complications after bariatric surgery.* J Am Coll Surg, 2008. 206(5): p. 935-8; discussion 938-9.
[54] Manta, R., et al., *Endoscopic treatment of gastrointestinal fistulas using an over-the-scope clip (OTSC) device: Case series from a tertiary referral center.* Endoscopy, 2011.
[55] Iacopini, F., et al., *Over-the-scope clip closure of two chronic fistulas after gastric band penetration.* World J Gastroenterol, 2010. 16(13): p. 1665-9.
[56] von Renteln, D., M.C. Vassiliou, and R.I. Rothstein, *Randomized controlled trial comparing endoscopic clips and over-the-scope clips for closure of natural orifice transluminal endoscopic surgery gastrotomies.* Endoscopy, 2009. 41(12): p. 1056-61.
[57] Repici, A., et al., *Clinical experience with a new endoscopic over-the-scope clip system for use in the GI tract.* Dig Liver Dis, 2009. 41(6): p. 406-10.
[58] Ito, K., et al., *Percutaneous cholecystostomy versus gallbladder aspiration for acute cholecystitis: a prospective randomized controlled trial.* AJR Am J Roentgenol, 2004. 183(1): p. 193-6.
[59] Itoi, T., et al., *Endoscopic transpapillary gallbladder drainage in patients with acute cholecystitis in whom percutaneous transhepatic approach is contraindicated or anatomically impossible (with video).* Gastrointest Endosc, 2008. 68(3): p. 455-60.

[60] Comin, J.M., R.J. Cade, and A.F. Little, *Percutaneous cystic duct stent placement in the treatment of acute cholecystitis.* J Med Imaging Radiat Oncol, 2010. 54(5): p. 457-61.
[61] Mutignani, M., et al., *Endoscopic gallbladder drainage for acute cholecystitis: technical and clinical results.* Endoscopy, 2009. 41(6): p. 539-46.
[62] Chen, D., et al., *Systematic review of endoscopic treatments for gastro-oesophageal reflux disease.* Br J Surg, 2009. 96(2): p. 128-36.
[63] Romagnuolo, J., *Endoscopic "antireflux" procedures: not yet ready for prime time.* Can J Gastroenterol, 2004. 18(9): p. 573-7.
[64] Thomson, M., et al., *Endoluminal gastroplication in children with significant gastro-oesophageal reflux disease.* Gut, 2004. 53(12): p. 1745-50.
[65] Chuttani, R., et al., *A novel endoscopic full-thickness plicator for the treatment of GERD: A pilot study.* Gastrointest Endosc, 2003. 58(5): p. 770-6.
[66] Schiefke, I., et al., *Use of an endoscopic suturing device (the "ESD") to treat patients with gastroesophageal reflux disease, after unsuccessful EndoCinch endoluminal gastroplication: another failure.* Endoscopy, 2005. 37(8): p. 700-5.
[67] Wong, R.F., T.V. Davis, and K.A. Peterson, *Complications involving the mediastinum after injection of Enteryx for GERD.* Gastrointest Endosc, 2005. 61(6): p. 753-6.
[68] Veerappan, G.R., J.M. Koff, and M.T. Smith, *Enteryx polymer migration to lymph nodes and beyond.* Endoscopy, 2008. 40 Suppl 2: p. E10-1.
[69] Noh, K.W., et al., *Pneumomediastinum following Enteryx injection for the treatment of gastroesophageal reflux disease.* Am J Gastroenterol, 2005. 100(3): p. 723-6.
[70] Urbach, D.R., et al., *A decision analysis of the optimal initial approach to achalasia: laparoscopic Heller myotomy with partial fundoplication, thoracoscopic Heller myotomy, pneumatic dilatation, or botulinum toxin injection.* J Gastrointest Surg, 2001. 5(2): p. 192-205.
[71] Pasricha, P.J., et al., *Submucosal endoscopic esophageal myotomy: a novel experimental approach for the treatment of achalasia.* Endoscopy, 2007. 39(9): p. 761-4.
[72] Inoue, H., et al., *Peroral endoscopic myotomy (POEM) for esophageal achalasia.* Endoscopy, 2010. 42(4): p. 265-71.
[73] Stavropoulos, S.N., et al., *Endoscopic submucosal myotomy for the treatment of achalasia (with video).* Gastrointest Endosc, 2010. 72(6): p. 1309-11.